SELF-STUDY COURSE FOR OPTOMETRIC ASSISTING

SELF-STUDY COURSE FOR OPTOMETRIC ASSISTING

Second Edition

Developed by the AOA Paraoptometric Section

Edited by

Mary Jameson

A.S., Opt. T., R.

Chair, Paraoptometric Section, American Optometric Association, St. Louis, Missouri; Laboratory Supervisor, Department of Clinical Sciences, Pennsylvania College of Optometry, Philadelphia

Butterworth–Heinemann
Boston Oxford Johannesburg Melbourne New Delhi Singapore

Copyright © 1997 by The American Optometric Association.

All rights reserved.

No part of this publication may be reproduced, stored in a retrieval system, or transmitted in any form or by any means, electronic, mechanical, photocopying, recording, or otherwise, without the prior written permission of the publisher.

Every effort has been made to ensure that the drug dosage schedules within this text are accurate and conform to standards accepted at time of publication. However, as treatment recommendations vary in the light of continuing research and clinical experience, the reader is advised to verify drug dosage schedules herein with information found on product information sheets. This is especially true in cases of new or infrequently used drugs.

 Recognizing the importance of preserving what has been written, Butterworth–Heinemann prints its books on acid-free paper whenever possible.

Library of Congress Cataloging-in-Publication Data

Self-study course for optometric assisting / developed by the AOA
    Paraoptometric Section ; edited by Mary Jameson. -- 2nd ed.
       p.   cm.
    Includes bibliographical references and index.
    ISBN 0-7506-9473-4 (alk. paper)
     1. Optometric assistants--Programmed instruction. 2. Optometry-
-Programmed instruction. I. Jameson, Mary, 1962- . II. AOA
Paraoptometric Section.
RE959.5.S45   1996
617.7'5--DC20   96-30878
                                                                       CIP

British Library Cataloguing-in-Publication Data
A catalogue record for this book is available from the British Library.

The publisher offers special discounts on bulk orders of this book.
For information, please contact:
Manager of Special Sales
Butterworth–Heinemann
313 Washington Street
Newton, MA 02158–1626
Tel: 617-928-2500
Fax: 617-928-2620

For information on all medical publications available, contact our World Wide Web home page at: http://www.bh.com/med

10 9 8 7 6 5 4 3 2 1

Printed in the United States of America

Contents

Contributing Authors   VII
Preface   IX

1. **Practice Management**   1
   Helen Noll and Pamela Capaldi-O'Brien

2. **Anatomy and Physiology of the Eye and Visual System**   39
   G. Timothy Petito

3. **Refractive Status**   63
   Catherine E. Muhr

4. **The Ophthalmic Prescription**   83
   Victoria B. Cipparrone and Rita M. Pierce

5. **Ophthalmic Lenses**   91
   Marian C. Welling and Lynn E. Konkel

6. **Neutralization and Verification**   105
   Gregory L. Stephens

7. **Ophthalmic Dispensing**   151
   Marian C. Welling

8. **Basic Pretesting Procedures**   161
   Mary Jameson

9. **Specialty Testing**   185
   Lynn E. Konkel and Sharon Overgaard

10. **Visual Fields**   199
    Kathryn J. Wood and Van B. Nakagawara

11. **Contact Lenses**   213
    E. S. Bennett and Bruce W. Morgan

12. **Low Vision Examination**   279
    Paul B. Freeman

13. Binocular Vision — 295
Karen Pollack

14. Sports Vision — 309
Shaun M. Ratchford

15. Ocular Emergencies and Triage — 315
Frank L. Galizia

Appendixes — 325
A: Infection Control Guidelines for the Optometric Practice — 327
B: Common Pharmaceuticals Used in Eye Care — 337

Glossary — 339

Index — 343

Contributing Authors

E. S. BENNETT, O.D., M.S.ED.
Associate Professor of Optometry, University of Missour–St. Louis School of Optometry, St. Louis

PAMELA CAPALDI-O'BRIEN, B.S., A.A.S., OPT. T., R.
Global Coordinator, International Association of Contact Lens Educators, Sydney, Australia

VICTORIA B. CIPPARRONE, OPT. T., R.
Lancaster, Ohio

PAUL B. FREEMAN, O.D., F.A.A.O., F.C.O.V.D., DIPLOMATE IN LOW VISION
Chief of Low Vision Services, Department of Ophthalmology, Allegheny General Hospital, Pittsburgh, Pennsylvania

FRANK L. GALIZIA, O.D.
Adjunct Clinical Professor of Optometry, Pacific University College of Optometry, Forest Grove, Oregon; Associate Health Profession Staff Member, Valley Hospital and Medical Center, Spokane, Washington

MARY JAMESON, A.S., OPT. T., R.
Chair, Paraoptometric Section, American Optometric Association, St. Louis, Missouri; Laboratory Supervisor, Department of Clinical Sciences, Pennsylvania College of Optometry, Philadelphia

LYNN E. KONKEL, B.S., OPT. T., R.
Program Director and Instructor of Optometric Technicians, Madison Area Technical College, Madison, Wisconsin

BRUCE W. MORGAN, O.D.
Clinical Assistant Professor of Optometry, University of Missouri–St. Louis School of Optometry, St. Louis

CATHERINE E. MUHR, A.A., OPT. T., R.
Educational Coordinator, Department of Clinical Sciences, Pennsylvania College of Optometry, Philadelphia

VAN B. NAKAGAWARA, O.D.
Research Optometrist, Vision Research Team, Aeromedical Research Division, Civil Aeromedical Institute, Oklahoma City, Oklahoma

HELEN NOLL, OPT. T., R.
Sun Lakes, Arizona

SHARON OVERGAARD, OPT. T., R., C.O.A.
Optometric Technician, Davis Duehr Dean, Madison, Wisconsin

G. TIMOTHY PETITO, O.D.
Private Practice, St. Petersburg, Florida; Director of Low Vision Services, Tampa Lighthouse for the Blind, Tampa, Florida

RITA M. PIERCE, M.A.
Director, Postgraduate and Continuing Education, Los Angeles College of Chiropractic, Whittier, California

KAREN POLLACK, OPT. A., R.
Therapist, Department of Pediatrics, The Eye Institute, Pennsylvania College of Optometry, Philadelphia

SHAUN M. RATCHFORD, B.S.
Sports Vision Therapist, Institute for Sports Vision, Ridgefield, Connecticut; Lecturer, International Academy of Sports Vision, Harrisburg, Pennsylvania

GREGORY L. STEPHENS, O.D., PH.D.
Associate Professor of Optometry, College of Optometry, University of Houston, Houston, Texas

MARIAN C. WELLING, J.D., B.S., A.S.
Instructor, University of Missouri–St. Louis School of Optometry, St. Louis

KATHRYN J. WOOD, OPT. T., R.
Health Technician, Vision Research Team, Aeromedical Research Division, Civil Aeromedical Institute, Oklahoma City, Oklahoma

Preface

The field of paraoptometry has developed into a challenging and ever-changing career. In an effort to address the educational needs of the profession, the *Self-Study Course for Optometric Assisting* has been recreated. This textbook should serve the paraoptometric in a number of ways. It can be used as an introduction to the field. It can be used in-office under the supervision of the optometrist or trainer as an educational tool as well. It has been used successfully as one of the study guides for the AOA Paraoptometric Section examinations for the assistant. As with any textbook, it is an indispensable reference book.

I would like to thank those individuals who volunteered their time and expertise on this project to see it to its completion. At the very top of the list is Karen Oberheim at Butterworth–Heinemann. She made the project a priority and kept up with it every step of the way. She provided me with the guidance I needed to develop the concept of a second edition.

I would also like to thank each of the authors for their dedication to the textbook and their patience throughout the process. I would like to thank Cheryl Bruce, Opt. T., R., who assigned me to chair the task force that led to this second edition during her term as Chair of the AOA Paraoptometric Section; Lynn Konkel, Opt. T., R., for her invaluable input and energy; Rita Pierce and the original "cast," who set the standards and provided a template for this edition; Carol Schartner, Opt. A., R., for reviewing an editing several chapters; and Catherine E. Muhr, Opt. T., R., who provided me with suggestions and support throughout the entire project.

Many thanks to members of the AOA legal department for their review of the chapters. Thanks also to Laura Baumstark, who served as the Section's administrative director during the development. A sincere thanks to Bruce Muchnick, O.D., who assisted in editing the chapters and artwork.

Most of all, I would like to thank all of the paraoptometrics who have communicated with us on this and other projects. It is with the support and the effort of paraoptometrics and those who support us that the AOA Paraoptometric Section will be able to continue to provide educational materials such as this textbook in the future.

MJ

1 / Practice Management

Helen Noll and Pamela Capaldi-O'Brien

This chapter presents the responsibilities and tasks performed by the paraoptometric to assist in the smooth and efficient business management of an optometric practice. The methods recommended are general guidelines. Duties and procedures will be outlined by your employer based on the optometrist's personal experience and preference. Specific procedures may vary due to the practice size or type. The solo practice will probably establish different procedures from those of a large group practice. In some areas, more than one paraoptometric will share or overlap in performing tasks.

WHAT IS A PARAOPTOMETRIC?

The American Optometric Association's definition of a paraoptometric is

> *a person who works under the direct supervision of a licensed doctor of optometry, collects patient data, administers routine, yet technical, tests of the patients' visual capabilities, and assists in office management. The paraoptometric may assist the optometrist in providing primary patient care examination and treatment services, including contact lenses, low vision, vision therapy and optical dispensing, and office management. State laws may limit, restrict, or otherwise affect the duties that may be performed by the paraoptometric.*

After deciding to enter the paraoptometric field, there are some important factors to consider when applying for a position in an optometric office. During the job interview, you and your prospective employer will discuss important guidelines that will be followed on a daily basis. Major points to discuss with the optometrist include hours worked per week (including specified lunch time), starting salary, vacation policy, sick leave, personal time off, performance and salary reviews, insurance benefits, dress code, and specific duties to be performed.

A written policy manual that includes position descriptions can eliminate misunderstandings. Policy and procedure manuals are discussed later in this chapter. It is important for the optometrist and paraoptometric to understand one another's expectations so that a harmonious atmosphere and happy working relationship can result.

THE PROFESSIONAL IMAGE

How you present yourself as a staff member will enhance your office's image. Appearance is one contributing factor in this image. It is important that you be perceived as a professional by exercising good taste to form a lasting impression.

Patient Contact

Since you provide the first personal contact when patients come into the office, you should acknowledge them immediately with a pleasant, courteous greeting that will make them feel welcome. It is important to acknowledge the patient's presence by a nod of the head or by

TABLE 1-1. Code of ethics of the American Optometric Association
It shall be the ideal, the resolve, and the duty of the members of the American Optometric Association
TO KEEP the visual welfare of the patient uppermost at all times;
TO PROMOTE in every possible way, in collaboration with this Association, better care of the visual needs of mankind;
TO ENHANCE continuously their educational and technical proficiency to the end that their patients shall receive the benefits of all acknowledged improvements in visual care;
TO SEE THAT no person shall lack for visual care, regardless of his or her financial status;
TO ADVISE the patient whenever consultation with an optometric colleague or reference for other professional care seems advisable;
TO HOLD in professional confidence all information concerning a patient and to use such data only for the benefit of the patient;
TO CONDUCT themselves as exemplary citizens;
TO MAINTAIN their offices and their practices in keeping with professional standards;
TO PROMOTE and maintain cordial and unselfish relationships with members of their own profession and of other professions for the exchange of information to the advantage of mankind.
Source: American Optometric Association, St. Louis, 1944.

saying, "I'll be with you in one moment. Thank you for your patience."

Use discretion when having a discussion with a patient when other patients are within hearing distance. This is especially important when discussing financial arrangements and other personal matters that might be embarrassing to the patient.

Phone Calls

Personal phone calls should be kept to a minimum at all times. If it is necessary to make a personal call, use a phone that is out of the patients' earshot. Try to take care of these calls at lunch time or in the evening, and save the business phone for business.

Patient Records

All patient records are confidential. Never discuss one patient's situation with another patient. Do not talk about patients when socializing outside of the office. Such a conversation could get back to the patient, and moreover, individuals overhearing your conversation may wonder if you would divulge information about them to other people.

When engaging in conversation with patients, use moderate voice levels both during telephone conversations and during face-to-face conversations. Use soft tones when talking to other staff members. Interoffice conversations should not be overheard by waiting patients. What you say is as important as the way you say it. Avoid using slang, and never call the optometrist by his or her first name in front of patients.

Patients are aware of many things that occur in the office. You will leave them with a better impression if they hear the busy hum of an office rather than chattering and giggles from the staff. This is particularly true if you are behind schedule and the patients are subject to a delay.

Your professional attitude both at work and socially will enhance the optometrist's practice and image in the community. You should be a goodwill ambassador for the practice at all times. Follow the principles as set forth in the Code of Ethics of the American Optometric Association (AOA) (Table 1-1). These guidelines will help build a successful professional practice.

Personal Appearance

A dress code will be established in each office. Uniforms may be required or a standard of dress established. Regardless of the dress code in your office, all attire should be clean, pressed, and tasteful. Keep your fingernails clean and manicured. Perfume and after-shave lotion should be worn sparingly. Many patients may be sensitive or allergic to these scents. Use deodorant daily and keep breath freshener handy at all times. Whatever the office policy, remember that your appearance says something about the quality of care provided by the practice. Therefore, you should appear professional at all times. Never smoke or eat in front of patients. If the staff is allowed to smoke, there should be a designated area of the office that is out of the patients' sight for this purpose (Figure 1-1).

FRONT OFFICE PROCEDURES

Reception Area

The reception area is the first room the patient sees when walking in the door (Figure 1-2). This first impression will affect the patient's judgment of the optometrist, the staff, and the practice.

The furniture must be clean and in good repair. Windows and floor coverings should be cleaned on a regular basis. Although your job may not be to do the actual cleaning, it may be your responsibility to see that the cleaning is done.

Opening the office at the beginning of the day should include a check of the systems that help ensure the patients' comfort when they visit. Regulate the temperature and air-circulating controls. Turn on the radio and tune it to a low, soft tone for background music. Never play music so loudly that it overpowers conversations with patients. Tidy up the reception area, and check the supply of magazines available for the patients (Figure 1-3). Repair or discard any old or torn magazines. Straighten up the children's corner. The children's area may need cleaning with a damp cloth to remove all the sticky fingerprints gathered during the previous day. Monitor the reception area throughout the day, and keep it as neat as possible. Plants should be watered on a regular schedule if they are part of your office decor.

Many offices have a bulletin board in their reception area where current activities of the optometrist, staff, and patients can be posted. Periodically check and update the bulletin board with new articles and pictures. Make a daily check of your local newspaper for articles of interest concerning accomplishments of

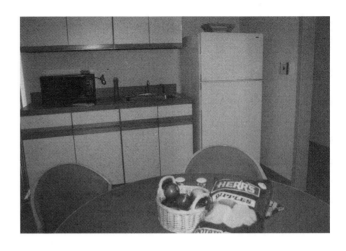

Figure 1-1—Eating area for staff.

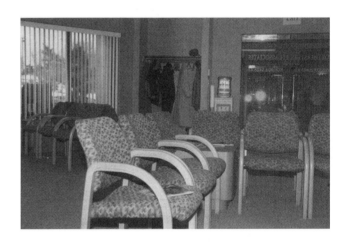

Figure 1-2—Reception area.

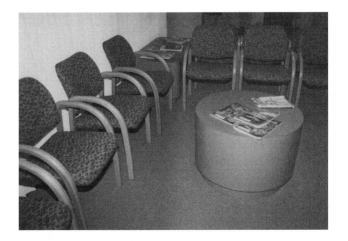

Figure 1-3—The magazine table in the reception area should be kept neat.

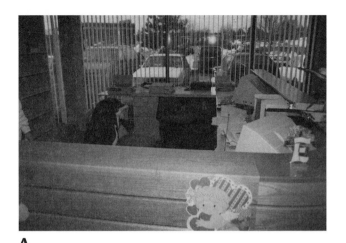
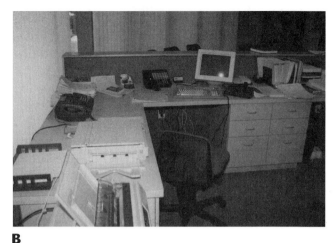

Figure 1-4—A. Patients' impressions of the front desk will affect their impression of the practice. B. A tidy front desk area will improve efficiency.

patients in the practice. During the check, also note patient births, deaths, and marriages, which may be useful in keeping your records up-to-date.

The front desk area must be kept clean and tidy (Figure 1-4A). Patients see this area clearly, and a cluttered desk indicates a disorderly and disorganized routine. Neatly stacked papers and patient records represent an efficient office staff and add a professional appearance to the practice (Figure 1-4B).

Typewriters and adding machines must be kept clean and in proper working order. Ribbons should be replaced periodically to ensure clean, clear typewritten letters and records that can be read easily. This equipment should be serviced at least once a year to keep it in proper condition. Cover the business machines at night to keep out dirt and dust.

Telephone Techniques

The telephone is the major access in and out of the practice. When talking on the telephone, you are the voice of the practice. Be pleasant and courteous and speak directly into the mouthpiece using a well modulated voice. Be attentive to the caller and listen politely. Do not interrupt the caller; wait for a break in the conversation before speaking.

The basic elements of telephone courtesy are politeness, kindness, consideration, and respect for others. Smile when talking on the phone. Even though the caller cannot see you, your smile can be sensed. The quality of you voice improves and gains a warm, pleasant tone when you speak with a smile. The use of "please" and "thank you" earns the cooperation and appreciation of the person calling. Using the patient's name several times during the conversation also gives the patient the feeling that he or she is valuable to you.

Screening Calls

Always answer the phone immediately. Many offices use the "three-ring" rule: The telephone is answered no later than the third time it rings. If you are on another line at the time, as soon as it is appropriate, ask the other party to hold for a moment and answer the incoming call. If you are talking directly to another patient, excuse yourself for a moment and answer the phone.

When answering the phone, use a moderate, unhurried voice, and speak distinctly. Keep a pad and pencil near the phone for messages and notes. A sample method of answering the phone might be, "Good morning [afternoon]. Dr. Smith's office, Carol speaking. How may I help you?" This has immediately identified the doctor's office and the person answering the phone. It has also created an opening for the party calling to proceed with the conversation.

If the call is for another staff member, politely ask, "May I tell him who is calling?" Always use the hold button when calling another staff member to the phone or when looking for information. Do not place your hand over the mouthpiece; it is ineffective and could be offensive to the party calling. If the staff member is busy with a patient, you may say, for example, "Joan is with a patient at the moment. May I have her return your call, or could someone else help you?" It is not advisable to have the calling party hold; try to route the call to someone else, or have the call returned. A staff member involved in direct patient care should not be interrupted with a telephone call unless it is an absolute emergency. If the staff member is on another telephone call, you may say, for example, "Joan is on another line at the moment. Would you care to hold, or may I have her return your call?" In a case like this, always give the party calling the choice of waiting. Remember to check back on the line approximately every 30 seconds. When checking on the line, you may say, for example, "Thank you for waiting. Joan is still on the other line. Would you care to keep holding, or could I have her return your call?" If the caller waits too long, he or she will probably elect to have the call returned.

The following is an example of the procedure to use for handling a patient requesting information over the phone. First, ask the patient to hold while you get his or her records. Use the hold button while locating the records. After finding the information, return to the line with "Thank you for holding, Mrs. Green. Your last vision examination was [date]." If you will need a few minutes to locate the information, indicate this to the patient: "It will take me a few minutes to get that information. Would you care to hold, or may I call you back?" The patient will not only be able to do something else with his or her time, but your telephone line will also be free for other calls if the caller chooses to be called back. Locate the information as soon as possible, and return the call promptly as promised.

The optometrist may have specific instructions on how to handle his or her calls. Screen the calls by saying, "Dr. Smith is with a patient now. May I ask who is calling?" The procedure you follow will probably depend on the caller. Consult with your optometrist for guidelines on which calls he or she will take while with patients. As a general rule, the optometrist will accept calls from family members, another doctor, or personal friends immediately or instruct you to tell the caller that he or she will be called right back. If a patient calls for the optometrist, determine if you or any other staff member can help. If not, indicate that you will have the optometrist return the call. A paraoptometric can handle many calls from laboratories or sales representatives, and the party calling can be told, "Dr. Smith is with a patient. May Joan or I help you?"

Never interrupt the optometrist when the caller refuses to identify him or herself. Simply say, "Dr. Smith is with a patient now. May I have him return your call?" These unidentified callers are probably solicitors. They will usually choose to call back at another time rather than having the optometrist return the call.

If expecting an important call, the optometrist will usually advise you in advance that he or she wants to speak to the caller immediately. Each office usually has its own methods and signals for informing the optometrist of a call waiting. One system that has been used with success has the paraoptometric write the name and message on a pad and take it into the examination room. The message is held so that the optometrist, but not the patient, can read it. This method may also be used when someone is waiting in the reception room to speak to the doctor.

When a call comes in while the optometrist is out of the office, say, "Dr. Smith is out of the office. May I have him return your call?" Do not indicate why the doctor is out of the office. If it is necessary to inform the caller of the time of the optometrist's expected return, say, "I expect him back at 2 this afternoon" or "He will be in the office Wednesday morning at 8:30." When the optometrist will be away from the office for a few days, you might say, "Dr. Smith is attending an educational seminar this week but will be back in the office Monday morning." In case of emergency, refer the patient to the optometrist who is covering your practice.

When taking a phone message, record the correct spelling of names and accurate phone numbers. Repeat the spelling and number to the caller to avoid errors. The phone message should be written legibly and completely. It should show the date and time of the call, as well as the name of the caller, phone number, and message.

If the caller is a patient, obtain the record and clip the phone message to the chart before giving it to the optometrist. The optometrist will then have an opportunity to review the patient's case before returning the call and will have all pertinent information available to answer questions that might arise during the call.

If the optometrist is out of the office when a visitor arrives, a message slip should also be filled out. Do not trust your memory for these types of messages. Always write them down and give them to the optometrist as soon as possible.

Many office supply and stationery stores have preprinted message forms in a variety of colors and formats. One design includes a carbon copy of the message. The original copy is torn out, and the carbon copy remains a part of the book. This is excellent to have if an original message with an important phone number is lost.

When placing or returning a call, exercise politeness and courtesy. Plan your professional calls before you place them. Have all pertinent information available so that you can answer questions intelligently. Immediately identify yourself with "Good morning [afternoon]. This is Joan at Dr. Smith's office. May I speak to Mrs. Green please?" Deliver your message, keeping the length of the conversation to a minimum.

Your optometrist may ask you to call patients to inquire about their visual care or progress or return calls to give the patient vision care information. Be sure that you have the correct information, making notes if necessary as the optometrist gives you instructions. Make notations on the patient's record indicating the date of and reason for the call.

Requests for Cost Information

Many of the requests for fees over the phone are from "shoppers," and these calls can be viewed as opportunities rather than nuisances. Think of all callers as prospective patients, and use tact and politeness when answering questions. The caller does not understand how difficult it is for you to answer questions for price information without having an idea of the exact visual needs. An examination fee can be quoted without too much difficulty. It is almost impossible, however, to arrive at an exact quote for a pair of glasses without knowing the prescription, lens materials, tint, and frame specifications.

Some offices prefer not to quote fees over the phone but are willing to schedule the patient for a fee consultation appointment.

When the caller insists on a price estimate, stress the fact that the prices are estimated, and explain that an accurate figure cannot be quoted until an examination has determined the exact services and specific type of lenses needed. If the party insists on knowing your price for contact lenses, stress again that the prices are estimated. Quote the price ranges for contact lenses and emphasize the importance of professional fitting fees and follow-up visits. Stress to the caller that patients receive professional care and that this quality of care will continue after the patient receives the lenses. Many callers are able to distinguish differences in quality and will select the office providing the best professional services.

When discussing fees with a caller, answer only one question at a time and avoid lengthy discussions of why fees are structured the way they are. One way to redirect the conversation is to determine the date of the caller's last examination and whether the caller is presently a contact lens wearer. Be sure to inquire about the patient's visual needs. There is a specific reason the patient is seeking eye care, and you will need to ask questions to establish that reason. Many shoppers are turned into patients when handled diplomatically.

Handling Complaints

Every office receives calls from time to time complaining about services or materials or a misunderstanding of charges for services. Handling complaints requires patience and understanding. Listen attentively and do not interrupt the patient who is expressing complaints. Always use a sincere tone of voice. Express concern for the patient's difficulty or problem. Do not, however, place blame on anyone else in the office. Your main concern should be solving the problem.

Offer solutions to resolve the complaint that will be beneficial to both the patient and the practice. Consult the optometrist or a senior paraoptometric if the problem is complex. Do not promise the patient anything that you will not be able to deliver. When the conversation is over, the patient should be satisfied with the solutions offered. The goal should be to solve the problem in an efficient manner and to retain the good will of the patient.

Mastering the Art of Making Appointments

Efficient appointment scheduling is essential to the smooth operation of any optometric practice. An efficient appointment system will prevent delays for the optometrist and the patient but will still allow time to handle emergencies with minimal disruption of the office routine.

The paraoptometric should consult with the optometrist to determine the length of time required for specific types of appointments. A complete vision examination will naturally require more time than a follow-up evaluation. Since paraoptometrics may spend time with the patients in data gathering and pretesting, optometrists will have more time available to see additional patients or to prepare consultation reports. Therefore, every staff member should have a thorough knowledge of the different types of appointments and the amount of time required by both the optometrist and the paraoptometric for each type.

All appointments should be written in the appointment book. Never rely on memory. When a patient calls requesting an appointment, determine what services will be needed to give you an indication of the amount of time needed for the appointment.

Appointments can be written in the appointment book in pencil and then erased in the event of rescheduling. If the optometrist prefers that you use pen, press-on adhesive strips can be applied over the rescheduled appointment, and the new appointment can be written legibly on them.

Depending on the size of the practice, the paraoptometric may be required to use a computerized appointment booking system. Many larger practices involving multiple optometrists require computerized booking of patients. In a solo practice or small practice of one or two optometrists, the handwritten appointment system may be the most efficient.

The first available appointment should be offered to the patient. Offering the patient a choice of two different appointments times may be effective. "Would you prefer Tuesday, January 12, at 10 A.M., or Thursday, January 14, at 2 P.M.?" By allowing the patient to choose the most convenient time, you are reducing the possibility of a "no show" or cancellation. Before ending the conversation with the patient, repeat the time and day of the appointment to eliminate misunderstandings.

If the situation is determined to be an emergency, work the patient's appointment into the schedule the same day. The optometrist may request that you inform the patient that his or her eyes will be dilated and he or she should therefore expect to have blurry vision after the examination. Suggest that the patient bring a pair of sunglasses to wear after dilation, and tell the patient that he or she may wish to have someone drive him or her home.

Emergency Appointments

The paraoptometric answering the phone will be in the position to determine whether a patient requires an emergency appointment. If in doubt, the paraoptometric should consult with the optometrist. Your office should have a system of assigning priority to emergencies that can be executed rapidly and efficiently.

Samples of emergency calls include painful symptoms from overwear of contact lenses; scratched eyes; red, itching eyes, possibly with a discharge; sudden blurred vision; severe headaches; trauma or a blow to the eye; excess tearing; broken glasses; and lost or damaged contact lenses. Other emergencies also include loss of vision, severe pain in the eye, no side or peripheral vision, double vision, seeing flashing lights, and seeing halos around lights.

Pain and loss of vision are critical and need to be taken care of immediately. If in doubt, consult with the optometrist for instruction as to how to handle the call. The optometrist may choose to talk to the patient personally. If the optometrist is out of town when an emergency call is received, immediately refer the caller to the practitioner who is covering the office while the optometrist is away.

When patients break their glasses or lose or damage a contact lens, they believe it is an emergency situation, even though the health of their eyes is not in immediate danger. Act swiftly to obtain suitable replacements or to make repairs. Although these situations would probably be called "urgent" rather than an emergency, patients are counting on your office to maintain their visual requirements.

When handling a call from a worried patient, use tact and express concern. The patient is calling the office for help, and to the patient the situation is an emergency. Respond to this need for help in a professional, considerate way. The patient will appreciate the quality of care you provide in an emergency or urgent situation.

Controlling the Appointment Book

Expertise and experience are required to keep the appointment book legible and under control. Each day, the next day's appointments should be confirmed. An example of a confirmation call might be, "Good morning, Mrs. Green. This is Carol at Dr. Smith's office. I am calling to confirm [Do not say "remind about"] your appointment tomorrow at 8 A.M. for a vision examination [contact lens check-up, etc.]." After confirmations are made, type the schedule, showing the time, name of the patient, and type of appointment. Often, a computer printout of the next day's schedule may be obtained by the simple push of a button if the office uses a computerized appointment system. Make a copy to be posted in the laboratory or any room that all staff have access to and a copy for the optometrist's private office or examination room.

Always keep a list of patients desiring to come in at the first available appointment. If there is a last-minute cancellation or a cancellation at the time the confirmation call is made, refer to this list. Call the patients who are waiting for an appointment and try to fill the empty spot in the schedule. Scattered and uneven scheduling wastes valuable staff time and can be as frustrating as an overcrowded schedule.

Most offices discourage patients from coming without an appointment. If patients drop in because they happened to be off work that day, broke their glasses, or showed up early by mistake for an appointment next week, carefully evaluate the schedule to see if there is an available time that day. It may be the office policy to check with the optometrist before scheduling the walk-in patient.

If a patient comes in without an appointment for a frame repair or adjustment, pull the records and check the date of his or her last examination. If the recall date has passed, then advise the patient that he or she is due for another examination. Ask the patient if he or she would like to schedule an appointment for a vision examination. In this way, you show patients you care about their vision needs, and you express the importance of regular eye care.

The appointment book is the controlling force in the office. A well organized book will govern an efficient, productive office. The appointment book can also create a dilemma in the office routine as well as inhibit the performance of staff members if it is disorganized.

The appointment system and type of book used will depend on the size of the practice and the number of doctors and paraoptometrics associated with the practice. Appointment systems may be simple or complex depending on the needs of the practice. Figure 1-5 illustrates simple appointment sheets for a one-optometrist or a one-paraoptometric practice. Complex appointment sheets for a multiple-optometrist or multiple-paraoptometric practice are shown in Figure 1-6.

Data Gathering

Individual offices vary in the amount of information to be obtained from the patient when making the appointment. Some optometrists want to know only the patient's name and phone number and whether the caller is a previous patient. Other optometrists require much more information.

The following list includes some questions that may be used in gathering information before the office visit:

- Do you need a vision examination? If not, what service do you require?
- Have you been to our office before? If not, how long has it been since your last eye examination?
- Which doctor examined you on your previous visit to our office (if applicable)?
- Do you wear contact lenses? If so, what type? How long have you worn them?
- Who referred you to the office? (Use this information to send a thank-you letter.)
- What is your date of birth? (Inform patients who are minors that a parent should accompany them to their initial visit.)

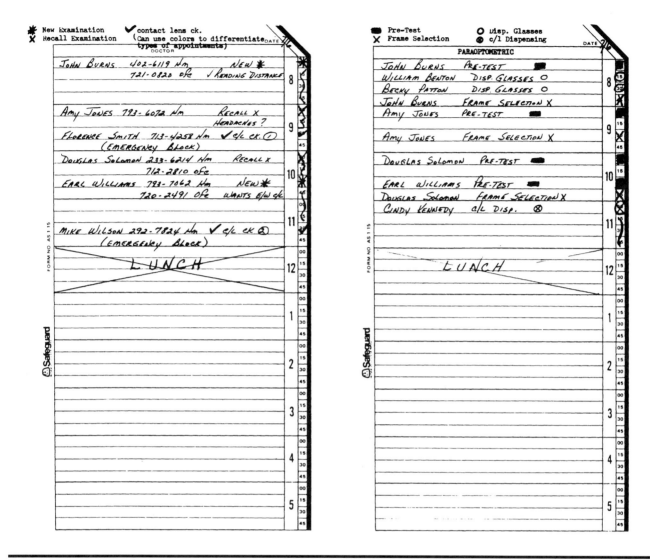

Figure 1-5—Appointment sheets for a one-optometrist or one-paraoptometric practice. (Courtesy of Safeguard Business Systems, Inc.)

- Are you covered by vision care or major medical insurance? (If yes, remind the patient to bring the form or insurance card to the visit.)

If this information is not requested over the phone before the appointment, it will be necessary to obtain it when the patient arrives for the appointment. Suggest to a new patient that he or she arrive a few minutes early to fill out a patient information sheet. The patient information sheet should include the following data: name, address, and phone number; occupation; employer name, address, and phone number; name of spouse; name, address, and phone number of spouse's employer; social security number; person responsible for the account; method of payment preferred (cash, check, credit card, etc.); name, address, phone number, and policy number of insurance company (if applicable); and chief complaint or reason for the visit.

The questions suggested are important to the business administration of the patient's records. The optometrist also might want included on this sheet (or a separate questionnaire) some information that could be considered part of a patient history.

Greeting the Patient

The role of the front office paraoptometric is to greet the patient, gather and prepare informa-

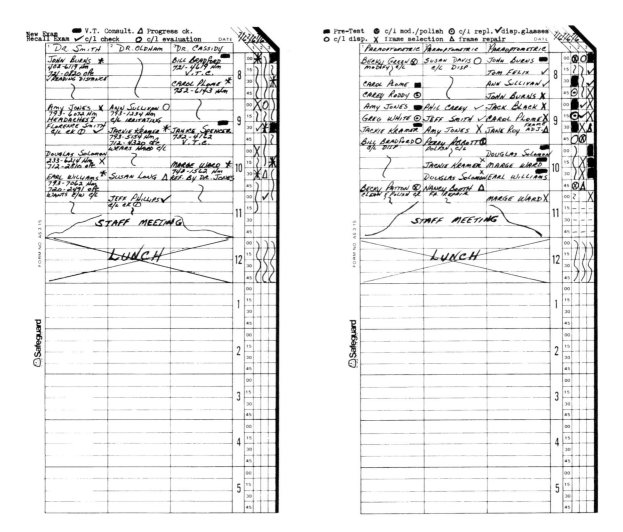

Figure 1-6—Appointment sheets for a multiple-optometrist or multiple-staff office. (Courtesy of Safeguard Business Systems, Inc.)

tion for the patient chart, and update the charts of patients. These procedures must be done efficiently so that the patient flow runs smoothly and the doctor or other staff members are not kept waiting.

If your office is running slightly behind schedule, advise the waiting patient of the delay. Be honest with the patient if your office is extremely behind schedule. Give your best estimate of how long it will be before the patient will be seen. Give the patient the option of running an errand or just relaxing. The patient will appreciate your honesty and courtesy. The patient's treatment at the front desk sets the atmosphere for the entire appointment.

Recalls

Recalls serve both the patient and the practice. An efficient and effective recall system will enhance the practice and, at the same time, help preserve the visual welfare of the patient. Most people are busy with their day-to-day activities and do not think of their vision care unless they develop a problem. An effective recall program can help maintain a regular vision care program for patients.

At the time of the appointment, the optometrist will indicate on the patient's chart when the recall is to be made. Begin programming for the next appointment when the patient is preparing to

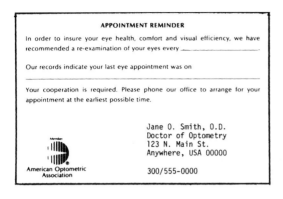

Figure 1-7—A sample recall card available from the American Optometric Association.

leave the office: "Dr. Smith will want to re-examine your eyes in a year. We will contact you at that time to make an appointment." Alternatively, "Dr. Smith would like to see you in 6 months to evaluate your contact lenses. We will be in touch with you then to schedule an appointment." Some offices schedule the appointment a year ahead of time and then send a card to the patient confirming the appointment about 2 weeks before the date.

Recalling patients may be done by card (Figure 1-7), letter, or telephone. Recall appointments may include eye examinations, contact lens evaluations, progress check-ups, and eye pressure checks, to name a few. Some offices send a letter for the annual vision examination and place a phone call for services needed in a shorter period of time, such as a 30-day contact lens recheck. When writing or calling any patient about a recall, always include the reason for the recall in the message.

Many offices find the telephone method of recall to be the most effective. If using the telephone recall method, the following example could be used: "Good morning, Mrs. Green. This is Carol at Dr. Smith's office. When you were in the office last month, the doctor indicated he would like to see you again to recheck the fit of your contact lenses. Would next Monday morning at 10:15 be convenient?"

The same basic approach may be used for rescheduling an appointment that has been missed: "Good morning, Mrs. Green. This is Carol at Dr. Smith's office. We missed seeing you yesterday for your eye examination. Would you like to come in next week at the same time, or would an afternoon appointment be more convenient?"

The recall system is important to the practice and is one of the easiest systems to manage. The following is one of many types of recall systems used. It is simple and effective. The optometrist may wish to include variations, but the basic principles will remain the same.

Make a 3 × 5-inch card at the time of the appointment and attach it to the patient record. The optometrist will indicate the recall date on the patient record, which will then be copied onto the recall card. When the patient is dismissed (glasses dispensed, etc.), the recall card is filed in a 3 × 5-inch drawer, first by month, and then alphabetically by the patient's last name. Each month, the following month's cards should be pulled and appointments made by whatever recall method (mailing, telephone call) the optometrist prefers. The cards should then be refiled in the drawer.

When the recall patient comes in for an appointment, pull the recall card and keep it with the rest of the patient records until the patient is again dismissed. At that point, a new recall date would be put on both the patient chart and the recall card. The recall date is shown on the general records of the patient so the recall card can be located immediately. The card is then filed under the new date.

All recall cards for patients who have not made a new appointment are left in the recall drawer under the original recall date. This drawer may then be reviewed by the optometrist to figure the percentages of patients that are not returning to the office. A study can be made of the type of patient and age group. This is also the source for pursuing a second and third recall effort.

When a patient comes into the office for an appointment, regardless of the type of appointment, the recall card should be pulled and attached to the patient's record. If the optometrist changes the recall date, the paraoptometric will be less likely to forget to change the date on the recall card.

Recall card drawers must be kept up-to-date. If a recall letter is returned from the post office stamped "moved, left no forwarding address," pull the recall card, combine it with the rest of the patient's records, and indicate on the records that the patient has moved. Check the general files for other members of the family and pull all their recall cards. This will save time and postage for sending undeliverable letters.

If a patient informs you of a name change, a new address, or a death in the family, pull the recall card and make the necessary changes to avoid embarrassing situations.

Computerized recall is easier than ever. Software packages are available that will list patients requiring recall based on a set of variables the paraoptometric introduces. Most often, the date will be the determining variable in generating a recall listing. A computerized system of recall operates on the same principal as the manual system; however, rather than jotting the date of recall on an index card, it is logged into the computer database.

Filing

Proper filing is vital to the efficient operation of the practice. The filing system used may vary with the size of the practice and with the number of professional services offered. There are advantages and disadvantages to every filing system, and selecting one will depend on how it can be adapted to the practice.

One of the simplest and most widely used systems is by alphabetical sequence according to the last name. Records are arranged in a drawer with A–Z index guides. Great care must be exercised to avoid misspelling a patient's name, which will result in misfiling of the record.

Another system of filing that is more complex than the alphabetical system is the numerical method. This system will decrease the chances of misfiling, since it is easier to spot a number out of sequence. It is more time-consuming, however, both when creating a file and when attempting to locate a file. A cross-index card is required for each file, indicating the patient's name and address and the number assigned to the file. It is best to use a number machine for numbering the files to avoid transpositions and accidentally using the same number for two patients. Keep a daily sheet of numbers to be assigned. Number the patient's chart, cross-index card, recall card, ledger card, and sheet all at the same time.

When a former patient comes in, assign a new number and cross out the old number. When assigning a new number, make sure all the records are changed to the new number. Allow the old number to remain legible in case the patient records should be misfiled by the old number.

The numerical system is better than the alphabetical system for keeping records up-to-date. Any old numbers still in the drawer will indicate immediately how long it has been since the patient was in the office. Old records can be pulled from the drawers and filed in a storage area.

Regardless of the system used, color coding will make it almost impossible to misfile a folder. If a folder is misfiled, the color code will make it easier to find the file that is out of sequence.

A simple method for coding the alphabetical filing system is to designate colors along with the letters such as red, A–C; blue, D–F; and so on. Some of the systems available have holding strips at the top of the file folders. This allows different shapes or color tabs to be inserted into the holding strip. Each color and shape of tab inserted at different areas on the holding strip represents a code. The folders can be identified by the first letter of the last name, type of patient (e.g., contact lens wearer, patient with low vision, etc.), year the patient was last seen, either or both month and year of recall, or bad credit risk. A special color tab can be inserted when a file is removed. This makes refiling easier. A quick glance will give information such as how many contact lens patients have been seen or how many recalls are due next month.

Every staff member should know how the filing system operates. The main responsibility for the refiling of patient records, however, should be assigned to one individual. At times, the optometrist may need a patient record immediately, and the staff member who is free at the time may locate the file, but refiling should be done by the individual responsible for that task.

Filing should be done every day to prevent records from being misplaced and scattered. It is easier to locate a file from an orderly file drawer than to leaf through a stack of cards and charts to find a patient's record.

Business files must also be maintained. The best procedure for arranging these files is alphabetical, either by name or by subject. These files will contain all the correspondence concerning business matters, as well as statements and invoices. The standard 8½ × 11-inch file folder system is recommended and should be kept separate from the patient files. A typed, standard gummed label is used for labeling folders.

Color Coding in the Laboratory

Color coding is an excellent method to use in the laboratory for monitoring prescriptions on order. After a patient has been examined, the record is put in a tray in the laboratory for ordering prescriptions. The trays can be color-coded to categorize contact lenses, glasses, and frame color. Coding can also be used to identify a special rush order.

The laboratory policy in the office might be to check on the progress of a prescription order after 2 or 3 days. At the time the prescription is ordered, the specific color label is put on the tray with the date ordered. For example, contact lenses (orange label) are ordered on Monday, June 20. The trays are then stacked on the shelf chronologically by date. By Thursday or Friday, it will be apparent at a glance which orders have not been received. The color of the label (orange) will indicate immediately the order was for contact lenses, which will aid the paraoptometric in determining where to call to check on the progress of the order.

Office Supplies on Hand

In most offices, a paraoptometric will be responsible for keeping track of office and optical supplies. The optometrist, with input from the paraoptometric, may decide on the various materials used in the office and perhaps even where to order them. Ongoing control of these materials will probably be delegated to the paraoptometric.

Always keep an adequate supply of all office materials on hand. There should be an added reserve of supplies and materials that are constantly being used. The materials should be stored in an area with easy access. Optical supplies and repair items should be stored in the laboratory and office supplies in or near the business office.

Business Supplies

The term "business supplies" covers all supplies used in the handling of the business affairs in the office.

A purchasing notebook should be prepared that lists all supplies and the company from which they were purchased. The notebook can include a reference in the back to all suppliers and a list of the supplies ordered from each of them.

In the notebook itself, note the quantity of the item ordered and the date received. This indicates how long each particular supply lasts and helps determine if it is advisable to order in a larger or smaller quantity. This is especially important for stationery and all other forms on which the name of the practice is imprinted. Imprinted forms take longer to obtain, so make the necessary allowances to ensure that new supplies arrive before the old ones are depleted. It is a good idea to indicate probable order delivery time, such as 4 weeks. Keep a checklist in the storage area listing the amount of each supply remaining and at what level it is time to reorder. When the supply gets close to your reserve figure, it is time to reorder. Check the supplies and this checklist about once a month. A good way to mark stationery and printed forms is to put a colored reminder in the box at the point where you will reorder. When supplies are taken out of the box and the colored reminder is exposed, it is time to reorder.

Review supply catalogs for price information. Some supplies are often less expensive when bought in quantities, and time may be saved by not having to order as often.

When receiving an order of supplies, check the packing slip or accompanying invoice against the items received. If the items are imprinted, check for accuracy. Make sure the quantity received is the quantity ordered and that the charges are correct. Place the invoice in a designated place until a statement is received at the end of the month.

Miscellaneous business office supplies, such as pencils, staples, and paper clips, are usually available immediately. Keeping a large supply of these items on hand is usually not necessary, although a reduced price is commonly available for purchases of large quantities.

Examination Room Supplies

Examination room supplies include everything used in the examination of a patient. To control the flow of these supplies, a checklist should be created with the input of both the optometrist and the paraoptometric in charge of supplies. Once the list is made, it will require tight control to ensure an adequate inventory of items ranging from projector bulbs to visual field paper and fluorescein strips. The checklist should be reviewed regularly, and the paraoptometric should maintain at least 1 month's reserve supply of these materials. The information contained in the purchasing notebook is valuable in this area in determining reserve quantities for projector bulbs (as an example) due to availability and length of life of the bulb.

Solutions and Drugs

The use of solutions and drugs can vary considerably from month to month; therefore, it is necessary to monitor the usage of these supplies carefully. Again, the purchasing notebook is valuable because of the information it contains regarding the availability and approximate usage.

A close watch over the appointment book will give a good indication of the types of patients scheduled for appointments. The number of contact lens patients seen will determine how quickly the care kits and solutions will be dispensed. The weather affects the amount of decongestants and artificial tears used. Factors such as these cannot always be anticipated.

Extra care must be exercised when ordering drugs and solutions, since most of them will have an expiration date. Do not order these items in such large quantities that the quantity on hand will become useless due to expiration of the solution. Check the expiration date on the bottles when the order is received, and make this notation in the purchasing notebook. The supply should be checked periodically and recorded properly, keeping expiration dates foremost in mind.

Proper storage of solutions is important for maintaining their effectiveness. Check labels on bottles and follow instructions regarding storage temperatures and other factors. This is especially true for pharmaceutical agents used during the examination or for treatment purposes.

Optical Supplies

The amount of optical supplies needed is often unpredictable. It requires careful monitoring, since the amount of reserves required cannot be determined easily due to constantly changing patient needs.

The optical laboratory that supplies the practice's prescription lenses may be the best source of materials needed to repair various optical items. It will be necessary to keep on hand an assortment of screws, nose pads, and lens liners. Although these items are not always difficult to replace, an adequate reserve supply should be maintained.

The supply of eyeglass cases requires a close watch. If the cases are imprinted with the practice name, they may take longer for delivery. Ordering imprinted spectacle cases in quantity has definite price advantages.

Frames

A separate purchasing notebook should be made for frames, showing the name, manufacturer, cost, and dispensing price to the patient. Some frame companies deliver quickly, whereas others may take 2 weeks or longer on frame orders. Delivery time is not as crucial when ordering a frame to replace depleted stock as it is when ordering for a patient.

The styles and number of frames dispensed at any given time are difficult to judge when ordering. The supply of styles may be supervised by the optometrist, but in most cases, it is the responsibility of the paraoptometric to keep accurate records on the purchase of frames. Occasionally, there are discounts offered by manufacturers when a certain dollar amount is purchased within a month.

The number of different frame types available through your optometrist's office must be rotated on a regular basis. If a frame is not dispensed within a certain period of time, return it to the manufacturer either for credit or an exchange for another style. There is usually a time limit on returns of this nature, so exercise diligence in this area. There are stock control sheets that can be purchased from office supply stores that will help in tracking the movement of frames in and out of the office. Information listed on the sheet includes the name of the frame, date purchased, and any reorders that are made. When the frame order is received, list it on the stock control sheet. When the frame is used for patient prescriptions, cross it off the sheet. By looking at the supply sheet, you can tell which frames are not moving and should be rotated and which frames need to be reordered.

The supply of frames should be checked thoroughly once every few weeks, comparing the stock control sheet against actual stock in the display area and in the stock drawers.

Contact Lens Supplies on Hand

The stock control sheet used for contact lenses should contain the same information as for frames, but types of contact lenses do not change quite as rapidly as styles of frames.

If the practice dictates a large supply of contact lenses, color coding may be used for quick identification of daily wear, extended wear, toric, and other types of lenses. A specific method may also be required for separating the lenses by manufacturer or by power and base curves.

Stock must be rotated, since some contact lenses have expiration dates. Check the expiration date and store the lenses so that the oldest lenses will be used first. If there are unopened lenses on hand that are approaching the expiration date, send them back to the manufacturer to exchange them for new ones.

Purchasing contact lenses in larger quantities gives a definite price advantage. With the introduction of frequent replacement and disposable lens types, contact lens inventory poses new challenges. Each lens manufacturer offers suggestions on how best to stock their lens types. The optometrist and the paraoptometric must examine the lens choices available and select a few to stock in the office using a simplified inventory system. Each practice must determine the adequate number of lenses to have on hand. Most contact lens manufacturers offer delivery of lenses within a day or two because they recognize the space limitations that may prevent an office from storing a large stock of lenses.

BUSINESS OFFICE PROCEDURES

Computerized Financial Records and Bookkeeping

Depending on the size of the practice, financial and business records may be handled either manually or by computer. The computerized practice offers definite advantages with regard to time saved in generating financial reports, as well as keeping daily financial records. An initial investment in time and equipment must be made when setting up the business records in a computer database; however, in the long term, this will prove to be time effective.

Financial record keeping plays an important role in the development of the practice. Records must be accurate and up-to-date. Records include an explanation of when and how much income is received and where and how the expenses are paid.

The optometrist will probably have an accountant who will prepare monthly balance sheets, profit and loss statements, quarterly payroll, tax reports, and year-end tax reports. The accountant will need precise, legible records from the paraoptometric keeping daily financial records to prepare all of these reports accurately.

Each cash receipt is recorded in a cash receipts book, and each check disbursed or cash paid out may be recorded in a cash disbursement book. Not every office will have a cash disbursement book. The accountant might take the information directly from the check stub and post it to the chart of accounts. The chart of accounts is the list of categories to which the expenses are posted, such as rent, office supplies, and telephone. If the office has a cash disbursement book, consult the accountant to set up the appropriate chart of accounts for the practice. Accurate posting to the chart of accounts is important since these figures are used by the accountant to prepare monthly financial statements and, at the end of the fiscal year, for income-tax preparation.

One check-writing system (Figure 1-8) works on a principle similar to the pegboard system used for income receipts. It is carbonized, and when a check is written, the information is transferred to the check register at the same time. The register then serves as the check stub. The register copy is headed with the chart of accounts, and the amount of the check is then extended out to the appropriate column. It includes a column for the bank balance, which should be brought forward as the checks are written. When the page becomes full, the columns are totaled. The total of the column showing the amount of the checks written should equal the combined total of all the columns headed with the chart of accounts.

If using a standard business checkbook, make sure the check stub is filled out com-

16 Chapter 1

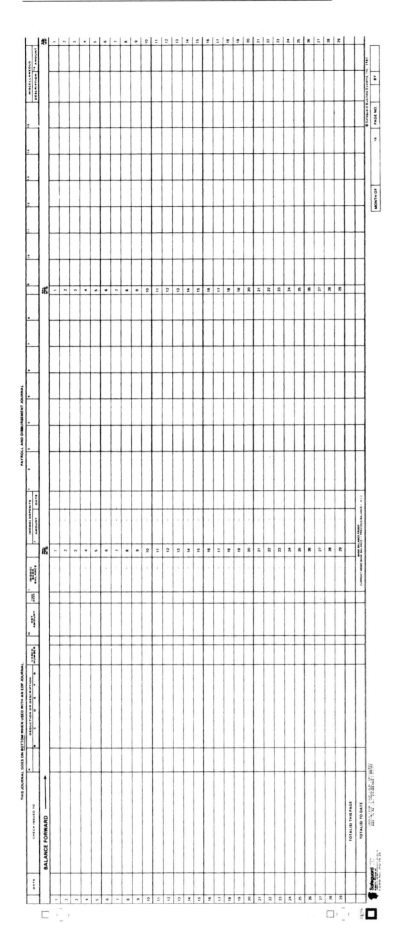

Figure 1-8—The Safeguard checkwriting system. (Courtesy of Safeguard Business Systems, Inc.)

Figure 1–8—(continued)

pletely so that the accountant will post it to the proper account.

Regardless of the type of system used, the balance should always be brought forward when writing the check. If there are charges to the balance by the bank, such as the service fees for credit cards, put a notation on the area beside the stub explaining the charge and deduct it from the balance.

Any bill owed by the doctor of optometry is an *accounts payable*. The credit rating of the optometrist's practice depends on the bills being paid on time. The time schedule for payment of bills will vary in different offices. Some offices use a system of paying on the first and fifteenth of each month. Immediate payment when the statement is received is a method used by other offices.

There should be a substantiating statement or invoice for almost every check that is written on the office account. The exceptions to this rule may be payroll and possibly rent payments.

For all regular payments made each month without an invoice, such as rent, a 3 × 5-inch tickler file can be made up for reminder cards. Use an index of 1–31 for the days of the month and put a card in back of the date due. The card should contain the following information: to whom the check is written, address, amount of check, and what kind of payment it represents. This file will also be valuable in training a new or substitute paraoptometric in procedures for payments of bills.

When a statement is received, all invoices should be matched to the statement. One check is written for the total amount of the statement. Make the proper deduction from the balance due if the company offers a discount for prompt payment. Staple the invoices and statement together and mark the statement with the date paid and the check number and file in the business files. The business files should be updated every year and, for accounting purposes, should coincide with the fiscal year of the practice. The old files should be stored in a file box and new files prepared each year. In the event of an audit, the records may be located quickly.

The law requires that certain records be kept for specified periods of time. The accountant can supply a list of what needs to be kept and for how long.

Payroll

All financial records of the practice are privileged information, and payroll is no exception. Never discuss any staff member's salary with anyone except for the doctor and the accountant.

When an employee is added to the staff, a W-4 form must be filled out. This form contains the employee's name, address, Social Security number, and withholding status to be applied when preparing the payroll check. The schedule for the amounts of Social Security and federal withholding taxes is available from the Internal Revenue Service. If state taxes are to be withheld, this schedule may be obtained from the individual state department of revenue.

The check stub should include the following information: gross salary; amount withheld for Social Security, federal tax, and state tax (if applicable); and net salary. Regardless of whether the employees are paid weekly, semimonthly, or monthly, the proper amount of tax must be withheld. Each check stub must contain all these figures for accounting procedures to record taxes accrued, which are then paid quarterly. The accountant will also instruct you as to the amount of tax due and the date it must be paid. There are no exceptions to the rules set out for payment of payroll tax deposits, and if the deadlines are not met, the Internal Revenue Service assesses penalties and fines for delinquent payments.

The figures contained on either or both the check stub and register are then posted to each individual employee's account and accrued to the end of the year. The totals are then transferred to the W-2 form, which is used for filing personal income tax.

Checks are available with a printed area for listing payroll information (Figure 1-9). This allows the employee to know immediately the exact amount of money withheld and for what purpose. Checks are also available with a detachable stub that can be removed and retained by the individual employee.

Petty Cash

Every office should have a petty cash fund. The amount of money kept in this fund is at the discretion of the optometrist. The size of the practice usually determines what expenses can be paid for out of petty cash. It is used mostly for postage due and small quantities of office supplies. It is a backup fund to use for a quick trip to the store for something you forgot to reorder. It is indeed used for making "petty" purchases.

A receipt must be put in the fund whenever money is taken out. At the end of each month, the fund must be balanced out and reimbursed. This is done by totaling all of the receipts and counting the remaining cash in the fund. The combination of the two totals should equal the starting amount at the beginning of the month.

A check is written for the total of the receipts, and the cash is put back into the fund.

Bank Statements

Bank statements are received each month and should be reconciled as soon as possible. Arrange all the canceled checks in numerical order. Mark off each check stub and corresponding check, listing all of the checks that have not cleared the bank. Compare the statement and check stubs, listing the deposits that were made but not posted by the bank in time for the cutoff period for that particular statement. Subtract any miscellaneous bank charges (as listed on the bank statement), such as check printing, from the balance shown in the checkbook.

To reconcile the bank statement with the checkbook, first list the "ending balance" figure from the bank statement, add any deposits made but not posted, and subtract the total outstanding checks. The figure should be the same as the figure in the checkbook.

	Amount	Description
	$2,646.00	Checkbook balance
−	23.00	Amount subtracted for printing checks
	$2,623.00	New checkbook balance
	$3,075.00	Ending balance taken from bank statement
+	200.00	Deposit made but not posted (add)
	$3,275.00	
−	652.00	Outstanding checks (subtract)
	$2,623.00	New reconciled bank statement figure

Recording Charges and Payments

An entry must be made on either or both the payment and ledger card whenever there is a charge for services performed or a payment is received from a patient. This financial record is an important procedure performed by the paraoptometric and must be accurate and legible.

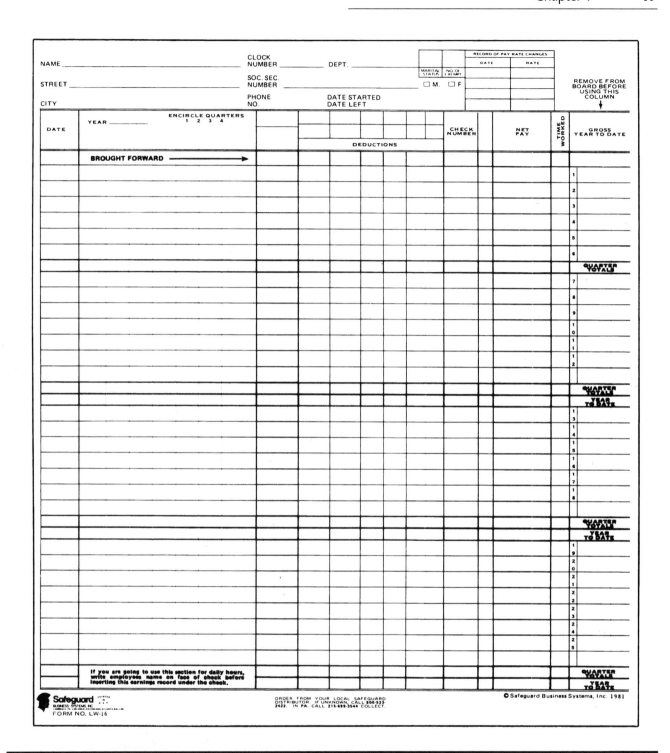

Figure 1-9— The Safeguard payroll check system. (Courtesy of Safeguard Business Systems, Inc.)

One widely used method for recording these transactions is the pegboard system (Figure 1-10). This system is one of the most error-free as well as the most efficient, since it uses either carbon or NCR (no carbon required) paper. It enables the paraoptometric to make entries on the charge/receipt slip, ledger card, and daily control sheet in one step.

When the patient arrives for the appointment, the ledger card is lined up between the charge/receipt slips and the daily control sheets. The date, patient name, receipt number, and balance due, if any, are posted in the appropriate spaces, and the detachable fee slip is torn off and placed with the patient's records. The fee slip will be returned to the front desk at the

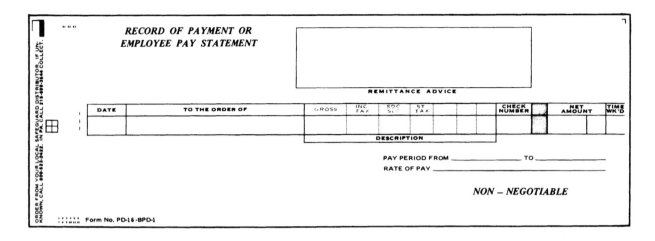

Figure 1-9—(continued)

completion of the patient visit, showing the services rendered and the charges. These items are then posted in the appropriate spaces on the charge/receipt slip, as well as payment received (if any) and the new balance due. The receipt is then given to the patient, and the ledger card is filed in the accounts receivable tray if there is a balance due. A photocopy of the ledger card can then serve as a statement when billing.

The ledger card and daily control sheet now have the information of previous balances, charges made, payments received, and new balance due on every financial transaction of that patient for that day. At the end of the day, these columns are totaled. The previous balance due total—plus the new charges made—minus payments received will equal the new balance due total. Errors may be found easily by a quick review of the daily control sheet. If an error is made on an entry, draw a single line through the entire entry (allowing it to remain legible) and make a complete new entry, being certain to insert the ledger card and ensuring that all records contain the new entry.

The new balance due total is now the total of all accounts receivable. This figure should be the same as the total of all ledger cards in the accounts receivable tray. These totals are usually checked against each other once a week.

A receipt is made for every payment received. If the payment is by check, stamp "for deposit only" on the back of the check immediately. Keep all payments in a locked drawer or in an area accessible only to authorized personnel. At the end of the day, the total payments and cash drawer must be balanced. The total payments received as shown on the daily control sheet should equal the amount of checks and cash in the money drawer. Prepare the bank deposit, making a duplicate for future reference in the event of a question on payment of an account or posting of the deposit by the bank. It is advisable to write the patient's last name and bank number on the deposit slip.

If the paraoptometric is involved in a solo or small private practice, it may be more efficient to continue to manage the business and financial records through standard bookkeeping systems. Even small practices, however, have converted most of these types of functions to a computerized system. There are many software packages available that perform a variety of tasks such as payroll, year-end tax reports, daily cash flow analysis, and so forth. The optometrist and the paraoptometric must examine the various systems available and select the one that best suits the needs of the practice.

Fees and Payment Policies

The amount charged to the patient must be carefully explained so that there are no misunderstandings about the cost of services rendered and the method of payment. An example explanation might be the following: "The new lenses are $X, and the examination today is $Y, for a total of $X + $Y."

Policy on payment varies from office to office. Some offices require full payment at the first visit. Others might require 50% at the first

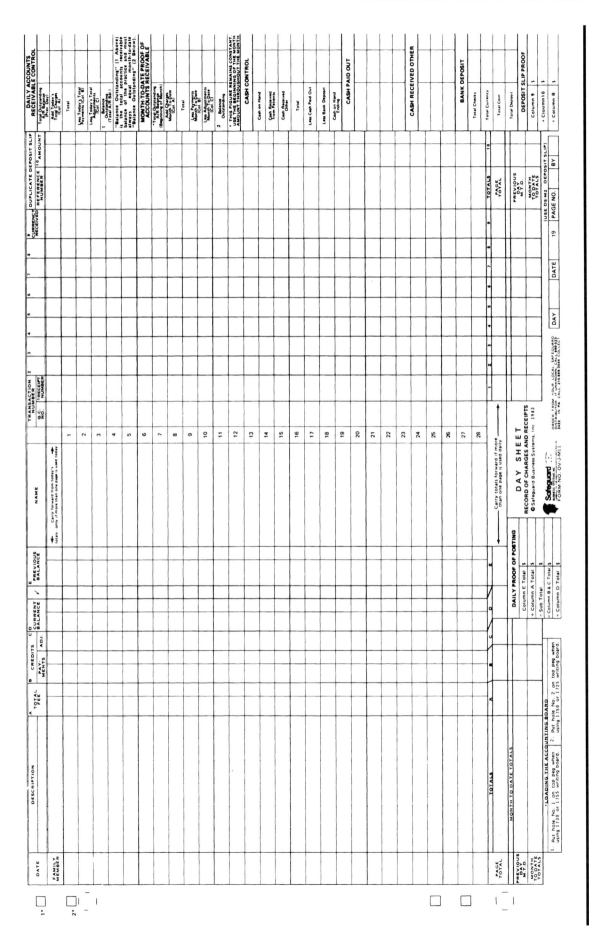

Figure 1-10—The Safeguard pegboard system. (Courtesy of Safeguard Business Systems, Inc.)

22 Chapter 1

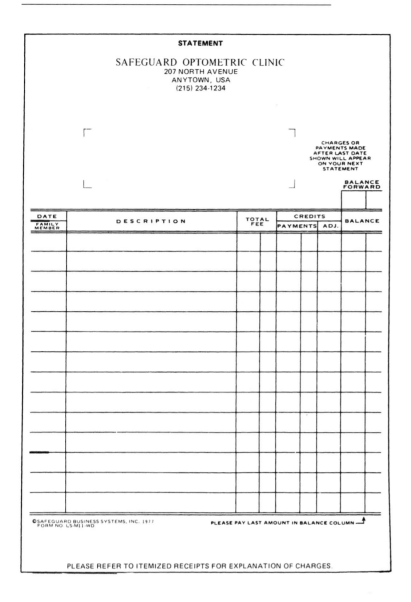

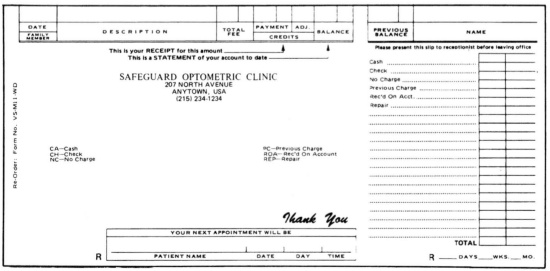

Figure 1-10—*(continued)*

visit, with the balance due at the last visit. Many variations are used, and the optometrist will specify the fee structure and payment policy to be used. A fee slip should be made out for each patient that indicates the type of professional service rendered and the amount charged for the service. If used with the pegboard system, this fee slip is the detachable stub of the receipt/charge slip (Figure 1-11). Also shown on the fee slip is a list of procedures and services available. An added item printed on the bottom could be "Your next appointment will be ____________." The fee slip is included with the patient's records during the examination, and the doctor will check off the services performed. The fee slip is then returned to the front desk for entering on the charge/receipt slip and for explanation of charges to the patient.

Some offices prefer to make up a fee slip for a more detailed explanation of charges (Figure 1-12). This type of fee slip can show a breakdown for lenses, frames, professional services and would include the service agreement. The slip allows the patient to see exactly what kind of lenses he or she is getting and the name of the frame. The slip is then signed by the patient and becomes a permanent part of the patient file. It eliminates any misunderstandings in ordering the materials. A separate fee slip can also be used for a breakdown of charges for contact lenses, such as examination, lenses, care kit, and service agreement.

The time to discuss payment policies is at the first visit. If the patient is a minor, parents must be consulted on professional fees before services are performed, and a payment policy must be established. When patients leave the office, they should be fully aware of their financial obligations. If a patient is unable to pay the full amount, a payment schedule must be set up.

The optometrist will set payment policy procedures but should not have to discuss financial matters with the patient. If the office offers a payment schedule, it is a delegated responsibility of the paraoptometric to use tact and diplomacy to explain the policy. Complete information must be obtained, including the name, address, and phone number of the person to be billed. This information is vital when patients are children, elderly dependents, and dependents in divorce situations. Judging a good credit risk is difficult. Appearance is misleading, and judgment must be

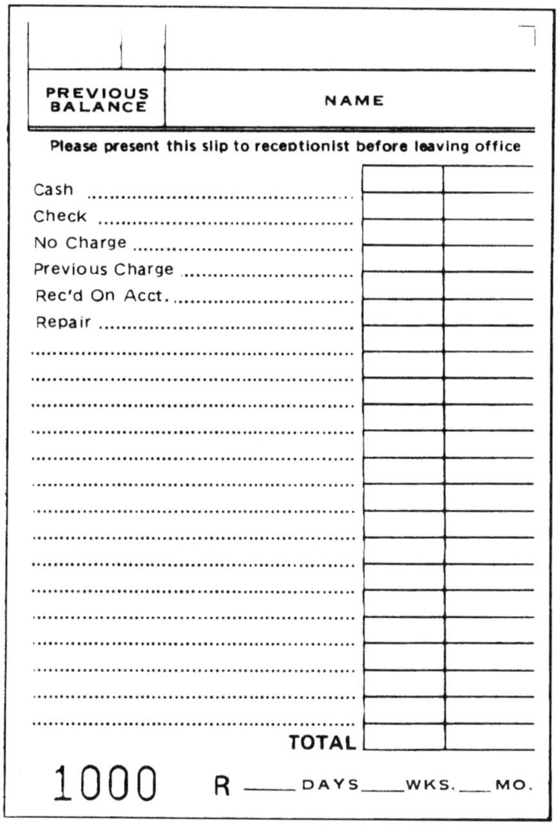
PREVIOUS BALANCE

NAME

Please present this slip to receptionist before leaving office

Cash

Check

No Charge

Previous Charge

Rec'd On Acct.

Repair

TOTAL

1000 R ____ DAYS____WKS.____MO.

Figure 1-11—Detachable stub of receipt/charge slip.

based on the information given by the patient. A reluctance or refusal to give information about employment is a good clue to a poor credit risk. The patient who acts insulted when asked for credit references or a definite date that payments can be expected could be a questionable risk.

Many offices find that allowing their patients to use a major credit card simplifies payments. Although a service fee is charged by the bank, the account is paid in full on the patient's ledger card. The bank instead of the doctor can collect the balance from the patient through the monthly billing.

If patients are not required to pay in full at the time of the visit, a schedule must be set up that will be beneficial to both the practice and the patient. The amount paid each month must be within a financial bracket the patient can afford, or partial and skipped payments may result. The schedule must also be compatible with the operation of the practice. Accounts receivable can accrue rapidly and become an expensive process due to the high cost of preparing statements and postage.

OPTOMETRY FEE SLIP

PROCEDURES (Refer to Optometric Procedures, Diagnostic and Treatment)

GENERAL DIAGNOSTIC & TREATMENT SERVICES

	NEW	ESTAB.	FEE
Minimal Service		90030	___
Brief Service	90000	90040	___
Limited Service	90010	90050	___
Intermediate Service	92002	92012	___
Comprehensive Service	92004	92014	___

INDEPENDENT DIAGNOSTIC PROCEDURES

Gonioscopy	92020	___
Visual Field Examination	92081	___
Provocative Test For Glaucoma	92140	___
Ophthalmoscopy, Extended	92225	___
Color Vision Exam, Extended	92283	___
External Ocular Photography	92285	___
Ophthalmoscopy, With Fundus Photography	92250	___
___	___	___

VISION THERAPY SERVICES

Administration and Interpretation of Developmental Tests	90775	___
Sensorimotor Examination	92060	___
Orthoptic/Pleoptic Training	92065	___
___	___	___

LOW VISION TREATMENT SERVICES

Spectacle Mounted Low Vision Aid	92354	___
Telescopic/Compound Lens System	92355	___
___	___	___

OPHTHALMIC LENS SERVICE (DISPENSING)

		FEE
Lenses, Monofocal	92340	___
Lenses, Bifocal	92341	___
Lenses, Multifocal	92342	___
Aphakic Lenses, Monofocal	92352	___
Aphakic Lenses, Multifocal	92353	___
Temporary Lenses, Aphakic	92358	___
___	___	___

CONTACT LENS SERVICES

Prescription and Management of Contact Lenses	92310	___
Prescription and Management of Contact Lenses for Aphakia, one eye	92311	___
Prescription and Management of Contact Lenses for Aphakia, two eyes	92312	___
Modification of Contact Lens	92325	___
Replacement of Contact Lens	92326	___
___	___	___

MATERIALS	**Rx#1**	**Rx#2**
Frame	___	___
Lenses	___	___
Contact Lenses	___	___
___	___	___
TOTAL FEE	___	___

PREVIOUS BALANCE	**NAME**

DIAGNOSIS (Refer to ICD-9-CM DIAGNOSIS CODES FOR OPTOMETRY)

Abrasion Cornea	918.1	Foreign Body Cornea	930.0
Accommodative Def.	367.5	Glaucoma suspect	365.00
Anomalous Corres.	368.34	Headache	784.0
Amblyopia	368.00	Hyperopia	367.0
Aniseikonia	367.32	Hyperphoria	378.43
Aphakia	379.31	Keratoconus	371.60
Astigmatism	367.20	Macular Degeneration	362.50
Binocular Vision Disorder	368.30	Myopia	367.1
Blepharitis	373.00	Normal (no problem)	V65.5
Blepharospasm	333.81	Nystagmus	379.50
Blindness, Legal	369.4	Paresis	378.55
Cataract	366.9	Photophobia	368.13
Color Vision Def.	368.5	Pinguecula	372.51
Convergence Excess	378.84	Presbyopia	370.4
Convergence Insuff.	378.83	Pterygium	372.40
Diplopia	368.20	Ptosis	374.30
Dry Eyes	375.15	Retinal Degeneration	362.60
Edema Corneal (CL)	371.24	Trichiasis	374.05
Esophoria	378.41	Visual Field Defect	368.40
Esotropia	378.00	Vitreous Floaters	379.24
Exophoria	378.42	Xanthelasma	374.51
Exotropia	378.10		

VISUAL ACUITY

Without treatment		**With treatment**	
Right eye	20/200	Right eye	20/20
Left eye	20/400	Left eye	20/20

Sphere	Cyl.	Axis	Prism
Add			

Pd. ______ Seg Type ______ Tint ______

Seg Ht: ______ Seg Wdth: ______ Type ______

ID #12345678
BC #67897654
Joe Doe, O.D.
1357 N.W. Main St.
Nicetown, SO 98765
789-234-8765

Figure 1-12—Sample fee slip.

The dollar amount owed is probably the primary factor in determining the schedule for payment. Some offices have a printed financial contract, allowing the dollar amounts and number of payments to be negotiated and entered on an individual basis.

Billing and Collections

Money owed to the practice is called *accounts receivable.* After the payment schedule has been set up with the patient, it is the responsibility of the paraoptometric to handle the billing. The terms of payment should be clearly written on the ledger card or payment card to ensure proper billing each month. The goodwill of the patient may depend on billing methods. Most offices will bill once a month, favoring the last week of the month as the most effective time.

The type of practice often determines the details to be included on billing the patient each month. Immediately after an office visit, the patient is aware of services received and the balance due the optometrist's office by the use of the fee slip and the charge/receipt slip. If the paraoptometric is using the pegboard system, a copy of the ledger card serves as an excellent statement. There are window envelopes available into which the folded ledger card copy will fit, exposing the name and address of the patient in the proper area.

If separate statements are prepared, the optometrist will determine the detail to be shown on the regular billing. For the most part, "balance due for __________ is __________" is sufficient (Figure 1-13). If there are two or more members of the same family being billed, they can be included on one statement. A separate listing should be shown for each member with a total due shown at the bottom, however (Figure 1-14).

Procedures used for billing delinquent accounts will be directly supervised by the optometrist. The older an account becomes, the

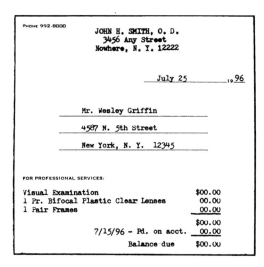

Figure 1-13—Individual fee statement.

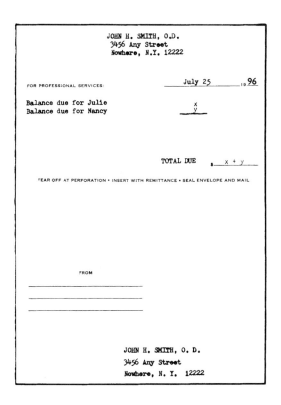

Figure 1-14—Fee statement for family.

more difficult it is to collect the outstanding balance. If an account is 30 days past due, a reminder (sticker or note) may be included on the statement. On an account 60 days past due, a more firm message may be included on the statement, and a phone call to the patient should be made. When using the telephone collection procedure, be friendly but firm, allowing the patient the opportunity to explain why the payment has not been made. Never become angry. Use tact and diplomacy when emphasizing office policy regarding delinquent accounts. Many offices use the following explanation: "The accountant has instructed me to get some type of payment on the account or it will have to be turned over for collection." This directs some of the unpleasant pressure from the optometrist's office to the accountant, maintaining good will for the practice. Skipped payments are not always intentional. There could be a very good reason that payments were not made and, if circumstances warrant, arranging a new type of schedule may be needed. Consult with your optometrist before making a definite commitment with the patient.

When an account is more than 90 days old, most offices consider it a bad debt. The optometrist determines the procedure for collection at this point. It may be referred to a collection agency or to an attorney for processing in small claims court. If the balance owed is relatively small, the account could be written off the books, since it would not warrant the cost of collection efforts. Always review 90-day-old accounts with the optometrist to assist him or her in deciding the final steps to be used for collection.

If a patient with an account receivable is known to have filed for bankruptcy, a letter should be sent immediately to the attorney handling the case along with a copy of the contract (if applicable) and the balance due.

Insurance

Many patients have some type of insurance (vision care, major medical, or both). It is the responsibility of the paraoptometric to fill out the insurance forms promptly and accurately.

Several options are available on acceptance of insurance payments. The optometrist may (1) accept payment directly from the insurance company as payment in full, (2) accept direct insurance payment as partial payments and have the patient responsible for the balance, or (3) not accept assignment of insurance payments at all. If the doctor accepts any part of the insurance payment, the patient must fully understand that the balance due is his or her obligation. The patient is responsible for full payment of the account. In some offices, the insurance forms are completed with the understanding that the patient is fully responsible for the total balance due, and reimbursement is between the patient and the insurance carrier. Some insurance carriers will pay only the patient directly. Insurance coverage may be lower than the usual or customary fee the optometrist charges. The patient is responsible for the total balance, and the insurance carrier will reimburse the patient for the benefits covered. This is advantageous to the practice since the account will be cleared entirely. If a benefit dispute occurs, it will be between the patient and the insurance carrier, without involving the practice.

When a claim is filed for a patient, it becomes an accounts receivable (if payment is accepted) and can remain outstanding for as long as 6–8 weeks. If the payment is not made by the insurance carrier within a reasonable time, the patient should be billed for the balance. A notation may be made on the statement, such as, "Have you heard from your insurance carrier?" This will remind the patient that the balance has not been paid and will re-emphasize the point that the patient is responsible for the total balance due.

A patient scheduling an appointment should be asked whether he or she is covered by insurance and, if so, to bring the proper insurance form or card on the first visit. When the patient arrives for the appointment, obtain the form, checking that the patient has completely filled out the sections required by the insurance company. If possible, figure the approximate coverage in order to advise the patient and to obtain payment at the completion of the visit.

The insurance claim form should be completed as soon as services are rendered. Fill out a separate form for each patient in a family. Never include two claims on one form. The form must be filled out completely, typewritten if possible, and all words must be spelled correctly. If diagnosis is required, make sure this is accurate, checking with the doctor if in doubt. Any question on the accuracy of information supplied on the form, or omissions will delay payment of the claim. Charge the usual and customary fee for services rendered, regardless of the amount the insurance company will pay. A notation should be made on the patient ledger card that indicates the date the claim is filed and the name of the insurance company.

Make a copy of the completed form and keep it in a pending folder until payment is received. If questions arise about payment of the claim, refer the patient to the insurance carrier. Even though the claim has been filed by the practice, the benefits allowed are a matter strictly between the patient and the insurance carrier.

Although many different types of claim forms exist, the average office will be exposed to only about six different forms of insurance carriers/employers in their area. Keep a notebook of sample insurance claim forms. Each insurance company pays different amounts for services, and it is to your advantage to know the approximate extent of coverage. Make a copy of the different insurance forms to use as a sample and obtain the name and phone number of someone at the insurance office you can contact to answer questions on eligibility benefits. If possible, obtain several blank forms from the insurance carrier to keep on hand in the event that the patient forgets to bring the form to the office.

There are service contracts, such as the Vision Service Plan, that operate in most states. These are plans whereby a panel of doctors provide professional services to patients for a predetermined fee. In these cases, each patient must have a personal benefit form when requesting professional services. A series of codes is used to determine eligibility benefits and overcharges, if any. Government programs such as Medicare and Medicaid also have special forms. These forms are filled out using codes to indicate services rendered. In many cases, optometrists' offices also attach an itemized statement of services that most insurance carriers will accept. A quick-claim form is available that serves as a receipt, as well as an itemized statement for all services performed (Figure 1-15). This completed form can be attached to the individual form supplied by the insurance carrier. Benefits change constantly because of the rising costs of materials and the renegotiation of contracts. The sample form notebook must be updated continually.

Incoming Mail

In most offices, paraoptometrics screen the daily mail. All checks received should immediately be stamped "for deposit only" and the proper accounting procedures performed. Frames or

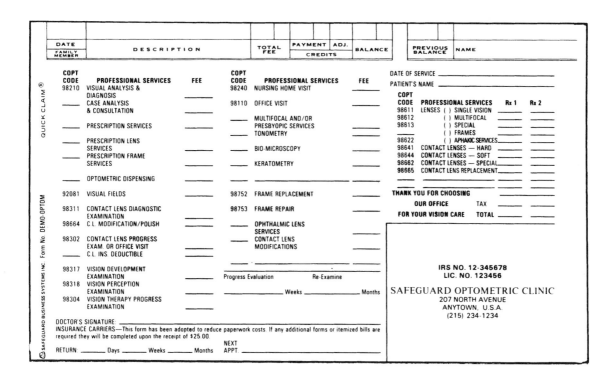

Figure 1-15—The Safeguard quick claim form receipt. (Courtesy of Safeguard Business Systems, Inc.)

laboratory supplies received in the mail may be distributed to the laboratory. The balance of the mail should be given to the optometrist. Never open the optometrist's personal mail, and never throw away any mail unless specifically directed to do so by the doctor. Trade and professional journals, after being read by the optometrist and staff, should be filed in the "Publications Library" for future reference.

Outgoing Correspondence

All office correspondence is confidential. Letters written on the optometrist's stationery immediately set the image of professionalism. Continue with this professionalism by typing letters neatly and correctly. With the introduction of word processing into many practices, error-free correspondence is easily achievable.

Letters may be typed using either the indented form or the block form, whichever the optometrist prefers. Be consistent in style throughout the letter. Allow two-line spaces between addressee and salutation, salutation and beginning of content of letter, paragraphs, and end of content of letter and closing, and allow four-line spaces for the signature. Proofread every letter. Check for correct spelling, punctuation, and balance of content on the page. Many word processors offer an automatic "spell check" function. The body of the letter should be centered on the page with even margins on both sides. Always make a file copy of every letter written for the office. A standard letter may be designed by yourself and the optometrist and stored in your computer's memory. Software packages are available to help you manage all outgoing correspondence.

Become familiar with terminology and definitions of words used in the field of optometry. Excellent references to use are *ICD-9-CM Diagnosis Codes for Optometry* and *Optometric Procedures, Diagnosis and Treatment*. Both of these publications are available (for a fee) from the AOA.

Consultation Letter

Consultations are often made with other health care providers (ophthalmologists, neurologists, internists) by telephone. This procedure can be handled by the paraoptometric while the patient is still in the office. The information conveyed to the other health care provider's office should include the patient's name, address, telephone number, age, and diagnosis. After an appointment is scheduled, the opto-

> Marshall Grimm, M.D.
> 4231 N. 10th Street
> New York, N.Y. 23521
>
> RE: James Cook—Age 59
> 6024 N. 21st Ave.
> New York, N.Y. 23510
>
> Dear Dr. Grimm:
>
> Mr. James Cook was in my office on June 10 for a routine vision examination. His vision is easily corrected to 20/20 in both eyes, and he reports no vision symptoms. The intraocular pressures are O.D. 29 and O.S. 27.
>
> At the present time he is scheduled for an appointment in your office on Monday, June 15 at 1:00 pm.
>
> Thank you for your consultation on this patient as a glaucoma suspect.
>
> Sincerely,
>
> John H. Smith, O.D.
>
> JHS:ab
> cc: Clinton Green, M.D.

Figure 1-16—Sample consultation letter to another health care provider.

metric practice should provide the patient with a letter that includes the provider's name and date and time of the appointment. The letter should indicate the reason the optometrist has arranged the appointment with the other health care provider and when the patient is scheduled to return to the optometrist.

The optometrist may write a follow-up letter to the other professional, confirming the appointment and stating the diagnosis of the patient and previous ocular history (Figure 1-16). A copy of the letter may be sent to the patient's family physician, and a copy is maintained in the patient's file. When sending a copy to another doctor, be sure it is printed on office letterhead.

On occasion a patient may move out of town and request that his or her vision records be forwarded to another optometrist. A patient referral form may be enclosed with the letter to the new optometrist (Figures 1-17 and 1-18). This form contains the ocular history of the patient, as well as the patient's signature granting permission to exchange this information. These forms are available (for a fee) from the AOA.

Thank-You Letter

The thank-you letter is an expression of gratitude from the optometrist for the referral of a new patient (Figure 1-19). This gesture is truly appreciated by the referring person and should be sent as soon as possible after the new patient is seen. The letter, note, or card should be short and simple; be sure to mention the name of the patient who has been referred.

Keep a notebook or a 3 x 5-inch card file, indexed A–Z, listing the name of the person referring the patient and the name of the new patient referred. The first entry in the notebook or on the card will indicate that the person has referred one patient. A notation should be made of the date the thank-you letter was mailed. This same information is efficiently managed in a computer database or word processor as well. If the same person refers another patient to the office, indicate this in the notebook or on the card, and send a second letter. This second letter should be worded slightly differently than the first. In some cases, the referring person may be a patient of several years, and the optometrist may want to use

> Joseph Green, O.D.
> 5678 Willow Drive
> Columbus, Ohio 72431
>
> Re: Janice Williams—Age 34
> 1240 Grant Street
> St. James, Ohio 72421
>
> Dear Dr. Green:
>
> Miss Janice Smith has been a patient of mine for the last five years. She has moved to your area and has requested that I forward her records to you.
>
> On July 15 of last year I performed a routine vision examination and found her prescription had not changed. She is presently wearing daily wear contact lenses and is interested in acquiring extended wear lenses. I am enclosing her ocular history.
>
> Janice has been a fine patient, and I am sure you will welcome her into your practice.
>
> Sincerely,
>
> John H. Smith, O.D.
>
> JHS:ab
> Enc.

Figure 1-17—Cover letter for patient referral form.

a first name in the salutation of the letter. Verify this with the optometrist before sending out the letter. After a certain number of referrals from the same person, the optometrist may wish to send a small token of appreciation.

School Reports

The optometrist may work closely with the local schools to maintain regular vision-care records for the children in the practice. Schools may have standard vision-report forms that they require be completed after an eye examination. It is the responsibility of the paraoptometric to see that these reports are returned to the school as soon as possible after completion of the appointment. The blank vision report can be inserted in the patient file when the patient is in for the vision examination. This will serve as a reminder for the doctor to fill out the form. Be sure to keep a photocopy of the report form for the patient record.

There are several forms that may be used to report the current ocular history of a child (Figure 1-20). Occasionally, the school nurse will send a request for the results of a child's vision examination. This type of request is usually prompted by a suspected vision problem found during a routine vision screening at school. A request could also be made by the teacher if a reading difficulty is thought to be caused by a vision disorder. Depending on the particular vision needs of a child, the teacher may elect to seat the child at a certain area in the classroom.

A vision report may be sent with the child on the first day of school, as well as an updated report to the school nurse whenever the prescription is changed. The school nurse can then keep these reports with the child's medical records for future reference.

Greeting Cards

Some offices use the practice-building technique of sending birthday cards to patients. This is especially appreciated by children and elderly patients. In the case of children, address the card directly to the child. Children are pleased to receive something in the mail that is

Member

American Optometric Association

CONTACT LENS PATIENT REFERRAL

This patient is being referred to you for contact lens care. Further information will be sent upon request.

Date ID #

Patient

This patient has come to our office for contact lens care. Please supply necessary information for our records.

THANK YOU

Telephone

To: From:

Pertinent Information

Original "K" O.D. Latest "K" O.D.

Date O.S. Date O.S.

Spectacle Rx O.D. 20/ Latest Refraction O.D. 20/

Date O.S. 20/ Date O.S. 20/

Bifocal Unaided VA Far O.D. O.S. O.U.

Add - Spectacles C.L.

Unaided VA Near O.D. O.S. O.U.

Current Contact Lens Specifications Original Date Date Replaced O.D. O.S.

Base	Power	Diam.	2nd	Peri.	PCW	O.Z.	C.T.	Tint	VA
									20/
									20/

Current Soft Lens Specifications Original Date Date Replaced O.D. O.S.

Base or Series	Power	Diam.	C.T.	Lot No.	Type	VA
						20/
						20/

Special Duplicating Instructions

Disinfecting Method

I hereby grant permission for the above named persons/optometrists to exchange information from my case records.

( ) Parent or ( ) Guardian Date Signed

A.O.A. L-9-483

PLEASE RETURN THIS COPY TO SENDER

Figure 1-18—Contact lens patient referral form. (Courtesy of American Optometric Association.)

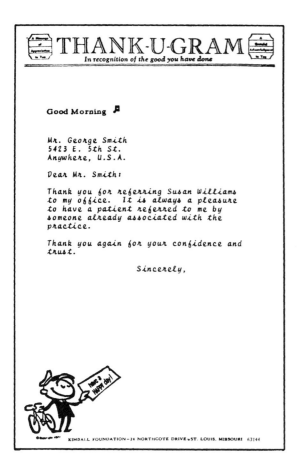

Figure 1-19—Thank-you letter for patient referral.

just for them. There are many different styles of birthday cards available. Keep several styles on hand if more than one member of the same family is a patient in the practice.

A special birthday file can be input into the computer or created using either a notebook or a 3 × 5-inch card file. The notebook or computer database should include the name, address, and birth date of the patient and be filed under the month of the birthday. The last week of the month is the time to address the following month's cards. If a computer is used, the paraoptometric should print out a listing of birth dates for the upcoming month. Have the optometrist and staff personally sign the cards and, if time permits, add a special touch by hand addressing the envelopes.

Other occasions such as weddings, births, and deaths could also warrant sending a card. Keep a supply of appropriate cards on hand for each type of occasion.

PATIENT EDUCATIONAL INFORMATION

Booklets and Pamphlets

The paraoptometric should be knowledgeable and prepared to answer many questions regarding eye conditions. One of the best aids in answering these inquiries is patient education materials available from the AOA. The doctor and paraoptometric may also develop in-office informational brochures or question-and-answer sheets specific to the most common questions asked by their patients.

Patient education materials typically explain eye conditions in a language that is easily understood by the patient. They may be displayed in the reception room, thereby becoming excellent reading material for those patients waiting to see the doctor. The pamphlets may also promote an interest in safety and sports vision and encourage the patient to ask the optometrist questions regarding the importance of these types of vision care. Educational brochures are an excellent tool to help you convey a great deal of information to the patient in a concise format, saving the paraoptometric time and effort in explaining ocular and visual conditions. More and more patients expect to be educated about their health and better understand their health status. These informational brochures provide the patient with excellent background information.

When scheduling a new patient examination, a "welcome" letter may be sent with a general eye care pamphlet explaining common vision conditions or something similar. If the appointment is for a child, the enclosure might be a pamphlet that explains children's vision. The pamphlets may also be included with recall letters, using the appropriate pamphlet for the specific needs of the particular patient.

Audiovisual Presentations

Audiovisual presentations are effective as instructional tools. They cover a large amount of information in a short time frame and provide consistent information from patient to patient. These presentations may cover contact lens instructions, provide explanation to the new wearer of multifocals, or provide information about other vision and ocular disease condition

STUDENT VISION REPORT FORM

Student's Name _____ Grade _____

Date of Birth _____ Address _____

Parent's Name _____

School _____ Teacher _____

This vision examination report is being sent to you so that you may be familiar with the student's vision needs and abilities. Please do not hesitate to ask for any further information that may be helpful.

Information For The Teacher and Parent

*Analysis of Vision: _____
_____
_____

Should Return for Further Care: _____

No Treatment Indicated _____ Present Prescription Satisfactory _____ New Glasses Prescribed _____

Contact Lenses Prescribed _____ Vision Therapy Prescribed _____

Purpose of Glasses: _____

Glasses Should be Worn: Constantly _____ Classroom _____ Desk Work _____ Reading _____

Homework _____ Distance _____ Movies _____ TV _____ Playing _____

Recommendations To Classroom Teacher (i.e., seating, lighting, etc.) _____
_____
_____

Summary of Findings

*Visual Acuity: At Distance   At Reading Distance _____ Inches

Without glasses:	R. Eye 20/	L. Eye 20/	Both 20/	R. Eye 20/	L. Eye 20/	Both 20/
With new glasses:	R. Eye 20/	L. Eye 20/	Both 20/	R. Eye 20/	L. Eye 20/	Both 20/

Binocular Efficiency: (Functioning of the two eyes to enable comfortable, efficient visual performance at all distances.)

1. Maintenance of Binocular Fixation: (Ability to look at the same object with both eyes for a sustained period of time.)

   Distance: Adequate _____ Remarks: _____
   _____

   Near: Adequate _____ Remarks: _____
   _____

*Defined on Reverse Side.

Figure 1-20—School report form. (Courtesy of American Optometric Association.)

Summary of Findings (Cont.)

2. Ability to Maintain Focus at Near:

    Adequate _____ Remarks: _____
    _____

3. Ability to Change Focus Quickly and Easily: (Example — chalkboard to book.)

    Adequate _____ Remarks: _____
    _____

4. Ocular Motility: (Ability of the eyes, both independent of each other and together as a team, to move freely in all directions.)

    Adequate _____ Remarks _____
    _____

5. Suppression of Vision: (Blocking out mentally of the image of either eye when it interfers with the fusing of the two ocular images into one.)

    Absent _____ Remarks: _____
    _____

6. Binocular Depth Perception: (The ability to perceive and judge depth or relative distances, using both eyes, rather than one.)

    Adequate _____ Remarks: _____
    _____

7. Color Perception: (The ability to distinguish colors)

    Normal _____ Remarks: _____
    _____

Date _____ Signed _____

　　　　　　　　　　　　　　　　　　　　　　　Address _____

VISION ANALYSIS — An adequate vision analysis includes the following:

   A. An examination of the eyes to determine the absence of disease.

   B. An examination of the eyes to insure visual acuteness at all distances. Primary consideration for the school child is the reading distance and of course the chalkboard distance.

   C. An evaluation of the visual skills necessary to insure adequate coordination and fusion of the eyes at all distances.

   D. An examination of the vision skills necessary to insure adequate focus of the eyes at all distances.

   E. An examination of the visual perceptual abilities of the individual.

VISION THERAPY — A physiopsychological procedure for re-educating the two eyes to function at a level of efficient and comfortable binocular vision and to enhance visual perception.

VISUAL ACUITY — Acuteness or keenness of vision. At distance: 20 feet or beyond (chalkboard, charts, movies, television, etc.) At near: within arm's reach.

This form has been prepared by:

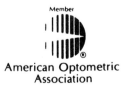

American Optometric Association

Printed in U.S.A.　　　　　　　　　　　　　　　　　　　　　　　　　　　　　　　　Form C18-R

Figure 1-20—*(continued)*

topics. The paraoptometric must be familiar with the presentations and be prepared to answer questions from the patient. If you are asked a question that you are unable to answer, seek out the answer from the optometrist and provide the patient with the answer during the course of the examination. In this way, you will be prepared and better educated if asked a similar question by another patient.

An audiovisual presentation on contact lenses, for example, is quite commonly used by the patient who is learning about the application and removal of the lenses, and instruction booklets are included in all care kits. The patient instruction for contact lenses may be performed by one specific staff member in the practice. Every paraoptometric in the office, however, should be familiar with the audiovisual presentations and all the kits used by the office in order to be able to answer patient questions.

COMPUTERS

The size of the optometrist's practice and the amount of information to be programmed and used will be the primary factors in making the decision to use a computer system. Although installing a computer system requires an initial investment of substantial time and money, modern practices find that the ease of data storage and retrieval offset the expense.

Many types of computers are available, ranging from the small, economy size, which can handle one or two tasks, to the large, more complex systems, which can be programmed to perform many tasks. These more versatile systems are capable of having additional programs entered into them at a future date with minimal effort and cost.

The physical components of the computer are called *hardware*; the collection of instructions that run the computer is called *software*. The software is the program that controls the computer and its peripheral equipment.

The video display terminal and keyboard are used by the paraoptometric for entering new data and for recalling information previously entered. The placement of the screen should be in an area free from glare, and the glass of the screen should be cleaned often to maintain clarity. The angle of the screen and the position of the keyboard are important for the user's comfort and for efficient computer operation. Maintenance contracts are available for computer systems, and it is the responsibility of the paraoptometric or office manager to see that the equipment is serviced regularly and also to maintain control of computer supplies.

Data are stored on magnetic disks. Proper storage of the disks is important to retain clarity of the records. Protect the disks from excess heat, cold, and humidity, as well as from magnetic forces that can alter their quality.

Each office must decide on the type of backup system that is needed. The computer manufacturer or sales representative can offer advice. Some offices transfer data to a duplicate disk or to a magnetic tape similar to a cassette to be used as a backup in case a disk is destroyed. Each office must determine how often backups should be run. One key question to ask when establishing backup protocol is how much information your office can afford to re-enter if data is lost (e.g., 1 day, 1 week, etc.).

The system can be programmed to handle many time-consuming tasks of the office, such as recall letters, newsletters, and monthly billings. The computer cannot think on its own, and it is the responsibility of the staff to update information as soon as it is collected. The computer will be only as effective as the data that is entered into the program. The data must be accurate and up-to-date.

A computer can be used to schedule appointments. An immediate report can be shown on the screen regarding the days and times available and showing the types of appointments that have been scheduled.

When patient records are programmed into the computer, reports can be made for the optometrist on practice statistics, such as number of contact lens patients, low-vision patients, age groups, or recall examinations.

The financial records of the practice can be keyed into the computer to provide an immediate report to the optometrist on the accounts receivable and accounts payable, as well as monthly financial statements and year-to-date totals for the practice. This is also an advantage if the practice's system is compatible with the system of the office accountant. All of the monthly financial records will be available immediately, along with all records for payroll and accrued taxes.

Monthly billing, as well as year-end statements for patients to use for income-tax purposes, can be prepared by the computer. The computer can also be programmed to send "special" statements on past-due accounts.

The computer can also be used for control of in-office supplies and materials. The amount of supplies on hand changes every day, and it is of utmost importance to input the new information into the system on a daily basis. The computer is excellent for the speed and accuracy of any report it can produce. Emphasis must again be placed on the importance of accurate and current information being supplied by the paraoptometric, however.

The updating of information can be a task specially assigned to one person; however, more than one staff member should be familiar with the operation of the computer. The office instruction manual should also be updated whenever a new computer program is added.

PATIENT COMMUNICATION

Patient communication is vitally important to the growth of the practice. The patient who is greeted warmly, treated fairly, and handled courteously during the office visit will be a happy patient. This communication with the patient is the responsibility of the entire staff of the practice.

Children

Handling children in the office often requires tact and patience. Encourage parents to bring children to the office before the appointment or when the parent has an appointment. At this time, the paraoptometric can get to know each child and show him or her around the office. Explain the instruments to the child. The child may also watch while the parent is being examined. If the practice includes many children, it is advisable to have a "children's corner" where they can amuse themselves with games and books. The area can be equipped with a small table and chairs.

During the examination, direct your conversation to the child. Use the child's name to build the youngster's feeling of importance. During pretesting procedures, it is recommended to keep the conversation steady because children become distracted quickly. Cartoons may be put on the projector to help amuse them.

Elderly and Disabled

Elderly and disabled patients may require special attention to make them feel comfortable and at ease. The parking area should have a ramp up to the sidewalk to accommodate wheelchairs. The reception room should have several chairs that can accommodate those with limited mobility. Elderly patients tend to have an easier time rising from a hard chair with arms than from a plush sofa.

Doorways and halls should be uncluttered and wide enough to accommodate wheelchairs, walkers, and unsteady steps down the hall with a cane. Make sure there is nothing in the pathway of the patient that could cause him or her to trip or stumble.

It will sometimes be necessary to give elderly and disabled patients extra attention. They may be eager to talk about their health. Let them be the leaders in this type of conversation.

There are times the elderly have difficulty hearing. In such a case, it might be advisable to take an elderly patient to a private area so that asking for information will not be embarrassing and questions may be repeated several times. If you encounter a patient who has difficulty with hearing, it is an added professional courtesy to refer them to another health care provider and assist them in obtaining a hearing aid. You may also discuss the patient's hearing difficulty with family members and assist them in obtaining a proper solution for their elderly loved ones.

OPTOMETRIST AND PATIENT COMMUNICATION

There are many ways the paraoptometric can assist the optometrist in communicating with the patient. If there is any information available about the patient that is not already contained on the patient information sheet, the paraoptometric should note it on the record for the optometrist's reference. A major accomplishment of the patient or the birth of a new grandchild, for example, could be points the doctor may wish to mention. Also include deaths in the family so that the optometrist may convey condolences.

At times, a paraoptometric may overhear a comment from a patient waiting in the reception room. If it is a question concerning vision care, make a note of it. Often the patient either will forget or will be afraid to ask the optometrist. The optometrist can explain the answer to the patient during the vision examination even if the patient does not remember to ask. As an added service, the patient could be given a pamphlet concerning the question, for example, one that explains astigmatism or presbyopia. The pamphlet could be included with the patient records, and the optometrist could then give it to the patient during the examination. If the patient has had a baby, a copy of the pamphlet "Your Baby's Eyes" could be included in the patient record. The optometrist could then congratulate the patient and present the pamphlet.

These added touches communicate to the patient that the optometrist and staff not only care about the visual needs of the patient, but also share in the pleasure of personal accomplishments.

Many optometrists send newsletters periodically to patients that discuss many aspects of the practice, such as informing them of new types of lenses available or perhaps of a new piece of equipment in the office. These types of materials and small tokens of thoughtfulness add a personal touch to patient communication and add to the practice-building efforts of the doctor and the staff.

OFFICE COMMUNICATION

The communication between the optometrist and staff is just as important to the practice as the communication with the patient. For the office to function smoothly with a minimal amount of friction, there must be an open line of communication among all staff members.

The size and type of practice will determine the methods by which this communication will be developed and maintained. The optometrist will determine the specific duties to be performed by each staff member, and these will be delegated as major areas of responsibility. In most offices, more than one staff member has a working knowledge of certain tasks; this allows for vacation, sick leave, and emergencies.

Office Manager

Many offices have an office manager who acts as a leader in the practice and makes sure that all the policies and procedures are carried out according to the optometrist's instructions. The office manager often screens new job applicants, schedules interviews for prospective staff members, and conducts exit interviews for employees leaving the practice. Other duties performed by the office manager may include keeping all personnel records for staff members, ordering supplies, tracking accounts payable, preparing the payroll, supervising patient flow, writing and interpreting the office procedure manual, acting as a liaison for the optometrist in handling patient complaints, and serving as a liaison between the staff and the doctor. The office manager may also act as an executive assistant to the optometrist, handling correspondence and personal appointments. The office manager is usually a paraoptometric who is highly qualified, has been in the field for several years, has a thorough knowledge of all aspects of the practice, and has leadership skills.

Staff Meetings

Every office should have staff meetings. The number of paraoptometrics in the practice will most likely determine the number and length of the staff meetings to be held. The staff meeting is an excellent way to allow each staff member to voice views and comments on happenings in the practice. The meetings should be held at a time when they will be uninterrupted. An agenda should be prepared by the staff, listing the items they would like discussed at the meeting. Each meeting should have a different moderator, and an effort should be made to see that each member has the opportunity to offer a comment or opinion. The addition of new policies, dropping of old policies, or explanation of a present policy or procedure are all items that should be put on an agenda for discussion at a staff meeting.

Office Procedure and Policy Manuals

The policies and procedures in effect for the office will be determined by the optometrist, many times with input from staff members.

Every office is different, and the optometrist and the staff can benefit by having a manual that specifically outlines the manner in which duties are to be performed for the particular office.

For every practice management procedure outlined in this chapter, there are at least one or two and sometimes many variations. The purpose of the office procedure manual is to set the exact procedure to be followed in the practice. The manual should include how, when, and by whom every procedure is performed. It should also cover rules, benefits, and other areas affecting the practice, such as vacation time, sick leave, lunch breaks, and so on. This manual can be a notebook or binder so that additions and deletions can be made easily. It is an excellent reference to be used by present staff members and as a training manual for new employees.

COMMUNITY INVOLVEMENT

The paraoptometric can be a very distinct asset to the practice by becoming involved in the community. The practice is enhanced by the fact that the public is educated in the field of optometry and, more specifically, the individual optometrist's practice. Accept invitations to speak at community groups, men's and women's clubs, and career and health programs. Many pamphlets and brochures that are available from the AOA can be distributed at these functions. Also available through the AOA are various audiovisual presentations. The introduction of vision health to smaller children can be done through the use of Seymour Safely promotional materials available from the AOA.

The paraoptometric can become involved with service organizations and community affairs. The assistant or technician can assist in health fairs and work with schools on screening children. Some paraoptometrics visit local hospitals or nursing homes to adjust patients' frames. The patients will be grateful for this special service and will certainly remember the paraoptometric and the optometrist.

CAREER INVOLVEMENT

To promote the field of optometry and the practice, the paraoptometric must have a sense of pride in the profession. There must be a continual upgrading of knowledge and personal development. Read optometric journals whenever possible to upgrade knowledge and learn new techniques. It is of great advantage to join local, state, and national associations in order to gain new knowledge and enhance the role of the paraoptometric in the optometric practice. Membership in the American Optometric Association Paraoptometric Section will provide you with information about when and where educational meetings are held, as well as fellowship among paraoptometrics from all over the country. The Section is able to offer answers to questions regarding membership in state associations and availability of continuing education and formal paraoptometric training programs. There are many benefits to be derived from membership in the Paraoptometric Section, and all paraoptometrics are encouraged to join.

To receive membership information or a brochure that describes the paraoptometric profession or to speak with an AOA representative, who will be able to answer your questions, please contact:

American Optometric Association
Paraoptometric Section
243 N. Lindbergh Boulevard
St. Louis, MO 63141
Telephone: (800) 365-2219
Fax: (314) 991-4101

The National Paraoptometric Registry is provided by the American Optometric Association Paraoptometric Section as a voluntary means of recognition for paraoptometrics who wish to be registered. The Optometric Assistant and Technician Registration Examinations are administered at many locations around the country to paraoptometrics trained on the job or in formal educational programs. After passing the exams, the title of Registered Optometric Assistant or Registered Optometric Technician is granted. Registration status can be maintained by submitting proof of completing continuing education at regular intervals. Handbooks with information concerning the examinations (e.g., infomation covered on the exam, tests dates) are available from the American Optometric Association's St. Louis office.

CONCLUSION

The paraoptometric plays an important role in the management of the optometric practice. As a team, the optometrist and paraoptometric work together to build a successful practice.

This chapter presents generalities. Although many policies and procedures presented here may apply, the day-to-day routine of each practice is determined by the applicable situation.

SUGGESTED READING

Baldwin RL, Christensen R, Melton JW. Rx for Success. St. Louis: Vision Publications, 1983.

Elmstrom G. Advanced Management Strategies. Chicago: Professional Press, 1982.

Sachs L. Do It Yourself Marketing. New York: Prentice-Hall, 1986.

2 / Anatomy and Physiology of the Eye and Visual System

G. Timothy Petito

Ocular anatomy is the study of the structures that constitute the eye and, for completeness, usually includes the study of related structures of the brain that make up the visual pathways. The knowledge of the tissues of the eye and visual pathway is the basis for differentiating normal from abnormal clinical presentations and understanding the pathogenesis and treatment of disease.

The purpose of this chapter is, first, to familiarize paraoptometrics with terms necessary for clinical communication with doctors of optometry and second, to provide them with the basis for testing they may be required to perform. Additionally, a working knowledge of ocular anatomy will allow the paraoptometric to provide the practitioner with insightful observations concerning patient health and function.

The chapter provides an overview of the eyes' structures and their functions. Structures are generally presented from the outside toward the inside and, where applicable, anterior to posterior (front to back) in the visual pathway. The exception to this general sequence of presentation is the orbit, which provides a basic reference point and is traditionally the first topic covered in the study of the visual system's anatomy. Where possible, pictures or sketches will be included to assist the reader in understanding the relationship of structure to function. Selected abnormalities and their clinical features will also be presented to illustrate the relative importance of the involved anatomy.

The orbital components are described in relation to general anatomic positions. The four principal anatomic directions are described in Figure 2-1 and are defined as follows: superior (toward the head), inferior (toward the feet), medial (toward the midline—the nose is on the midline), and lateral (away from the midline).

THE ORBIT

The orbits are the bony sockets containing the eye and most of its accessory organs. Specifically, each orbit contains an eyeball, orbital fat, fascia (connective tissue sheaths), levator muscle of the upper lids, lacrimal gland, extraocular muscles, and the nerves and circulatory supply (blood vessels) for the orbital contents and some of the face. Figure 2-2 shows the seven bones that contribute to the formation of the orbit: the *maxilla, frontal, zygomatic, ethmoid, lacrimal, palatine,* and *sphenoid* bones. The first three form the orbital rim at the front; the last one forms the apex at the back. All of these bones are fused together at lines called *sutures.* There are eight openings, called *foramen,* which allow arteries, veins, and nerves that serve the orbital contents and parts of the face to enter and leave the orbit. The major foramen of the orbit are also pictured in Figure 2-2. Specific foramen, the bones that contain them, and the structures passing through them are summarized in Table 2-1.

Many bones of the head, particularly those contributing to the formation of the orbit, have air spaces in them that connect to the nasal cavity. One effect of these air spaces is to reduce the weight of the skull significantly. Air spaces contained within bones are called *sinuses*; these are

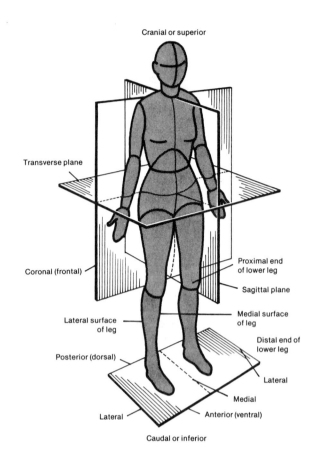

FIGURE 2-1—The anatomic planes and directions of the human body. Note particularly the anterior, posterior, superior, inferior, medial, and lateral directions. (Reprinted with permission from SS Bates. Fundamentals for Assisting in Primary Care Optometry. New York: Professional Press/Fairchild, 1983.)

specifically named for the bones that contain them—that is, the frontal, maxillary, ethmoid, and sphenoid air sinuses.

The orbit consists of four walls (see Figure 2-2). The superior wall, or roof, is formed by part of the sphenoid bone (2%) and the frontal bone (98%). Behind the orbital rim, the frontal bone is extremely thin and may be easily damaged by penetrating injuries. The frontal lobe of the brain is directly above the orbital roof and is subject to damage in injuries that puncture the frontal bone.

The medial wall (closest to the midline) is formed, from front to back, by the frontal process of the maxillary bone, the lacrimal bone, the ethmoid bone, and a small part of the sphenoid bone. The ethmoid is the largest medial surface and the thinnest bone of the orbit (0.2–0.4 mm thick). Because it is so thin, infection can extend into the orbit from the nasal cavity and ethmoid air sinuses with relative ease. Indeed, ethmoiditis (infection of the ethmoid air sinuses) is the major cause of infections of the orbit and orbital contents. Between the maxillary and lacrimal bones, in front of the ethmoid, a depression called the *lacrimal fossa* is formed. There are two depressions in the orbit that are each called the lacrimal fossa. The one in the medial wall contains the lacrimal sac, which allows for drainage of the tears from the eye into the nose.

The floor of the orbit is composed of three bones (front to back): the maxilla (largest portion), the zygomatic, and a small portion of the palatine bone. This floor is very thin (0.5–1.0 mm thick) and separates the orbital contents from the maxillary sinus. Because it is so thin, tumors from the maxillary sinus may erode the bone and extend into the orbit, causing proptosis (bulging) of an eye. Another consequence of this arrangement is evident when blunt trauma results in fracture of the orbital floor. This is called "blowout fracture," and the eye usually appears to be sunken. There may also be an inability to elevate the eye (look up) because the inferior rectus muscle may be trapped in the maxillary sinus by the fractured bone.

Laterally, the orbit is made of the zygomatic bone and the greater wing of the sphenoid bone. The lateral wall is the thickest orbital wall. This is fortunate, since it is exposed to the most external stress. It is also the only wall not associated with a paranasal sinus.

In addition to those conditions involving the paranasal sinuses already mentioned, the sinuses may be clinically significant as a cause of facial pain. Poor drainage, infection, or neoplastic (cancerous) enlargement of the sinuses may cause headaches or pain described as periorbital (located around the eye), or referred directly to the eye. Because of this, questions about sinus conditions are usually included in the complete medical history, particularly when headache is a presenting symptom.

THE EXTERNAL STRUCTURES

The eyes and orbits are protected by reinforced folds of skin called the *palpebrae*, or eyelids. Figures 2-3 and 2-4 show an external view of the eyelids and the anterior structures of the eye-

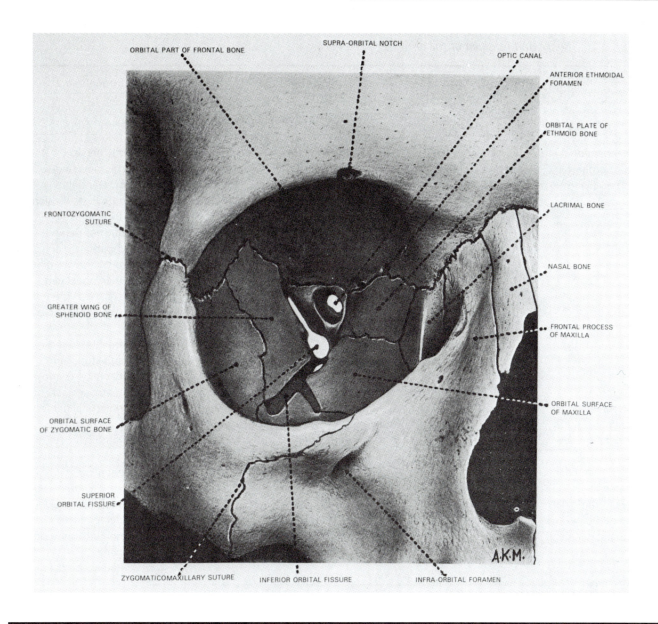

FIGURE 2-2—The bones of the orbit and the major foramen they contain. (Reprinted with permission from WJ Hamilton [ed]. Textbook of Human Anatomy [2nd ed]. London: Macmillan, 1976.)

ball. The eyelids serve three basic functions. First, by the rhythmic opening and closing of the eyelids (spontaneous blinking), the tear film is replenished and spread evenly across the front surface of the eye. This provides a smooth optical surface and cleanses the front of the eye. Second, the action of the eyelids pumps the tears through the lacrimal sac for drainage from the eye and in this way regulates the amount of tear fluid in the eye. Finally, the eyelids protect the eyes from small foreign bodies and excessive light by rapidly and forcefully closing when danger is apparent. This rapid, forceful closure is called *reflex blinking*. The condition in which the eyes are so tightly closed that they cannot be opened is called a *blepharospasm*.

When the eyelids are open, the upper lid usually covers a small portion of the superior cornea, which is the clear covering in front of the colored part of the eye (see Figure 2-3). The lower lid usually covers the globe up to the area of the inferior limbus, which is the junction of the cornea and sclera—the "white of the eye" (see Figure 2-4). The space between the lids is called the *palpebral aperture* or *fissure* and measures approximately 10 mm wide at its widest

TABLE 2-1. Bones and foramen of the orbit

Name (foramen)	Bone(s) foramen is contained in	Allows for the passage of these structures through skull		
		Arteries	Veins	Nerves
Optic foramen	Aphenoid (lesser wing)	Ophthalmic artery	—	Optic nerve
Superior orbital fissure	Between the greater and lesser wings of the sphenoid	Recurrent branch of lacrimal artery	Superior ophthalmic vein	Oculomotor nerve Trochlear nerve Ophthalmic division of trigeminal nerve Abducens nerve Sympathetic nerves Orbital branch middle meningeal nerve
Inferior orbital fissure	Sphenoid and maxilla	Infraorbital artery	Infraorbital vein Branches of the inferior ophthalmic vein	Maxillary division of trigeminal nerve Zygomatic nerve Filaments from the sphenopalatine ganglion (sympathetic nerves)
Supraorbital notch (foramen)	Frontal bone	Supraorbital artery	Supraorbital vein	Supraorbital nerves
Infraorbital groove (canal)	Maxilla	Infraorbital artery	Infraorbital vein	Infraorbital nerve
Anterior ethmoidal foramen	Ethmoid/frontal bones	Anterior ethmoid arteries	—	Nasal nerve
Posterior ethmoidal foramen	Ethmoid/frontal bones	Posterior ethmoid arteries	—	Posterior ethmoidal nerve
Zygomatic foramen	Zygomatic bone	—	—	Zygomaticotemporal nerve Zygomaticofacial nerve

point. If the palpebral aperture is too small (i.e., the upper lid "droops"), the condition is called *ptosis* (pronounced *toe-sis*), and if severe, can impair vision by blocking the pupil, which is the black "hole" in the colored part of the eye. Conversely, the palpebral fissure may be larger than normal (i.e., the upper lid is retracted), leading to a "staring" appearance. Generally, if the palpebral fissures of the two eyes are not equal, a pathologic condition must be suspected and investigated.

Normally, the eyelids are in very close proximity to the globe, being separated only by the very thin layer of tears. This results in scratches on the surface of the globe when foreign matter is trapped under the eyelids. Scratches on the front of the eye may also occur when eyelashes are directed toward it because of the lids turning in toward the globe. This condition is called *entropion* and may be the result of trauma, scarring secondary to inflammation, or a loss of elasticity of the lid tissues. When the eyelid tissues lose their elasticity, they may droop away from the eye rather than turn in towards it, resulting in a condition called *ectropion*. The clinical consequence of ectropion is the fact that the tears cannot drain effectively without the lid close to the eye and may spill onto the cheek. If this happens, the patient may complain of "crying" as a symptom.

The eyelids are constructed of seven layers of tissue. The outermost layer, the skin, contains all

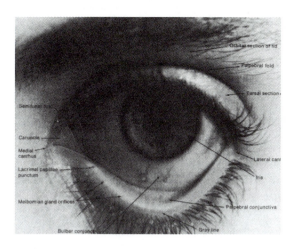

FIGURE 2-3—External structure of the eyelids and anterior eyeball viewed from the front. (Reprinted with permission from SS Bates. Fundamentals for Assisting in Primary Care Optometry. New York: Professional Press/Fairchild, 1983.)

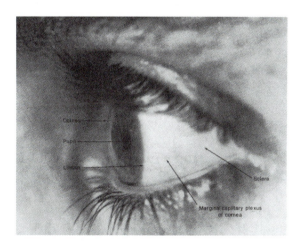

FIGURE 2-4—External structure of the anterior globe viewed from the side. (Reprinted with permission from SS Bates. Fundamentals for Assisting in Primary Care Optometry. New York: Professional Press/Fairchild, 1983.)

the layers typical of skin anywhere on the body but has the distinction of being the thinnest (less than 1 mm thick). There are, however, some subtle differences between the skin of the lids and the rest of the body. These are related to the sweat glands, hair, and melanocytes (the cells that give skin its coloration). The skin of the nasal portion of the lid is smoother, greasier, and almost devoid of hair, compared with the temporal portion. As the skin of the lid approaches its junction with the conjunctiva (the deepest layer of the lid, next to the eye) at the lid mar-

gin, it becomes thicker and contains more elastic tissue. This junction of the skin and conjunctiva is called the *gray line* because of its color and represents the boundary between the parts of the lid that remain "wet," that is, in contact with the tear film, and the outside parts that remain "dry," that is, not in contact with the tears under normal conditions (see Figure 2-3). This line is considered the demarcation line. Growths of the lid closer to the eye are considered dangerous and require immediate removal, whereas growths outside this line can be watched to see if removal is imperative.

Immediately below the skin is an area of loose connective tissue called the *subcutaneous areolar layer*. This layer normally contains no fat. It is loosely connected over the extent of the lid. Because of this loose attachment, the eyelids easily demonstrate edema and frequently appear "puffy" in conditions in which general edema is a feature (e.g., thyroid conditions, kidney failure, congestive heart failure, etc.).

Under this layer of connective tissue, there is a muscle, the *orbicularis oculi*, which occupies the entire length of the eyelid. The orbicularis muscle is responsible for eyelid closure and is controlled by the facial nerve (cranial nerve [CN] VII). Its position over the tarsal plates helps it to hold the lids back against the globe. Any time a weakness of closure is noted, the integrity of the facial (seventh cranial) nerve and muscle must be checked.

Below the orbicularis is another layer of connective tissue, the *submuscular areolar layer*. This layer is similar to the subcutaneous layer and contains most of the major nervous and circulatory supplies for the lids.

The *levator palpebrae superioris* is another muscle in the eyelid occupying the space under the areolar tissue. It extends from its origin at the back of the orbit (on the sphenoid bone) to its insertions in the lid. The levator muscle occupies the entire width of the lid and is the major muscle responsible for eyelid retraction (eye opening). The paraoptometric should look for drooping of the upper lid (ptosis) or abnormal head posture and report them to the doctor for further investigation.

Continuing through the lid from outside to inside, the next major structure is the *tarsal plate*. Both the upper and lower lid have a plate, but the tarsal plate in the lower lid is much smaller than that of the upper lid. Tarsal plates are composed of dense fibrous and elastic connective tissue and are responsible for the shape and rigidity of the eyelids. The tarsal plates have large parallel sebaceous glands, called *meibomian* or *tarsal glands*, running down their length. These glands (approximately 25 in the upper and 20 in the lower) have openings on the lid margins and produce the oil that floats on the watery layer of the tear film to retard evaporation of the tears and prevent tear overflow onto the cheek (see Figure 2-3). This oily layer also promotes a tight seal between the lids when the eyes are closed, which helps prevent drying of the cornea. Occasionally, these glands become blocked by their secretions or due to an infection. When this happens, the oil cannot be excreted by the meibomian glands. Typically, patients with this condition will complain of dry eye symptoms—that is, the eye feels "gritty," stings, burns, and produces excessive tear fluid. If an infection is the reason for the blockage, the gland becomes irritated and swollen, which appears as a red painful bump on the lid. This bump is an internal hordeolum, commonly known as a *sty*. When a sty has resolved, without the gland's adequately draining, it becomes hard and no longer painful or red. This hard, painless bump is called a *chalazion*. Usually, the chalazion can be felt through the lid and frequently is described as feeling like a "pellet" in the lid. These observations may be part of the intake procedure expected of the paraoptometric by the optometrist, or they may be reported to the paraoptometric during preliminary testing or history and should be reported to the optometrist.

A muscle lying below the orbital septum is also involved in the retraction of the lid. This muscle is called *Mueller's muscle*. This muscle takes its origin from the levator in the upper lid and an extension of the inferior rectus muscle in the lower lid. The insertion is at the orbital margin of the upper and lower tarsal plates, respectively. Because of this muscle's role in opening the eye and maintaining the size of the palpebral fissure, anything that interrupts the innervation to the muscle results in ptosis. The severity of ptosis from weakness of Mueller's muscle is less than that resulting from problems with the levator muscle. Again, the presence of a ptosis may indicate neurologic disease and should be pointed out to the optometrist for further investigation.

The deepest layer of the palpebrae (eyelids) is the *conjunctiva*. This is the mucous membrane that covers the inside of the eyelids and the outside of the globe. The conjunctiva is very thin, but is actually composed of several layers of cells. The conjunctiva begins at the gray line, where it is called the marginal conjunctiva, and covers the entire surface of the inside of the lids. The part of the conjunctiva lining the inside of the lid and covering the tarsal palates is called the *tarsal conjunctiva*; the part of the conjunctiva above (or in the lower lid, below) the tarsal plates is called the *orbital conjunctiva*. The marginal, tarsal, and orbital portions are collectively called the *palpebral conjunctiva*, since they line the inside of the eyelids (palpebrae). The conjunctiva is also reflected back onto the globe at the upper and lower fornices, where the eyelids are connected to the eye. The conjunctiva covering the eyeball is called the *bulbar conjunctiva*. It covers the eyeball from the fornices (*fornix* is singular for *fornices*) to the cornea, where it becomes continuous with the most superficial corneal layer (see Figures 2-3 and 2-4). The conjunctiva is loosely connected inside the lids and outside the globe and may become distended and puffy as a result of infection, injury, or hemorrhage. This edema of the conjunctiva is called *chemosis*. The conjunctiva itself is a clear layer, with blood vessels lying in and just below it. When these blood vessels become engorged with blood because of irritation or infections of the eye, the eye appears red. Inflammation of the conjunctiva is called *conjunctivitis*.

Several important glands are situated in the conjunctiva. The epithelium is the most superficial layer of the conjunctiva and contains glands called *goblet cells*, which produce mucous that covers the entire surface of the conjunctiva and cornea. This mucous allows the tear film to remain stable on the otherwise nonwettable surfaces of the eye. Deep in the layers of the conjunctiva are the accessory lacrimal *glands of Krause and Wolfring*. These glands produce the watery layer of the tear film in conjunction with the lacrimal gland.

The other glands present in the lids, thus far, are the sebaceous glands of Zeis and Moll. The *glands of Zeis* are attached to the follicles of the eyelashes, producing an oil that protects the hair from drying out and becoming brittle. Follicles are holes through which hairs protrude through the skin. The eyelashes (and eyebrows) serve to protect the eye from foreign matter falling toward it from above. The tarsal, or ciliary, *glands of Moll* are sweat glands located at the lid margin. When the glands of Moll or Zeis become blocked and infected, the result is an external hordeolum, a sty. If the hair shafts and glands of Zeis become infected, the entire lid margin may also become inflamed. This inflammation is called a *blepharitis*. If the conjunctiva adjacent to the lid margin is also involved, the condition is called *blepharoconjunctivitis*.

Many other conditions also present as "lumps and bumps" of the eyelids. Generally, the paraoptometric involved with external examination of the patient should pay attention to the shape of the lids, the equality and size of the palpebral apertures, the coloration of the skin and conjunctiva, and any swelling or distention of the lids. Any findings should be reported to the doctor.

THE LACRIMAL SYSTEM

The lacrimal system is responsible for the production, maintenance, and elimination of the tear film. The major components of the lacrimal system are depicted in Figure 2-5. The tear film itself is composed of three layers (superficial to deep): the superficial oily layer; the tear fluid, or watery layer; and the mucin layer. The oily layer is produced mostly by the meibomian glands and serves to prevent spillover and evaporation of the tear film. The watery layer is produced by the lacrimal and accessory lacrimal glands (Krause and Wolfring) and serves several functions. First, the tears provide a smooth, optically clear surface for the cornea. Second, the tear fluid "washes" away debris and cellular waste products that are continually produced by the epithelium (most superficial layer) of the conjunctiva and cornea. Additional purposes served by the tear fluid are the transport of oxygen to the cornea and the inhibition of bacterial growth because of natural antibiotics present within the fluid. The deepest layer of the tear film, the mucin layer, is in contact with the epithelium of the conjunctiva and cornea and is produced by the goblet cells of the conjunctiva. This layer allows the tear fluid layer to remain stable on the surface of the epithelial cells, which normally (i.e., without the mucin layer) would not wet. A disturbance of any of these layers compromises the tear film and may lead to dry eye symptoms. An inadequate tear film also endangers the health of the cornea and conjunctiva.

The neural control of the glands that produce the fluid layer of tears is part of the autonomic nervous system. This system is responsible for the functions within the body that do not require our conscious control. Tearing is one of the functions controlled by the autonomic system.

The glands of Krause and Wolfring are considered *basic secretors*. They are called "basic" because the rate of production from these glands is relatively constant. The specific control of these glands is indirect since the more blood that flows through them, the more tears they produce. The lacrimal gland is a major factor in the overall volume of tear fluid only during reflex or psychogenic tearing (weeping). During normal (basic) tear production, the lacrimal gland is a minor factor. The clinical significance of these differences in control of the tear secretors is apparent when a patient presents with either symptoms or signs of inadequate tear production (dry eye).

The lacrimal gland rests in a depression (called the lacrimal fossa) in the temporal process of the frontal bone (see Figure 2-5). Because it is temporally located, it usually discharges in the upper temporal fornix, although occasionally some of the discharge is in the lower temporal fornix. The tears run along the margin of the lid toward the nasal canthus as the marginal tear strip (or prism). The *nasal canthus* is the angle created where the upper and lower lid are joined near the nose. At the nasal canthus, tears fall because of the effects of gravity to the lower lid margin, forming the lower marginal tear strip. The action of blinking squeezes these two tear strips together across the eye, wetting the entire front surface, smoothing the mucin layer, and spreading the oily layer over the tear fluid in the process. From the front of the eye, approximately 25% of the tear volume is evaporated. The rest of the tears are eliminated via the *puncta*, which are small holes in the upper and lower lid margin near the nasal canthus (see Figure 2-5). From the punc-

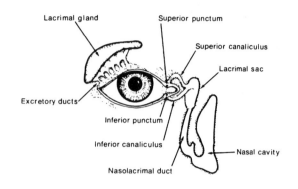

FIGURE 2-5—Schematic representation of the lacrimal apparatus, not including the accessory lacrimal glands of Krause and Wolfring. (Reprinted with permission from SS Bates. Fundamentals for Assisting in Primary Care Optometry. New York: Professional Press/Fairchild, 1983.)

ta, the tears are drawn into small tubes (called the *canaliculi*), which then empty into the *lacrimal sac*. (This sac is located nasally, in the first "lacrimal fossa" presented in the section on the orbit; see Figure 2-2.) The tear fluid is collected here and is periodically "pumped" into the nasolacrimal duct (another, slightly larger tube leading to the nose: see Figure 2-5). Obviously, if the tear volume is to be maintained, the total amount of tears leaving the eye via the evacuation system just described and through evaporation mentioned earlier must equal the amount produced by the accessory and lacrimal glands. If the tear drainage system is blocked or if the puncta are not in contact with the tear strip (as in the case of ectropion), the result would be too much tear fluid in the eye at any one time, which would then spill over onto the cheek. Tears spilling onto the cheek is called *epiphora*. Of course, epiphora could also result from the overproduction of tears, with the drainage system being normal.

THE GLOBE

The eyeball itself, also called the globe, is essentially three concentric spheres, or *tunics,* filled with fluids. Figure 2-6 shows the eyeball "cut in half." The spheres are (from outside to inside) the fibrous tunic, the vascular tunic, and the nervous tunic. The globe is divided into the anterior and posterior chambers by the iris, the colored part of the eye. Both chambers are fluid-filled. The anterior chamber and the posterior chamber in front of the lens are filled with aqueous humor. This fluid was named "aqueous" because it has the consistency of water. The posterior chamber behind the lens is filled with vitreous humor, which is also known as the vitreous body. This fluid was called "vitreous" because it has the consistency of egg whites. Both aqueous and vitreous humors help maintain the eye's shape as a ball.

The *fibrous tunic*, which is outermost, is comprised of the cornea (the anterior one-sixth) and the sclera (the posterior five-sixths). The *vascular tunic*, which is also called the uvea, is the "middle layer" of the globe and consists (from front to back) of the iris, ciliary body, and choroid. The innermost layer is the *nervous tunic*, which includes the retina and retinal pigment epithelium (RPE). Each of these tunics will be described in detail in the following sections.

Fibrous Tunic
Cornea

The cornea functions as the major refracting (light-focusing) surface of the eye and is unique among body tissues in that it is transparent. It is approximately circular and is thinner in the center than at the edges. The cornea is approximately spherical over the central 4 mm and becomes flatter in the periphery.

The cornea has five layers and normally contains no blood vessels. The oxygen and nutrients used by the cornea are absorbed from the vessels of the conjunctiva and sclera at the limbus and from the fluid in front and behind the cornea. When conditions exist that do not allow adequate circulatory support for the cornea (such as edema, inflammation, or inadequate tear film oxygen content), new vessels will grow into the cornea, disturbing its transparency. This is called *corneal neovascularization*, and its cause should be diagnosed as quickly as possible.

The innervation (nervous supply) of the cornea is mainly sensory branches of the trigeminal nerve (ophthalmic branch, CN V). Sensory nerves are those nerves responsible for pain, temperature, and touch sensations.

Figure 2-7 shows the layers of a monkey cornea, which is virtually identical to the structure of a human cornea. The front surface

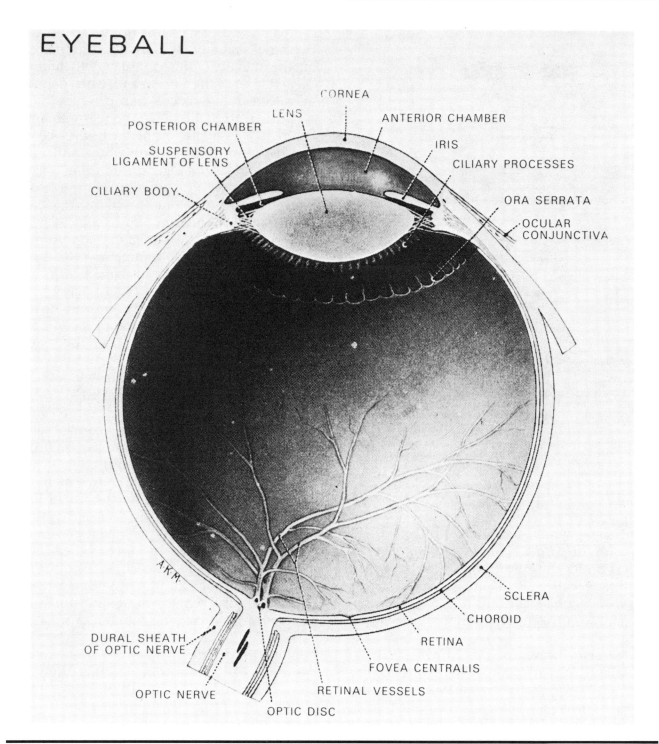

FIGURE 2-6—Cross section of the human eyeball from front to back. (Reprinted with permission from WJ Hamilton [ed]. Textbook of Human Anatomy [2nd ed]. London: Macmillan, 1976.)

of the cornea is covered by epithelial cells continuous with, but not identical to, the epithelial cells of the conjunctiva. These cells basically prevent water from entering the front of the cornea and provide several layers of protection from abrasion as a result of foreign matter getting into the eye. When the epithelium is damaged, the cells slide into the area of damage and then begin to regenerate, quickly regaining the number of cells lost due to injury or disease. The nerves of the cornea terminate freely as bare nerve endings between the cells

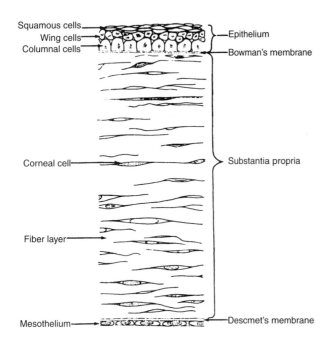

Figure 2-7—Schematic representation of a section of a monkey cornea showing the layers of tissue. The human cornea is very similar to a monkey sclera, but the deepest layer of the human cornea is the endothelium, not mesothelium. (Reprinted with permission from SS Bates. Fundamentals for Assisting in Primary Care Optometry. New York: Professional Press/Fairchild, 1983.)

of this layer, which accounts for the great sensitivity of the cornea to very slight stimulation.

Just under the epithelium, there is a tough membrane called *Bowman's membrane*. This layer does not have the capability to repair itself when cut or broken and therefore scars when damaged.

The center layer of the cornea (also the largest layer, approximately 90% of the corneal thickness) is called the *stroma*, which is composed of collagen. Collagen is a specific type of connective tissue that is very tough and does not stretch. These corneal layers are precisely arranged and lined up so that they do not interfere with the transmission of light. This is the reason the cornea is clear. If the layers are altered or damaged, the stroma does not allow light to pass through, and corneal opacity is the result.

The posterior border of the stroma is another membrane (*Descemet's membrane*), which is very thin and does have the capacity to regenerate when damaged. This membrane is not as resistant to damage as Bowman's membrane and is often affected by trauma (injuries) to the eye. Descemet's membrane is involved in maintaining the integrity of the corneal endothelium (the deepest layer of the cornea) and, when damaged, may decrease the corneal transparency.

The *endothelium* (called the mesothelium in Figure 2-7) is a single-thickness layer of cells (consisting of approximately 500,000 cells at birth) that does not regenerate throughout life. Any damage to this layer results in the remaining cells "spreading out" to fill in for the cells that were lost. The function of this layer is to keep water out of the cornea so that the stroma is not disturbed. If the number of cells is sufficiently reduced because of damage or normal cell death through life, the cornea may begin to "soak up" water; when this happens, it is no longer clear. Another function of the endothelium is to transport nutrients from the aqueous humor into the cornea.

Several different forms of mechanical damage can occur to the cornea; each type usually involves a particular layer. For example, abrasions (which may be caused by contact lenses, fingers in the eye, or blunt trauma) are usually confined to the epithelium, although at times they may be deeper. These are normally not considered serious except for the risk of infection, and they heal quickly, usually within 24 hours. Lacerations may damage Bowman's membrane and possibly some of the stroma, usually resulting in a scar. These are more serious than abrasions but not as serious as a penetrating injury, which, by definition, causes perforation involving the entire thickness of the cornea. Perforation of the globe is very serious because the fluid contents of the globe that maintain its shape can be lost, and the increased chance of intraocular infection threatens the loss of the eye.

In addition to the mechanical injuries that can be inflicted on the cornea, several degenerations and dystrophies can be involved with corneal abnormality. One of the most common of these is *keratoconus*. In this condition, the stroma of the cornea is thinned, and the intraocular pressure causes the cornea to bulge forward. This bulging stretches the endothelium, which eventually loses its capacity to maintain the water-free condition of the cornea. Damage to Descemet's membrane from the resultant edema can be seen before irreversible scarring of the

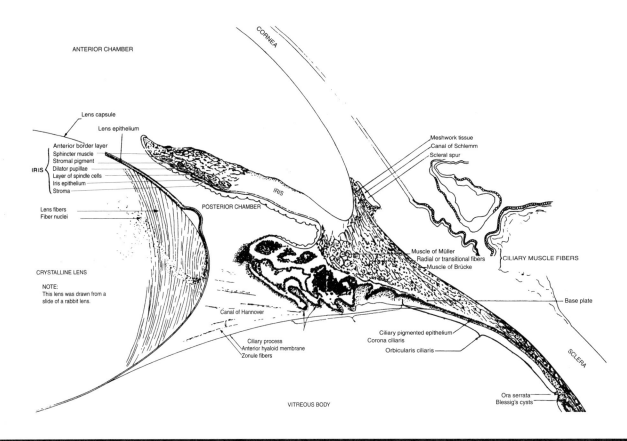

Figure 2-8—Schematic drawing of a cross section of the human eye at the junction of the cornea and sclera. This view shows the internal structures of this area in greater detail than in Figure 2-6. (Reprinted with permission from SS Bates. Fundamentals for Assisting in Primary Care Optometry. New York: Professional Press/Fairchild, 1983.)

corneal epithelium and stroma occurs. The treatment of this condition prior to the scarring stage is to fit the patient with rigid contact lenses. If the cornea is scarred significantly, a penetrating keratoplasty operation (also known as a *corneal transplant*) must be performed in order to regain good vision. Corneal transplant involves the replacement of a scarred cornea with a donor cornea from an eye bank. The probability of the paraoptometric's having contact with patients who have keratoconus is high. Therefore, there is also a great need for clear explanations of it, illustrating the need for basic understanding of anatomical terms and relationships.

Sclera

The posterior five-sixths of the fibrous tunic consists of the sclera and episcleral connective tissue (see Figure 2-6). The sclera is commonly called the "white" of the eye because it is white in color (see Figure 2-4). It begins at the cornea as an extension past the iris called the *scleral spur* (Figure 2-8). At the back of the eye, it is pierced by the fibers of the optic nerve. The sclera is made of collagen fibers very similar to the fibers of the corneal stroma. The main difference between these two structures is that the cornea's fibers are regularly arranged, whereas the scleral collagen is randomly arranged. For that reason, the sclera is opaque and appears white in the normal adult eye. Most of the blood and nerve supply for the front of the eye runs from the back of the eye to the front. Even though there are many vessels in the sclera, the sclera itself gets most of its nourishment from the episclera lying just above it (exterior to it) and the choroid just below it (interior to it). The functions of the sclera are to provide a rigid protective shell for the intraocular contents while allowing for variations in intraocular pressure, as well as to provide a relatively elastic insertion point for the extraocular muscles.

The *episclera* is a layer of connective tissue lying just outside the sclera. It is between the sclera and the bulbar conjunctiva. As mentioned, it supplies most of the nutrients to the sclera and has a rich blood supply. Because of this, the episclera reacts quite vigorously to inflammations of the sclera. *Scleritis* and *episcleritis* are among the more perplexing clinical conditions encountered by the optometrist. These conditions are present as red eyes that may or may not be painful. Since the conjunctiva loosely overlies the episclera, which is more tightly bound to the sclera, inflammation of any of these layers results in similar clinical appearances. A patient's eye that is red because of a conjunctivitis (inflammation of the conjunctiva) may look similar to an eye that is red because of a scleritis (inflammation of the sclera), but these two conditions have very different etiologies (causes), clinical time course (which means they last for differing periods of time), and treatments. Conjunctivitis is the most common cause of red eyes, episcleritis is less frequent, and scleritis is almost rare. In other words, the deeper the layer, the less frequently it is inflamed. When blood vessels in these layers break, the blood usually pools between the conjunctiva and episclera because these two layers have the loosest attachment. When this happens, it is called a *subconjunctival hemorrhage* and should be noted along with any discoloration of the sclera and adjacent tissues.

Vascular Tunic

The layer just interior to the sclera and providing some of the vascular support for it is called the *choroid*. This represents the majority of the vascular tunic of the eye. The vascular tunic (also called the *uvea* or *uveal tract*) has three main parts: the choroid, the ciliary body, and the iris. The part that is the most anterior (toward the front) in the eye is the iris. At the junction of the uvea (just anterior to the iris), cornea, and sclera, there is a specialized structure called the *trabecular mesh* (or meshwork), which acts as a drain for the intraocular fluid that is continually produced in the eye.

Iris

The iris is referred to as the "colored part" of the eye by laypeople. It gets its color from the amount of melanin (brown pigment) it contains. Irides (singular: iris) with a small amount of melanin are blue; irides with a lot of melanin are dark brown. All the colors of eyes between these two extremes have intermediate amounts of pigment. The iris divides the eye's internal space into the anterior chamber, which is in front of the iris, and the posterior chamber, which is behind the iris (see Figure 2-8). The iris has three main layers, and all three layers are perforated in the center, creating the pupil (see Figure 2-4 for a description of pupil and Figure 2-8 for a description of layers). The front of the iris, the *stroma*, is made up of loosely structured collagen fibers. The iris stroma contains the melanocytes (pigment cells); the *sphincter*, or constrictor muscle, which makes the pupil get smaller in bright light; and the blood vessels of the iris. The blood vessels take up the majority of the stroma. The central layer of the iris is the *nonpigmented epithelium*, which is basically the *dilator muscle* that is responsible for opening the pupil in the dark.

Since the dilator and sphincter have opposite functions, the control of these two muscles must be accurately coordinated by the body for proper light regulation into the eye. The functions of these muscles are not controlled voluntarily. Rather, the nervous control of these two muscles is part of the autonomic (nonvoluntary) nervous system, with one of them under the control of the sympathetic ("fight or flight") system and the other muscle under the control of the parasympathetic ("normal" control) system. The sphincter is the one controlled by the parasympathetic nerves and is the weaker of the two muscles throughout most of life. The dilator is sympathetically controlled. Because of the delicate balance between the actions of these two nervous systems, any disturbance of that balance is rapidly reflected in pupil size changes and errors in the normal reactivity of the pupils. This fact makes pupillary testing one of the most sensitive methods of examining the integrity of the nervous system. Pupillary testing should be done carefully on every patient. Optometrists may also use the dual innervation system for clinical benefit by influencing the balance with topically applied drugs. For example, if the doctor wants to examine the retina more completely, he or she may instill a mydriatic drug. These drugs make the pupil larger by stimulating the dilator muscle (acting as the sympathetic nerves do) or by paralyzing the sphincter muscle ("knocking out" the parasympathetic system), allowing the dilator muscle to open the pupil without the opposition of the other muscle.

The deepest layer of the iris is the *pigmented epithelium*. This layer is very darkly pigmented and extends around the edge of the pupil as the *pupillary frill*. It may be stuck to the lens as a result of inflammation of the iris (iritis). When the iris sticks to the lens, it is called a *posterior synechia*. If a posterior synechia is broken, the pigmented epithelium may pull away from the nonpigmented epithelium and remain stuck to the lens. The small pieces of pigmented epithelium stuck on the front of the lens give the doctor evidence that the person had an iritis in that eye sometime in the past.

Ciliary Body

The ciliary body is located immediately behind the iris and just inside the sclera (see Figure 2-8). It begins anteriorly at the scleral spur and ends posteriorly where it joins the retina. As is the iris, it is composed of several layers. The most external layer is the *ciliary muscle*. The ciliary muscle lies just under the sclera and is responsible for the triangular shape of the ciliary body when examined in cross section. This muscle also makes up most of the bulk of the ciliary body. Inside the ciliary muscle is a layer called the *stroma*, which contains the blood vessels and ciliary processes. The blood vessels of this area are responsible for the production of *aqueous humor* (the fluid that fills the anterior chamber). Aqueous is produced by filtration mechanisms similar to those for plasma filtration in the kidney.

The ciliary body has several very important functions. First, as mentioned above, it is the structure that produces aqueous humor, which fills the front part of the posterior chamber (between the lens and the iris) and the entire anterior chamber. The aqueous humor enters the posterior chamber in front of the lens and flows through the pupil into the anterior chamber. In the anterior chamber, it comes in contact with and filters through the trabecular meshwork to the canal of Schlemm. From the canal of Schlemm, it empties into the aqueous veins of Ascher in the sclera and is mixed with blood and removed from the eye (see Figure 2-8).

Aqueous humor provides the nutrients for the lens and posterior cornea (endothelium) and carries away waste products. It is also responsible for maintaining the intraocular pressure, since it is the only fluid continually produced in the eye. Because it is produced continually, the rate of drainage out of the eye must be equal to the rate of production, or the pressure inside the eye will not remain constant. If the rate of production is too high or the rate of drainage is too low, the pressure in the eye increases; this is called *ocular hypertension*. If the pressure becomes high enough to cause damage to the optic nerve, *glaucoma* results. It is also possible for the pressure to be too low (*ocular hypotension*); this is a threat to the maintenance of the shape of the eye. Ocular hypotension is usually due to penetrating injury; sometimes, it is the result of a decrease in aqueous production because of an inflammation of the ciliary body. These inflammations are part of *anterior uveitis*. Anterior uveitis is usually painful and associated with "red eyes," photophobia (light sensitivity), and possibly blurred vision. The blurring of vision is the result of the inflammatory cells and proteins from the iris blood vessels often seen in the anterior chamber of eyes with anterior uveitis. These findings are called "cells" and "flare," respectively.

The second major function of the ciliary body is accommodation. The smooth muscle of the ciliary body, called the *ciliary muscle*, is responsible for the change in focus when a person looks from far away to near targets, and from near to far. This muscle is also under the control of the parasympathetic system, which means that the function of the ciliary muscle can be influenced with drugs that prevent the activation of those nerve types. These drugs are called *cycloplegics* when they are used to paralyze the ciliary muscle so that accommodation cannot affect the outcome of certain tests. The reader should remember that drugs of this type can also be used for their effect on the pupil (mydriatics, mentioned earlier, act on the parasympathetic nerves). Even though the ciliary muscle is controlled by one of the same systems as the pupil, this does not mean it is as sensitive a measure of nervous integrity as pupil reactions. This is because the ability of humans to focus continually decreases with advancing age. The lens of the eye loses its elasticity as it ages, resulting in a lack of focusing ability, called *presbyopia*. Therefore, measuring the ability to accommodate is not always a good way to measure the health of the nerves that control it.

Other functions of the ciliary body include (1) secretion of one component of vitreous humor, (2) preventing the passage of materials into the aqueous humor from the blood (the so-called blood-aqueous barrier), and (3) helping to control the flow of aqueous humor through the trabecular meshwork through the action of some of the fibers of the ciliary muscles.

Choroid

Posterior to the ciliary body, the uvea (vascular tunic) consists of the choroid (see Figures 2-6 and 2-8). The choroid is a network of blood vessels that functions to provide vascular support to the structures around it. Vascular support mainly includes bringing blood with oxygen and nutrients to the tissues and carrying blood with waste products away from the tissues. The choroid lies between the sclera (which is external to the choroid) and the retina (which is internal to the choroid). From this location it provides vascular support for the outer retinal layers as well as the inner layers of the sclera. All of the blood supply to the eye comes through the ophthalmic artery, which fills the choroid through two sets of smaller vessels. At the back of the eye, the blood vessels of the choroid are supplied by the short posterior ciliary arteries, whereas the anterior choroid is supplied by the long posterior ciliary arteries. Both the long and short ciliary arteries are branches of the *ophthalmic artery*. These vessels branch off before the ophthalmic artery actually enters the eye. After the long and short ciliary arteries have branched off, the ophthalmic artery enters the eye, where it is renamed the *central retinal artery*. The central retinal artery supplies the internal layers of the retina, whereas the choroid supplies the external layers. This differentiation in blood supply is important in cases of retinal artery occlusion or any condition that decreases the blood flow through the internal retinal circulation. In these cases, the parts of the retina served by the choroidal circulation are not affected, but the portion that depends on the retinal circulation may be permanently damaged. This dual retinal blood supply explains the clinical signs and symptoms often encountered in these disorders.

The outermost layer of the choroid, called *Haller's layer*, is made up of large vessels. The caliber of the arteries and veins of the choroid become progressively smaller the closer they get to the retina. The next distinct change in vessel size occurs in *Sattler's layer*; its vessels are considered to be medium-sized. The vessels of both Haller's and Sattler's layers are classified as arterioles and venules because of the construction of their walls. The next layer, which lies next to the retina, is called the *choriocapillaris*. Its vessels are primarily capillaries. Because of the obvious differentiation between this capillary layer and those layers external to it, Haller's and Sattler's layers are usually considered together, and the choriocapillaris is considered separately.

Pigment cells called *melanocytes* are scattered throughout the choroid and give it a very dark coloration. There are also nerves that travel through the choroid that are named for the arteries they accompany. The long and short posterior ciliary nerves accompany the long and short ciliary arteries. The choriocapillaris is separated from the retina by a thin membrane called *Bruch's membrane*. This thin layer of connective tissue is the most internal part of the choroid and provides for the insertion of the ciliary muscle, which is responsible for accommodation. This is also the site of some retinal detachments where the entire thickness of the retina may separate from the inside of Bruch's membrane. Such detachments are called *RPE detachments*.

Just as the anterior uvea (the ciliary body and iris) may be inflamed because of infection, trauma, or allergic responses, the posterior uvea can also be inflamed. When this occurs, it is called a *posterior uveitis*. This condition usually develops very slowly and is difficult to treat. There usually is no pain, and it may not even be noticed by the patient until it is quite well developed and causes a significant decrease in vision. This condition is associated with many autoimmune diseases such as sarcoidosis, tuberculosis, and arthritis. For this reason, questions regarding the patient's general health are usually included in the preexamination history. Occasionally, both anterior and posterior uveitis occur at the same time to the same eye. This is called *panuveitis,* and it is considered a serious condition, requiring aggressive systemic treatment and, at times, hospitalization.

Nervous Tunic: Retina

As mentioned earlier, the retina is located just inside Bruch's membrane, the inner membranous layer of the choroid. The retina is the internal covering of three concentric tunics. It starts at the *ora serrata*, which marks the end of the choroid, and is continuous over the posterior five-sixths of the globe except for the optic nerve head (see Figure 2-8). The fact that the retina does not extend over the optic nerve head means that there is no visual sensation there—that is, light hitting this part of the eye is not registered. When plotted with a visual field tester, this area is called the *blind spot*. When considering the inside of the eye, the area anterior to the ora serrata (the inside of the ciliary body) is called the *pars ceca*, and the area behind the ora serrata (the retina) is called the *pars optica*.

There are ten layers in the retina, depicted in Figure 2-9. They are numbered such that the outermost layer (next to the choroid) is number one, and the innermost layer (next to the vitreous) is number 10. The retina is divided into two general sections: the outer layer, which is the RPE, and the inner, or neural, retina. There is a "potential" space between these two retinal regions, and this is the site of retinal detachment (as opposed to RPE detachment described earlier). In a potential space, two tissues meet that normally have no space between them; however, they do have the potential to separate from each other, creating a space. The retina's general function is to convert the light energy falling onto it into electrical impulses that can be analyzed by the brain. There are many interconnections between retinal elements. These provide for efficient processing of the information contained in the light patterns that the retina registers. These processes will be briefly explained with the anatomic description of the retinal element responsible for it.

Layer one, the RPE, is the most external of the retinal layers and is in contact with Bruch's membrane of the choroid. This layer performs several major functions necessary for proper retinal physiology. For example, it is involved with the regeneration of the chemicals used in the conversion of light to electrical energy. Specifically, it provides the photoreceptors, the retinal elements that actually convert light to electrical impulses, with vitamin A. Vitamin A is a major

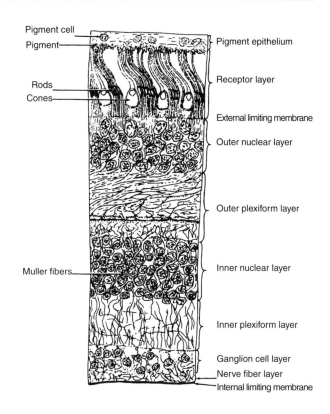

Figure 2-9—Schematic drawing of the retina, showing the ten layers detailed in the text. The top of this picture is the outside the retina near the choroid; the bottom is the inside layer of the retina near the vitreous humor. (Reprinted with permission from SS Bates. Fundamentals for Assisting in Primary Care Optometry. New York: Professional Press/Fairchild, 1983.)

component of the chemicals that "capture" the light energy for conversion to electrical energy. It is found in high concentrations in carrots—which is why the "eat your carrots" cliché has persisted for so long. The chemicals that are used to collect the light energy in the photoreceptors are called *photopigments*. The RPE must also transport nutrients into the retina, since the choroid supplies the outer retina. The RPE cells also phagocytize ("eat") the used-up portions of the photoreceptor cells so that the area near the photoreceptors is not cluttered with cellular debris that would interfere with the proper reception of incident light. (Retinitis pigmentosa is a genetic defect that results in the RPEs not performing this function adequately; it starts as night blindness and can progress to total blindness.) Finally, the RPE prevents the intraocular reflection of stray light. The cells of this layer have large amounts of melanin and therefore absorb light that has not been converted to electrical impulses before it can reflect back toward another part of the retina. This also increases the efficiency of the retina in detection of small amounts of light.

The next layer begins the *neural retina*. A brief description of the typical anatomy and physiology of a nerve cell will be helpful. Nerve cells are usually long, with the ends specialized to perform certain functions. One end, the *axon*, is specialized for transmitting neural impulses; the other end, the *dendrite*, is specialized to receive neural impulses. Because of these specialized ends, the nerve always transmits impulses in the proper direction. Between the axon of one cell and the dendrite of the next cell there is a small gap called a *synapse*; in order for the nerve impulse to cross this gap, a chemical must be released from the axon. The chemical, called a *neurotransmitter* floats across the synapse and stimulates the dendrite of the next nerve cell in line. The receptive end (dendrite) of the next cell in line has sites that can be stimulated by the neurotransmitter to recreate the electrical impulse that is the neural signal.

Since the RPE is involved in alignment and maintenance of the photoreceptors, it should be obvious that the next layer (number two) is the photoreceptor layer. There are two classes of photoreceptors in the human eye: *rods* and *cones*. These two types differ in their anatomy, physiologic response characteristics, and distribution throughout the retina. Among other anatomic differences, the rods have flat outer segments, called the receptors, whereas the cones have pointed (cone-shaped) outer segments. The outer segments of the photoreceptors are the ends closest to the RPE. Regardless of their differences, the rods and cones perform the same general function, that is, converting light energy into neural impulses. This is accomplished through a series of chemical reactions involving the photopigments that are present in their outer segments.

Functionally, the response of the rods is based on the presence or absence of light energy; the cones are additionally responsible for color discrimination. The cones require much higher light levels to be stimulated than do rods; therefore, when there is minimal light, the rods do the seeing and the cones are relatively inactive. That is why people cannot see color in dim illumination. Two important clinical correlations are drawn from these facts. First, conditions of color deficiency are predominately errors of the cones. Second, problems in seeing in dim illumination are usually because of rod dysfunctions (one exception is retinitis pigmentosa). The differential responses of the rods and cones to color and darkness form the basis of clinical testing to investigate this layer of the retina. For example, dark adaptometry looks at the time it takes for a person to see in the dark after a bright flash. The rods are quicker to recover, and therefore the integrity of the rods can be investigated separately from the cones. The rods and cones also differ in the time it takes for them to respond to lights bright enough to stimulate both (the rods are slower). This is the basis for using rapid flashes of light in electroretinogram and critical flicker frequency testing.

The rods and cones are not evenly distributed throughout the retina. The retina is divided into concentric zones based on anatomical or physiological characteristics. The central 1 cm of the retina is called the *macula lutea* or *macula* because it has a pigment that gives it a yellow color. In this region, the photoreceptors (mainly cones) are the most dense, and in the very center of this region (the central 1.5 mm of the macula), there is a depressed area called the *fovea*. In the fovea, there is a region that has only cones called the *foveola*. This area is responsible for fine discriminations and high visual acuity.

Outside the macula, the density of rods increases, and the density of cones decreases toward the periphery (toward the ora serrata). This provides another way to separate the functions of the rods from the cones. The peripheral retina and the central retina rods can be preferentially tested without involving the cones, and vice versa.

The layer that lies just interior to the photoreceptor layer is the *external limiting membrane* of the retina. This structure is not really a membrane; it is the point at which the photoreceptors are joined together by a specific type of cellular junction called a *zonula adherens*. It basically marks the midpoint of the length of the rods and cones.

Internal to this layer is the location of the cell bodies of the photoreceptors. These cell bodies contain the nuclei; therefore, this layer (number four) is called the *outer nuclear layer*. The cell body of photoreceptors, as in all cells, is the site where metabolic functions of the cell are carried out, usually near the nucleus. The electrical response started in the outer segments is also conducted through this part of the cell.

Layer number five is one that contains the first synapses in the visual pathway. *Synapses* are the junctions between nerve cells. This layer is also the last layer (most internal) to be supported by the choroidal circulation. Actually, it gets some nutrients from the retinal circulation in the next layer and some from the choroid. The term given to layers without cell bodies that contain synaptic sites is *plexiform*, so this layer is called the *outer plexiform layer*. In this layer, the terminal ends of the photoreceptors that transmit neural impulses via chemical neurotransmitters (like axons) synapse with the dendrites (specialized receiving ends) of bipolar cells and horizontal cells. The *bipolar cells* provide for the transmission of the visual signal up the visual pathway (toward the brain), acting like a relay or "wire" in the pathway of visual information; this is called "vertical" transmission of information. Some bipolar cells only receive input from one photoreceptor, whereas others receive input from several receptors. In this way, the input from several receptors is combined at some bipolars and not at others. Therefore, the information passed along by the bipolar may be from any one or from several of the receptors synapsing with it. In addition to the higher density of cones in the fovea, this unbranched transmission of information through the bipolar cells accounts for the high spatial resolution, and therefore good visual acuity, of the fovea, as compared with the poor resolution of the peripheral retina. Bipolar cells are not the only ones at this layer with multiple connections; the *horizontal cells* connect receptors to other receptors and to other horizontal cells. These connections are involved in integrating the input from groups of cells into receptive fields and represent horizontal processing of visual information. This organization allows for contrast and border enhancement by the visual system. The horizontal cells have also been implicated in the processing of color information to a small degree.

The cell bodies of bipolar and horizontal cells, Mueller cells, and amacrine cells are found in the *inner nuclear layer* (number six). *Mueller cells* are nutritional support cells that are actually scattered throughout all the layers internal to the outer nuclear layer, specifically layers five to nine. This layer represents the first (i.e., the most external) layer, which is completely supported by the circulation of the retina, as opposed to the choroidal circulation. Blood vessels can also be found in all the layers internal to this. Amacrine cells have no apparent axons or dendrites. Instead, they have processes that allow for bidirectional transmission of neural signals. In this way, amacrine cells are unique, since typical nerve cells conduct impulses in only one direction. The amacrine cells function much as the bipolar cells do, but instead of integrating information from retinal receptors, they integrate the information of ganglion cells. This provides further enhancement of border detection and may also be involved in the processing of temporal information, such as movement sensation. This is another example of horizontal, rather than vertical, processing.

The amacrine cells' processes and the axons of the bipolar cells connect to ganglion cells in the *inner plexiform layer* (layer seven). The ganglion cells are the next step in the transmission of the visual impulses to the brain. This is another example of vertical processing.

Layer eight consists of the cell bodies of the ganglion cells, which are all collected at this level of the retina. This is called the *ganglion cell layer*. Visual information is carried via the axons of the ganglion cells out of the eye. The axons themselves collect as a bundle that is properly called the *optic nerve* (CN II). On their way to form this bundle, the axons run across the inside of the retina and constitute the ninth layer, which is called the *nerve fiber layer*.

The tenth layer of the retina is the *internal limiting membrane*, which separates the ganglion cell layer from the face of the vitreous, which fills the posterior chamber. This membrane is composed of collagen fibers that connect the Mueller cells.

Summary

The retina is divided into two sections that have a total of ten layers that are numbered from the outside to the inside. Layers one to five are supported by the circulation of the choroid and layers six to ten by the retinal circulation. The RPE (layer one) is the outer retina, whereas the inner, or neural, retina comprises layers two through 10. Generally, the signals generated are combined such that the input from 126 million photoreceptors are contained in, and transmitted through, 1 million optic nerve fibers that are actually the ganglion cell axons.

LENS

The lens is a structure composed mostly of elongated epithelial cells that are arranged in concentric layers, similar to the way an onion is constructed around its nucleus (see Figures 2-6 and 2-8). These elongated cells, or fibers, are collectively called the *cortex*. The cortex is surrounded by a single layer of epithelium, some cells of which elongate to form new cortical fibers. Because of this process, the lens continues to grow throughout life. The entire lens is surrounded by a tough elastic membrane called the *capsule*. The regular pattern and tight adherence of the lens fibers to each other are responsible for the lens' transparency. The lens is suspended by the *zonular fibers*, or *zonules*, from its edge to the *ciliary muscle* (see Figure 2-8). It is the second most important refracting, or light-focusing, component of the eye. (The cornea is the most important refracting surface of the eye.) The lens is not normally a rigid structure in a young person. It is bendable and can change shape in response to the ciliary muscle's contraction. The mechanism by which people focus their eyes on near targets is a complex interaction between the muscle, the zonules, and the lens capsule. A simplified explanation of the process is as follows: The ciliary muscle tightens, allowing the zonules to loosen, and the elasticity of the capsule makes the lens bulge in the center so that it becomes a more powerful lens.

If the lens fibers become separated from each other because of mechanical swelling of the lens, damage from radiation, or some metabolic disturbance, the space between them is called a *vacuole*. Vacuoles usually lead to clouding of the lens in that area. This clouding is called a *cataract*. Several different kinds of cataracts exist. They are named for their location, cause, size, density, or time of occurrence. These methods of classification are somewhat arbitrary, and the important clinical feature is the fact that vision is reduced (sometimes significantly) if the cataract prevents enough light from entering the eye. The only treatment for a cataract is surgical removal of the clouded lens. After a clouded lens has been removed, the power of the lens for refracting the light entering the eye must be replaced if clear vision is to be attained. This is done in one of three ways: spectacle correction, contact lens correction, or intraocular lens implants. In all three cases, patients usually require glasses for near visual activities because they cannot focus near with the lens removed. Cataracts are discussed in greater detail in Chapter 3.

THE VISUAL PATHWAY

In the section titled "Nervous Tunic: Retina," the first part of the visual pathway, which involves the structures from the rods and cones to the optic nerve, is explained. This section discusses the rest of the pathway, from the eye, specifically the optic nerve, to the visual cortex (Figure 2-10). The visual cortex is the part of the brain responsible for analyzing the neural signals representing sight. The visual pathway basically runs a horizontal path from the front of the head to the back of the head.

The amount of the world a person can see at any one time without eye or head movements is called the *visual field* or simply the *field*. To trace the visual pathway systematically and correlate it to the visual field, the retina must be divided so that the information from retinal elements stimulated by any part of the field can be followed throughout the visual pathway. To accomplish this, the retina is usually considered in quarters, or sectors. The sectors are created by dividing the retina into halves by imagining a vertical line through the fovea, separating the nasal (toward the nose) from the temporal (toward the temple) retinal halves. By imagining a horizontal line through the fovea, the nasal and temporal retinal halves are each divided into the superior (upper) and inferior (lower) quarters. The retinal quarters created by these imaginary lines are called *quadrants*. Light from the part of the world that is physically temporal to the fovea of an eye strikes the nasal retina, and vice versa, for light from objects nasal to the fovea strikes the temporal retina (see Figure 2-10). Likewise, the objects above the fovea strike

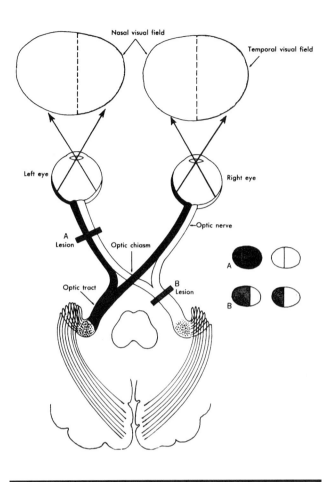

Figure 2-10—Representation of the visual pathway, showing the left visual field in white and the right visual field shaded. The field defects caused by damage at A and B are represented. (Reprinted with permission from SS Bates. Fundamentals for Assisting in Primary Care Optometry. New York: Professional Press/Fairfield, 1983.)

the inferior retina; the opposite relationship holds for the part of the visual field below the foveal level. In other words, the retinal elements in any quadrant actually are representing the visual field that is opposite to it in the real world. For example, the superior nasal quadrant is stimulated by light from the inferior temporal field. Therefore, visual information about the area below and temporal to a person's eye would be gathered by the retinal elements in the superior nasal retina and transmitted to the visual cortex by the elements of the visual pathway connected to those retinal elements. These concepts form the basis of visual field testing, as well as much of the diagnosis of retinal and neurologic disease that involves the visual pathway.

The fibers in the optic nerve—actually, the axons of the ganglion cells—are arranged such that fibers originating in a specific quadrant of the retina are grouped together rather than haphazardly intermingled. Therefore, all the visual information from that quadrant is contained in a group of optic nerve fibers. All the visual information from one eye is carried by that eye's optic nerve as far as the *optic chiasm*. The optic chiasm, also called simply the chiasm, is formed by the fusion of the optic nerves inside the skull near the pituitary gland. At this point, the fibers from the nasal retina of each eye cross to join the temporal fibers of the other eye (see Figure 2-10). This puts the nasal fibers of the right eye, which represent the right half of that eye's visual field, together with the temporal fibers of the left eye, which also represent the right half of the visual field. Therefore, the fibers that represent the right half of the visual field from both eyes are grouped together from the chiasm back to the cortex. This combination of fiber bundles from the two optic nerves continues from the left side of the chiasm as the *left optic tract*. The fibers from both eyes that represent the left field are also together and become the *right optic tract*. Thus, the left optic tract represents the right visual field, and the right optic tract represents the left visual field (see Figure 2-10). Because the visual information is organized in this way, any disease or lesion involving the visual pathway behind the chiasm results in a loss of sensitivity or visual sensation in part of the field of both eyes. These losses are called field defects, or *scotomas*. A field defect that affects approximately a quarter of the visual field in either eye is called a *quadrantanopsia* or *quadrantanopia*. A loss of half of the visual field of either eye is called a *hemianopsia* or *hemianopia*. If a field defect such as a hemianopsia exists in both eyes and affects the same field in each eye, it is called *homonymous*. For example, a scotoma involving the right half of the visual field in both eyes is homonymous. A field loss that involves the right half of the visual field in the right eye and the left half of the visual field of the left eye is not homonymous. Lesions involving the retina or the optic nerve (prechiasmal) result in unilateral (one-eye) field defects, whereas bilateral, often homonymous, losses occur with chiasmal and postchiasmal lesions (see Figure 2-10). These facts give the doctor information regarding the segment of the pathway that is involved in conditions that affect the visual pathway. If the lesion is at the chiasm, the resultant visual field defects are usually bilateral. Combining this knowledge with the area of the field affected helps pinpoint the insult to the chiasm. For example, pituitary adenomas (a type of cancer of the pituitary gland), because of their location directly above the chiasm, destroy the crossing nasal fibers, which results in a characteristic loss of the temporal field in both eyes. This type of field defect, known as a *bitemporal hemianopsia*, indicates a lesion either pressing down from above the chiasm or pressing up from below it. The temporal fibers can be damaged by the chiasm being compressed from the sides. This can occur in cases of an internal carotid artery aneurysm. (An *aneurysm* is a bulge in the wall of an artery.) Because the internal carotid arteries run vertically up the sides of the chiasm, a bulge in the wall of the internal carotid artery may push against the side of the chiasm where the fibers representing the temporal field are located. The field defect that results from the damage to the temporal fibers is a *binasal hemianopsia*, since the temporal fibers convey the information from the nasal field. Binasal and bitemporal scotomas are not homonymous, since they do not affect the same side of the visual field in each eye.

The optic tract runs from the chiasm, approximately halfway back to the visual cortex. The optic tracts end at a structure called the *lateral geniculate nucleus* (LGN), or the *lateral geniculate body*. Lesions of the optic tract produce homonymous hemianopsias that affect the field on the opposite side. For example, an injury to the left optic tract produces a right homonymous hemianopsia; the vision in the right half of the visual field in both eyes is lost.

The LGN is a pyramid-shaped mass of cells where a synapse occurs between the terminal ends of the ganglion cell axons and the dendrites of the nerve fibers, which carry the visual information the rest of the way to the visual cortex. Lesions of the LGN or further back in the pathway will create identical defects in each eye. All such defects are homonymous and identical. Identical defects in each eye are *congruous*. This again helps to localize lesions in the postchiasmal part of the pathway, since lesions between the chiasm and the LGN produce similar (but usually not identical) defects in the two eyes. The axons of the cells of the LGN continue to the visual cortex as the *optic radiations*.

Once they reach the cortex, these fibers synapse with cortical cells in the part of the brain known as Brodman's area 17, located at the very back tip of the brain. Lesions of the cortex always produce congruous homonymous hemianopsias, either left or right, depending on the side of the brain that is damaged. Damage to the right side of the cortex causes a congruous left homonymous hemianopia. An unusual feature of the congruous homonymous hemianopias due to cortical injury is *macular sparing*, the term given to a visual field when a complete hemianopsia exists except for the central 2–5 degrees, where the field is intact. This phenomenon has not been adequately explained but does serve to localize the lesion at the cortical level. From area 17 the visual information is distributed throughout the brain by cortical fibers that are called *association fibers*. These fibers distribute the visual information throughout the cortex for analysis and for association with other sensory data and motor coordination.

One of the major pathways of the association fibers is from the visual cortex to the area of the brain known as the motor eye fields. This area of the brain, also called Brodman's area 8, is responsible for planning eye movements. Anatomically, it is located in the frontal lobe, which may be damaged in injuries that penetrate the roof of the orbit.

THE EXTRAOCULAR MUSCLES

Eye movements, regardless of the stimulus for them, are necessary for the eyes to be coordinated with each other and accurately aimed at visual targets. This is accomplished through the coordinated manipulation of six distinct muscles, the extraocular muscles, attached to the globe (Figure 2-11). They include *rectus muscles*—the medial rectus, the lateral rectus, the superior rectus, and the inferior rectus; and the *oblique muscles*—the superior oblique and the inferior oblique. These muscles are unique in that the number of muscle fibers controlled by each nerve fiber is very small, allowing for very accurate control of eye movements. All of the extraocular muscles are striated muscles—that is, they are under voluntary control. The recti and the superior oblique muscles originate from a tendon that surrounds the optic fora-

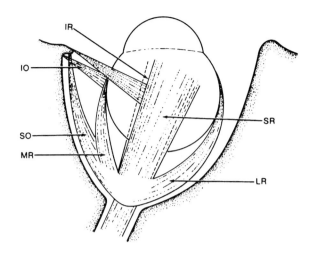

Figure 2-11—Drawing of the extraocular muscles in position within the orbit. Note the angle made between the medial wall of the orbit (left side of picture) and the superior and inferior recti and obliques. (Reprinted with permission from SS Bates. Fundamentals for Assisting in Primary Care Optometry. New York: Professional Press/Fairchild, 1983.)

men at the back of the orbit. This tendon, called the *common tendinous ring* or the *annulus of Zinn*, is connected to the sphenoid bone. The recti muscles insert into the sclera in front of the equator. The superior and inferior obliques insert into the sclera behind the equator. The term *equator* is used to refer to that area that is roughly halfway from the cornea to the macula along the sclera or retina—that is, it is the midpoint of the eye. Each muscle will be presented in terms of its location, actions, and neural control. Table 2-2 summarizes the anatomic and physiologic facts associated with the individual muscles.

Medial Rectus

The medial rectus runs from its origin at the optic foramen, along the medial wall of the orbit, to its insertion onto the sclera. It is the most powerful of the extraocular muscles and has only one action: adduction (turning the eye toward the nose). It is controlled by the inferior branch of the oculomotor nerve (CN III).

Inferior Rectus

The inferior rectus runs along the floor of the orbit from the orbital apex to its insertion. Its path is such that it makes a 23-degree angle with the medial wall of the orbit. Because of this angle, contraction of the inferior rectus makes the eye move in more than one direction. The primary action of this muscle is the depression of the eyeball, rotating the eye toward the maxillary bone. In addition to this effect, the inferior rectus also adducts the eye (secondary action) and extorts it slightly (tertiary action). Extorsion means that the top of the eye rotates out toward the temple and that the bottom of the eye rotates in toward the nose. It is also controlled by the inferior division of the oculomotor nerve (CN III).

Lateral Rectus

The lateral rectus runs along the lateral wall of the orbit and, similar to the medial rectus, only has one action. The lateral rectus abducts the eye—that is, it moves the eye away from the midline. The lateral rectus is controlled by the abducens nerve (CN VI).

Superior Rectus

This muscle, like the inferior rectus, also makes a 23-degree angle with the medial wall. It also has several actions that are directly opposite those of the inferior rectus. The primary action of the superior rectus is one of elevation, which means that it rotates the eyeball toward the frontal bone. The secondary action of the superior rectus is abduction, and the tertiary action is intorsion. It is also controlled by a branch of the oculomotor nerve (CN III).

Superior Oblique

The superior oblique has its origin on the annulus of Zinn or very near it on the sphenoid bone. It runs along the superior medial wall to a small bony loop at the front of the orbit called the *trochlea*, which acts as its functional origin. The ligament of the muscle passes through the trochlea and is reflected back onto the globe to its insertion behind the equator. This ligament makes an angle of 51–53 degrees with the medial wall. Therefore, this muscle also has several actions. The primary action is depression (turning the eye down) toward the maxillary bone. Abduction is its secondary action, turning the

TABLE 2-2. Extraocular muscle facts

	Medial rectus	Inferior rectus	Lateral rectus	Superior rectus	Superior oblique	Inferior oblique	Levator palpebral superiorous
Origin	Annulus of Zinn	Annulus of Zinn	Annulus of Zinn	Annulus of Zinn	Near or on annulus	Fossa near lacrimal duct	Sphenoid bone above annulus
Insertion	Sclera anterior to equator	Sclera interior to equator	Sclera anterior to equator	Sclera anterior to equator	Sclera posterior to equator	Sclera posterior to equator	1 mm anterior and 1–2 mm below macula
Limbus insertion	5.5 mm	6.6 mm	7.0 mm	7.7 mm	13.8 mm	—	—
Innervation	Inferior branch (cranial nerve III)	Inferior branch (cranial nerve III)	Abducens (cranial nerve IV)	Superior branch (cranial nerve III)	Trochlear nerve (cranial nerve VI)	Inferior branch (cranial nerve III)	Superior branch (cranial nerve III)
Arterial blood supply	Medial ophthalmic	Infraorbital, medial ophthalmic, or both	Lacrimal, lateral ophthalmic, or both	Lateral ophthalmic	Lateral ophthalmic	Medial ophthalmic	Supraorbital
Venous drainage	Inferior orbital vein	Inferior orbital vein	Superior orbital vein	Superior orbital vein	Superior orbital vein	Inferior orbital vein	Superior orbital vein

TABLE 2-3.	Antagonist muscle pairs in one eye
Muscle	Antagonist
Medial rectus	Lateral rectus
Lateral rectus	Medial rectus
Superior rectus	Inferior rectus
Inferior rectus	Superior rectus
Superior oblique	Inferior oblique
Inferior oblique	Superior oblique

TABLE 2-4.	Agonist muscle pairs in the two eyes
Right eye	Left eye
Medial rectus	Lateral rectus
Lateral rectus	Medial rectus
Superior rectus	Inferior oblique
Inferior rectus	Superior oblique
Superior oblique	Inferior rectus
Inferior oblique	Superior rectus

eye away from the nose. The tertiary actions of the superior oblique are intorsion (rotating the top of the eyeball in) toward the nose and that of rotating the bottom of the eyeball out, away from the nose. The superior oblique is controlled by the trochlear nerve (CN IV).

Inferior Oblique

The inferior oblique is the only extraocular muscle that has an origin at the front of the orbit. It begins at a fossa (depression) in the maxillary bone near the lacrimal sac and runs between the eye and the inferior rectus. It makes the same angle as the superior oblique tendon to its insertion at the back of the eye near the macular area. The actions of this muscle are opposite those of the superior oblique. Its primary action is elevation, with adduction and extorsion being the secondary and tertiary actions. It is innervated by a division of the oculomotor nerve (CN III).

The six muscles of each eye are set up as three opponent pairs, with the action of one of the muscles of a pair being directly opposed by the action of the other one. These pairs are called *antagonists*. The antagonist pairs for one eye are listed in Table 2-3. Another association that is important is the pairing of muscles of the two eyes that move the eyes in the same direction (i.e., to the left, or up); these are called *agonists*. The agonists are listed in Table 2-4. The agonists must respond properly to the neural signal to move the eyes if proper binocular alignment is to be maintained. If one muscle does not fully respond to its neural signals for contraction, it is called a *paretic muscle*. If the muscle does not respond to the neural signals for contraction at all, it is called a *paralytic muscle*. Paretic muscles appear to be weakened, whereas paralytic muscles are not functioning at all. When, for any reason, one of the pair of agonists is not properly controlled, when either one muscle overacts or the other underacts, *strabismus* is the result. Strabismus, also known as "squint," is the condition present when both eyes cannot be directed to an object of regard at the same time; it is often called "cross-eye" or "wall-eye." The condition in which there is a tendency for the eyes to misalign but the person can overcome that tendency so that both of his or her eyes do point at objects of regard is called a *heterophoria*, or simply phoria.

To determine whether the existence of strabismus or phoria is the result of neurologic deficit or muscular damage, the evaluation of strabismus must include the assessment of eye-movement control. All examinations should include this. Eye movements should be tested monocularly; these are called *ductions*. Binocular eye movements in the same direction are called *versions*. Testing with the eyes moving in opposite directions is called *vergence testing*. There are three types of vergences. An eye movement in which both eyes turn toward the nose (the right eye turns left and the left eye turns right) is called *convergence*. Both eyes turning away from the nose (right eye to the right, left eye to the left), it is called *divergence*. The third type of vergence involves one eye turning up and the other eye turning down. This is called *vertical divergence* or simply vertical vergence.

SUGGESTED READING

Bates SS. Fundamentals for Assisting in Primary Care Optometry. New York: Professional Press/Fairchild, 1983.

Hamilton WJ (ed). Textbook of Human Anatomy (2nd ed). St. Louis: Mosby, 1976.

Moses R (ed). Adler's Physiology of the Eye: Clinical Application (7th ed). St. Louis: Mosby, 1981.

Pavan-Langston D (ed). Manual of Ocular Diagnosis. Boston: Little, Brown, 1980.

Schapero M, Cline D, Hofstetter HW (eds). Dictionary of Visual Science. Radnor, PA: Chilton, 1968.

Warwick R. Eugene Wolff's Anatomy of the Eye and Orbit (7th ed). Philadelphia: Saunders, 1976.

3 / Refractive Status

Catherine E. Muhr

The refractive status of the eye relates to the manner in which light rays entering the eye are brought to a focus. When light rays pass through the optical components of the eye, such as the cornea and the crystalline lens, and are brought to a single-point focus on a healthy retina, they produce a clear visual image. When light rays are not bent properly to allow this focus, clear vision does not result, and the eye is said to have a refractive error.

The purpose of this chapter is to review the refractive status of the eye through a basic discussion of the optics of light, the structure and function of the optical components of the eye, and various refractive errors. A more detailed discussion of ocular anatomy and physiology and of ophthalmic lenses used to correct refractive errors may be found in Chapters 2 and 5, respectively.

BASIC OPTICS OF LIGHT

Some basic principles of optics are fundamental to understanding the characteristics of light and lenses. Perhaps the most elementary principle is that what we see is light. It can be direct light, as projected from a light source, such as the sun, a lamp, a television, and so forth, or it can be reflected light from a wall, a car, a person, or any other surface.

Light travels through space in straight lines, which are often referred to as *light rays*. As light rays are emitted from a source, they diverge, or spread. While they actually continue to diverge, the amount of divergence gradually decreases. At a distance of approximately 20 feet, or 6 m, the light rays assume a virtually parallel course, which is continuous to infinity. Twenty feet, or 6 m, therefore, may be considered *optical infinity* due to the virtually parallel course of the light rays at that point. In most illustrations in this chapter of light rays entering a lens or the eye, a light source at infinity will be assumed, and parallel light rays will be drawn.

When light rays encounter an object such as a wall or a window, they are absorbed, reflected, or refracted. When light strikes a wall, for example, some of the light is reflected and some is absorbed, depending on the color and texture of the wall. When light strikes a transparent medium, such as a window, some of the light is reflected from the surface, some is absorbed within the medium, and most of the light continues through the medium.

The path a light ray takes as it passes through a transparent medium depends on two factors: angle of incidence and index of refraction.

The *angle of incidence* is formed by the light ray and the surface of the medium. For example, light rays striking a flat pane of glass straight on, or perpendicular to the surface, form a right angle, or a 90-degree angle, with the surface. The angle of incidence in this case is 90 degrees. Light rays could strike the glass from any direction, and the angle between the light ray and the surface of the glass can be measured. For the purposes of this chapter, however, the measurement of that angle is not important.

In geometry, a line perpendicular to another line is referred to as the *normal*. In optics,

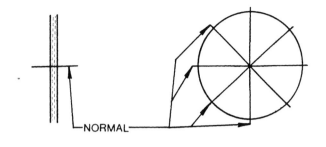

FIGURE 3-1—The optical normal.

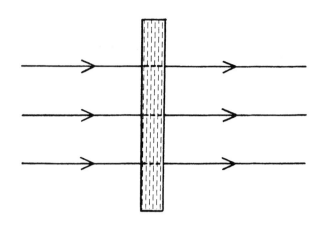

FIGURE 3-2—A plane or plano lens has no refracting effect.

every surface, flat or curved, has a normal (Figure 3-1), a theoretical line at right angles to the surface. A light ray traveling from one medium to another, such as from air to glass, will be bent or refracted toward or away from the normal depending on the index of refraction of each medium.

The *index of refraction* is a number that indicates the speed of light through a medium compared with the speed of light in a vacuum. It is calculated by dividing the speed of light in a vacuum, which is 186,000 miles per second (mps), by the speed of light in the medium. Two examples follow that illustrate this principle.

Example 1: The index of refraction of air. Light travels through air at virtually the same speed as light through a vacuum, or 186,000 mps. 186,000 divided by 186,000 equals 1.00. The index of refraction of air is therefore 1.00.

Example 2: The index of refraction of water. Light travels through water at approximately 140,000 mps. 186,000 divided by 140,000 equals 1.33. The index of refraction of water is therefore 1.33.

The slower the light travels, the higher the index of refraction. Index of refraction is abbreviated by the symbol n. As shown above, water has an index of refraction of 1.33. This can also be stated as "n water = 1.33."

Light rays traveling from air to water are slowed as they pass into the water. This change of speed contributes to the change in direction of incident light rays. This can be illustrated by observing a pencil dipped into a glass of water or an oar dipped into a body of water. Light rays that are seen and perceived to represent the pencil or the oar travel slower through water and cause the submerged portion of the pencil or the oar to appear bent.

The relationship between the index of refraction and the geometric normal is key to the refraction of light. A light ray traveling from one medium to another medium with a higher index of refraction will be bent toward the normal. Conversely, a light ray traveling from one medium to another medium with a lower index of refraction will be bent away from the normal.

We can now tie in the relationship between angle of incidence and index of refraction.

Assume that the first medium is air (n = 1.00) and that the second medium is flat glass (n = 1.54). If the light ray strikes the surface of the glass at a 90-degree angle, or perpendicular to the glass, its angle of incidence is the same as normal. It will be bent neither toward nor away from the normal but will travel straight through the glass (Figure 3-2).

If the angle of incidence of the light ray is not perpendicular to the glass, the effect of the change in the index of refraction from air to glass (from lower to higher index) will cause the light ray to be bent or refracted toward the normal. The glass also has a second surface that must be considered. When the light ray exits the glass, it is in effect striking air, a medium of lower index of refraction than the glass. The light ray will therefore be bent away from the normal. The result is no ultimate deviation in the direction the light travels through this piece of flat glass (Figure 3-3).

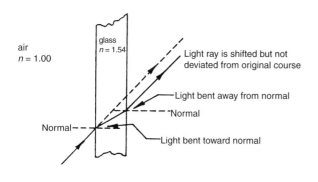

FIGURE 3-3—The path of light traveling through a piece of flat glass.

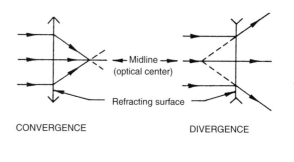

FIGURE 3-4—Principles of convergence and divergence.

Because this flat glass does not ultimately change the direction of the light ray, the glass has no refracting power. "No power" is also called *plano* when one refers to lenses. Most ophthalmic lenses, as well as the optical components of the eye, cause an ultimate change in the direction of the light rays, except at the midline.

The *midline* is that point where light is traveling along the normal. There is no refraction of light at this point, and it is called the *optical center*. Light rays parallel to, but not on, the midline will be refracted. Light rays refracted toward the midline converge (con = with; verge = to bend), and light rays refracted away from the midline diverge (dis = against or opposed to) (Figure 3-4).

Two major types of lenses change the direction of light rays. The first type of lens is *convex*. Its curves are such that the lens is thicker in the center and thinner at the edges. Parallel light rays passing through a convex lens are refracted by each surface so that they converge toward the midline behind the lens. The point at which the light rays meet at the midline is considered the focus point of the lens. Convex lenses are also referred to as *plus* lenses, and the refractive action of a plus lens is convergence. The more curved the surface of a plus lens, the more the light rays will be converged (Figure 3-5).

The second type of lens is *concave*. Its center is thinner than its edges. Parallel light rays passing through a concave lens are refracted away from the midline. In a concave lens, the focus point is at a virtual point in front of the lens. Concave lenses are also referred to as *minus* lenses, and the refractive action of a minus lens is divergence. The more curved the surface of a minus lens, the more the light rays will be diverged (Figure 3-6).

The power of a lens is measured in *diopters* (abbreviated D) and is equal to the reciprocal of the focal length of a lens in meters. In other words, diopters = 1 divided by focal length in meters. The focal length is measured from the lens to the point at which the light rays meet on the midline.

If a lens has a focal length of 1 m, the reciprocal would be $\frac{1}{1}$, or 1, and the lens would have a power of 1.00 D. A lens with a focal length of 0.50 m, or 50 cm, would have a power of 2.00 D ($\frac{1}{0.50}$). A lens that has a focal length of 40 cm (a distance roughly equivalent to 16 inches and frequently used as an average near point for reading) has a power of 2.50 D ($\frac{1}{0.40}$).

The reverse equation is useful in determining the focal length of a lens whose power is known. A 2.00 D lens will have focal distance of 50 cm ($\frac{1}{2.00}$ = 0.50 m = 50 cm). A 3.00 D lens will have a focal length of 33 cm ($\frac{1}{3.00}$ = 0.33 m = 33 cm).

This brief review has covered five points regarding light and lenses:

1. Light travels in straight lines, and 20 feet, or 6 m, is considered optical infinity, at which point light travels in parallel lines.
2. The medium must be transparent to allow light through.
3. Refraction of light depends on the angle of incidence of the light rays and the index of refraction of each medium.
4. Curved surfaces can cause a change in direction of the light rays, and the more curved the surfaces, the more the light will be converged or diverged.

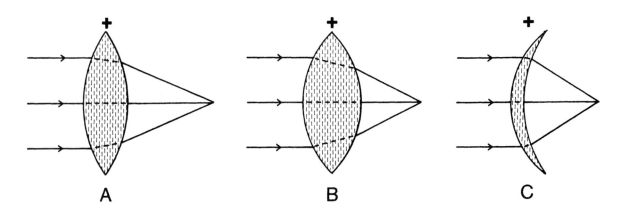

FIGURE 3-5—Convex or plus lenses converge light rays. A and B are biconvex lenses, B having greater power than A. C is a convex lens in meniscus form, such as those used in ophthalmic lenses.

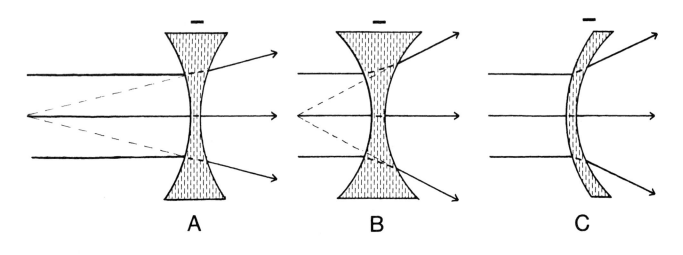

FIGURE 3-6—Concave or minus lenses diverge light rays. A and B are biconcave lenses, B having greater power than A. C is a concave lens in meniscus form, such as those used in ophthalmic lenses.

5. The power of lenses is related to the focal length. These factors are integral to understanding how the eye functions as an optical system to direct light to the point of focus and how ophthalmic lenses are used to redirect the light when necessary.

OPTICAL COMPONENTS OF THE EYE

Some of the structures of the eye directly contribute to its ability to see. Others are involved in nourishment, protection, and moving the eye to the direction of gaze. This section discusses three ocular structures that relate to vision: the cornea, the lens, and the retina.

The Cornea

Light rays entering the eye pass first through the cornea. It is a clear, transparent, steeply curved structure that contributes approximately 70% of the optical power of the eye. The refracting power of the cornea is the result of the combined effects of its curvature, its index of refraction, and the index of refraction of its adjacent media (air on the anterior or front side and the watery aqueous humor on the posterior or back side). Light rays traveling from air

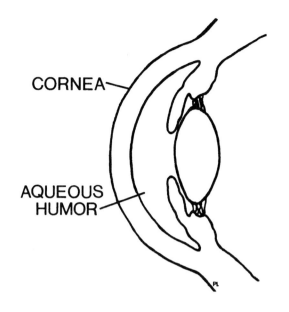

FIGURE 3-7—The cornea is surrounded by air on its anterior surface and by aqueous humor on its posterior surface.

into the cornea are refracted as a result of anterior corneal curvature combined with the change in their speed as they pass from air into the cornea. As these light rays emerge from the back of the cornea, they are again refracted because of posterior corneal curvature combined with the change in their speed as they pass from the cornea into the aqueous humor. Combining front and back surface powers, the total power of the cornea averages approximately 42.00 D, which is very strong plus power (Figure 3-7).

Corneal curvature can be measured using an instrument called a *keratometer* or ophthalmometer. Keratometry measurements are usually readings of just the central anterior portion of the cornea. Clinically, the average corneal curvature measures approximately 44.00 D on the keratometer.

Acting similarly to a very strong plus lens, the cornea and aqueous humor converge light rays entering the eye. The cornea's curvature is a factor in determining where the light rays focus in the eye and therefore plays a role in refractive errors. A steeply curved cornea will refract light rays more than an average cornea, and a flatter-than-average cornea will refract light rays less. A cornea that is not round, or spherical, in curvature will cause a certain distortion of emergent light rays, not bringing them to a single-point focus in the eye.

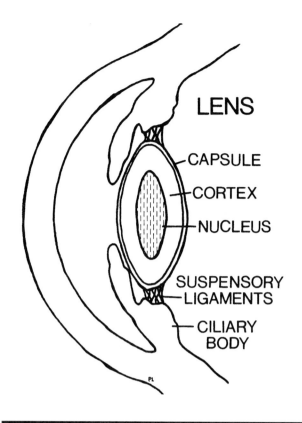

FIGURE 3-8—The crystalline lens.

The Crystalline Lens

The crystalline lens is a biconvex, normally transparent, resilient structure that lies just behind the iris in the eye. It is approximately 10 mm in diameter and is surrounded on its anterior side by aqueous humor (a watery fluid) and on its posterior side by vitreous humor (a gelatin-like substance). It is held in place by the suspensory ligaments, attached at one end to the ciliary body and at the other end to the lens at its edge or equator. Three major layers of the lens are the highly elastic outer capsule, the cortex, and the nucleus in the center (Figure 3-8).

The curvatures of the surfaces of the crystalline lens, combined with the average index of refraction of its media, calculate to an average power of approximately +18.00 D. The structure of the lens is such that the central nucleus consists of more densely packed cells, and it has a higher index of refraction than the surrounding cortex. This structure allows the lens to be a very efficient refracting medium.

Changes in tension on the suspensory ligaments allow the lens to change its shape. When

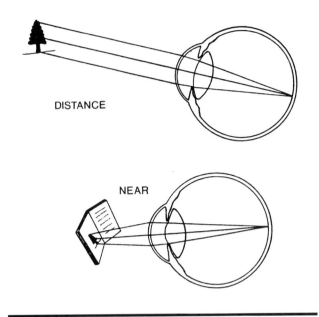

FIGURE 3-9—Accommodation. The lens is at rest when viewing at distance, and it bulges to focus at near.

at rest, the lens is in its least curved configuration. When focusing on a near object, the central anterior portion of the lens capsule bulges to create greater surface curvature and more refracting power. The act of the crystalline lens changing its shape to focus is called *accommodation* (Figure 3-9).

Accommodation is necessary to focus objects at varying distances within optical infinity, or 20 feet. Light rays that form the images of objects viewed at near are divergent rather than parallel. The increase in lens power is required to focus these light rays.

It is not known exactly what triggers accommodation. It is probably safe to say that the brain recognizes the difference between a clear, sharp image and a blurry one. When presented with a blurry image, the sensory nerves in the brain react by prompting innervation of the motor nerves that control the focusing process until a clear image is achieved.

The ability of the eye to accommodate depends on many factors, including age, refractive error, and overall physical health. Accommodation plays an integral role in defining refractive errors, particularly hyperopia, presbyopia, and accommodative insufficiency.

The first concept is *amplitude of accommodation*, or the ability of the crystalline lens in the eye to focus. There are a few ways to measure amplitude of accommodation. One is the "push up" method. A near point target is presented to the patient and brought toward the eyes until it blurs. The distance between the target and the eye is measured in centimeters and converted into diopters by dividing the measurement into 100. For example, if the target blurs at 8 cm, the accommodative amplitude is 12.50 D ($^{100}/_{8}$). The closer the target is to the patient, the higher the amplitude of accommodation.

The second principle is that accommodation is generally greatest in children and decreases with age. Studies have indicated that accommodative amplitude norms relate to age. A formula has been developed to calculate the average expected amplitude of accommodation. Using this formula, the average expected amplitude of accommodation is 14.00 D for a 15-year-old, 6.50 D for a 40-year-old, and 0.50 D for a 60-year-old.

Finally, *accommodative reserve* is the difference between supply and demand. The 20-year-old with no refractive error should have approximately 10.00 D of accommodative amplitude. Reading at 40 cm requires 2.50 D of accommodation ($^{100\,cm}/_{40\,cm} = 2.5$). In this example, supply equals 10.00 D, demand equals 2.50 D, and reserve equals 7.50 D. Visual discomfort usually occurs when the accommodative reserve is less than the demand. In this case, three times the demand is in reserve, so this person should not have a problem focusing for near and sustaining that amount of accommodation. The 44-year-old with no distance refractive error should have approximately 4.00 D of accommodative amplitude. Given a 40-cm reading distance and a 2.50 D demand, the reserve is 1.50 D, which is less than the demand. This person may be able to see an object clearly at 40 cm, but prolonged near work will probably cause discomfort.

The significance of these numbers to this discussion is to illustrate that there are mathematic and physiologic limits to what the eye can do and to clarify certain characteristics of refractive errors that can be more fully understood with future application of these principles. For example, one visual condition is accommodative insufficiency. Whereas a 20-year-old should possess about 10.00 D of accommodative amplitude, less than 10.00 D could possibly cause some difficulty with prolonged near work. Further examples will be given later in this chapter.

The Retina

The third structure that relates to the refractive status of the eye is the retina. The retina receives light rays; translates them into electrophysiologic impulses; and transmits these impulses to the brain, where they are interpreted as a visual image. When the light rays come to a point focus on the back of the retina, a clear image results.

The photoreceptors, or light receivers, are the rods and cones, which are named because of their shape. The rods are more prevalent, numbering about 130 million in the human retina, and they are mainly responsible for scotopic vision (dark-adapted or vision in dim light), for peripheral vision, and for detection of movement. There are approximately 7 million cones in the human retina. They provide photopic vision (light-adapted or vision in bright illumination), acute visual acuity, color vision, and central vision. The rods and cones are specialized cells that respond to the amount and color of light. When stimulated, they begin a chain reaction through the retinal layers, where the pattern they receive is perceived by the brain as a visual image.

The area of the retina that provides the most acute vision is the *fovea centralis*, a small depression in the center of the *macula lutea*, which is located at the back of the retina. At the fovea, there are only specially designed cones. In the macular area surrounding the fovea, the cones become more tapered, and rods begin to appear. The number of cones decreases away from the macula until, in the periphery of the retina, only rods are present.

Length of the Eyeball

In addition to the functions of the cornea and the lens to bend light rays and of the retina to receive and transmit them, another factor may be involved in the refractive status of the eye: eyeball length. The length of the eyeball from the cornea to the posterior pole is called *axial length*. The average axial length is 23–25 mm, about the size of a quarter.

Although not part of a routine eye exam, axial length may be measured by A-Scan ultra-

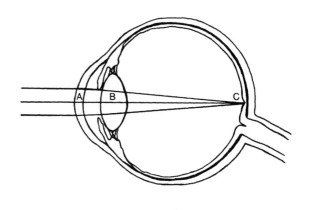

FIGURE 3-10—In a "normal" eye, light rays are refracted by the cornea, A, and by the crystalline lens, B, to focus on the retina at the fovea, C.

sonography. This procedure is usually performed to calculate the power of an intraocular lens (IOL) before cataract surgery. This is discussed later in this chapter in the section on aphakia.

Given an average refracting system (cornea/aqueous humor/lens) and an average axial length, light rays entering the eye should focus at the fovea on the retina (Figure 3-10). Axial length discrepancies result in light focusing either in front of the retina or behind the retina, producing a refractive error.

REFRACTIVE ERRORS OF VISION

Emmetropia Versus Ametropia

In the emmetropic eye the power of the cornea and the lens at rest corresponds with the axial length of the eye, so parallel light rays are appropriately refracted to focus on the retina.

This does not necessarily assume that all emmetropic eyes have the same refractive power and axial length. A more powerful refracting system (i.e., steep cornea) combined with a relatively short axial length will yield emmetropia. Conversely, a weaker refracting system (i.e., flat cornea) combined with a relatively long axial length will also result in emmetropia (Figure 3-11).

Ametropia may be defined as the refractive condition in which, when accommodation is relaxed, parallel light rays entering the eye do not focus on the retina. Myopia, hyperopia, and astigmatism are all types of ametropia. Ametropia can be either refractive or axial. In

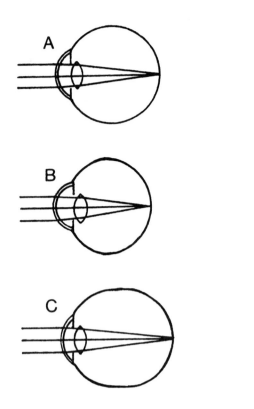

FIGURE 3-11—Emmetropia. A represents an average eye. B represents a steep cornea combined with a short eye. C represents a flat cornea combined with a long eye.

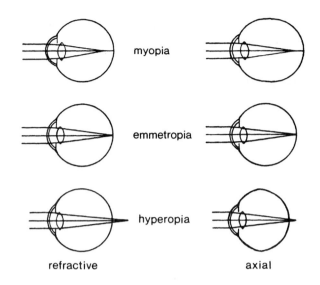

FIGURE 3-12—Emmetropia versus ametropia. Refractive and axial illustrations of myopia, emmetropia, and hyperopia.

refractive ametropia, the axial length of the eye is normal, whereas the refractive power of the eye (either or both the cornea and the lens) is either too strong or too weak to focus light rays on the retina. In axial ametropia, the refractive power of the eye is normal, and the axial length is either too long or too short to place the retina at the point of focus (Figure 3-12).

Myopia

Myopia may be defined as the refractive condition in which, when accommodation is relaxed, parallel light rays entering the eye focus in front of the retina. It is commonly called *nearsightedness*. The most common symptom of myopia is blurred distance vision or the need to squint to clear vision at distance. Very young myopes may not recognize their potential for clear vision and therefore may not complain of blurred distance vision. Myopia is often readily detected in routine vision screenings because visual acuity for distance objects is reduced.

The lay term nearsightedness derives from the fact that myopic individuals may be capable of clear near vision without correction. They may develop near skills early, such as reading and fine motor tasks; they may sit close to an object of regard; and they may hesitate to participate in outdoor activities. Squinting and reduced night vision may be signs of myopia because a smaller pupil size usually results in a sharper visual image.

Few people are born myopic. Whether myopia can be attributed to normal physical changes in the body as it grows or to adaptive or functional changes incurred by increased visual demand at near is an unresolved and highly debated topic. No conclusion will be drawn here, but evidence of higher proportions of myopes in urban than in rural populations, in certain races and cultures, and among professionals than among artisans, and of increased myopia correlated with increased schooling, suggests that some adaptive changes have been made, either in individuals or over generations, that result in myopia.

Myopia is usually physiologic, referring simply to the shape of the eye, involving particularly either or both a steep corneal curvature and long axial length. The onset of physiologic myopia is usually during childhood or adolescence. Although the amount of myopia may increase during adolescence, it usually stabilizes by early adulthood, and it may decrease later in life.

Pathologic myopia is not as common. Causes include diabetes, which causes changes in the body's blood sugar level that affects the index of refraction of either or both the cornea and the lens, and degenerative changes in the eyeball. Complications associated with high myopia include keratoconus (a progressive thinning of the corneal apex) and a number of retinal anomalies (tears, holes, peripheral retinal degeneration, and retinal detachment) that may be due to the stretching of retinal fibers that eventually separate in an elongated eyeball.

Treatment of physiologic myopia may take many forms. The most common treatment is application of spectacle or contact lenses. Concave, or minus, lenses are used to diverge incident light rays, thereby moving the focus point of the light back to the retina (Figure 3-13).

If the refractive component of the average eye is considered 60.00 D of power, the myopic eye might have more than 60.00 D. A 62.00 D eye might need a –2.00 D ophthalmic lens to bring the whole system back to 60.00 D. Although this is a rather simplistic computation, it is generally concurrent with the basic principle of correcting refractive errors.

Many myopes can see at near and therefore can simply remove their glasses for reading. In most cases, however, it is recommended that they leave their glasses on to affect normal stimulation of the accommodative mechanism. Exceptions might be presbyopic myopes and those who have convergence anomalies at near that are compounded by accommodation.

Minus lenses have a minifying effect, causing objects viewed through them to appear smaller. First-time minus lens wearers and those who receive a substantial increase in minus power may remark that things look smaller or farther away. This is a normal reaction, and adaptation can be expedited by advising myopes to view mostly distant objects for several hours, avoiding near work and close spaces. The curvature of minus lenses may also cause a "barrel" distortion, where straight lines appear rounded. This will also disappear in time.

Another form of lens therapy involves reading glasses or bifocals for young children who are diagnosed or suspected to be emerging myopes.

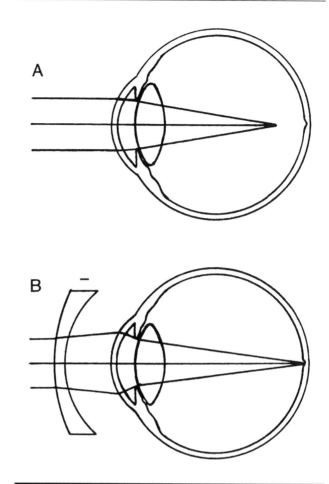

FIGURE 3-13—Use of minus lens to redirect light rays in myopia.

The theory is that relaxation of accommodation achieved with lenses prescribed for near work will reduce or eliminate the onset or progression of myopia. This is a much-debated theory. The classic/anatomic view is that myopes will become myopes whatever treatment is prescribed. The developmental/functional view is that myopia is largely a product of an environment that includes an unnatural near demand that, if alleviated, does not have to lead to myopia.

Orthokeratology is another treatment for myopia. It is based on the theory that refractive myopia can be corrected by flattening a steep cornea to the point where corneal curvature/power correlates with axial length, so the focus of light rays falls on the retina. Orthokeratology has its roots with the ancient Chinese, who, it is said, slept with stones on their eyes to flatten their corneas. Instead of stones, orthokeratology uses a series of progressively flatter contact lenses to flatten the cornea.

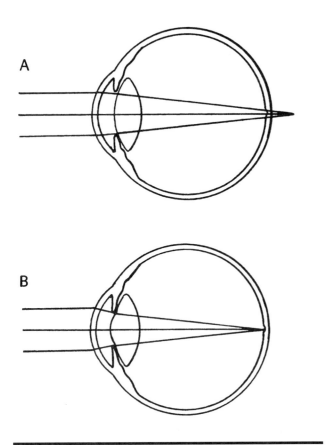

FIGURE 3-14—Hyperopic eye accommodating to move focus point to the retina.

Hyperopia

Hyperopia may be defined as the refractive condition in which, when accommodation is relaxed, parallel light rays entering the eye focus behind the retina. It is commonly called *farsightedness*. It is also sometimes referred to clinically as *hypermetropia*. Hyperopia is closely connected to accommodation.

In the hyperopic eye, either the cornea is too flat, not having enough power to bring the focus to the retina, or the axial length is too short, causing light rays to overshoot the retina. Through the normal process of accommodation, the crystalline lens can make up for at least some of the difference by increasing its power and bringing the focus point to the retina. As discussed earlier, the brain can distinguish the blurry object of regard of the hyperopic eye and can automatically stimulate accommodation without the hyperope even knowing what is happening (Figure 3-14).

Because of this phenomenon, the term *farsighted* may be misleading. One may infer from the term alone that the hyperope can see at distance but not at near. The young hyperope, however, may be able to see clearly at all distances, whereas the older hyperope may not be able to see clearly at any distance. The quality of vision in a healthy hyperopic eye at any given distance depends on the combination of refractive error and accommodative ability.

The 8-year-old 4.00 D hyperope should have 14.00 D of accommodative amplitude, so he or she should be able to clear the far point of vision by accommodating for the 4.00 D. Even adding the additional 3.00 D required for the individual to read at 33 cm, he or she has 7.00 D of accommodation in reserve. At age 20, the individual's reading distance may have increased to 40 cm, and he or she has 11.00 D of accommodative ability, leaving only 4.50 D in reserve. By age 30, the individual is pushing the limit of accommodative ability, and anything within 40 cm would be difficult if not impossible to see clearly. Any accommodative insufficiency would compound the effort and the difficulty experienced by a person with hyperopia.

When accommodation is at its usual peak in childhood, the hyperopic child can often function relatively well. Although there is no physical sensation of accommodation occurring, this constant effort can cause certain side effects. Physical signs may include rubbing the eyes, tearing, closing one eye for near work, and low-grade blepharitis. Behavioral manifestations may include poor attention span, reluctance to read, poor reading skills, and an affinity for gross motor tasks and outdoor games rather than for fine near point tasks. Because Johnny may not know *why* he does not like to read, his behavior may be misconstrued as lazy rather than as being symptomatic of a potential vision problem.

The hyperopic child may not be referred to an eye doctor from a routine school screening because the child can read all the letters on the chart at 20 feet. The hyperopic individual, usually a child or adolescent who accommodates constantly to compensate for refractive error, is called a *latent hyperope*. Routine subjective refraction on this individual frequently may reveal only low hyperopia. This component of the refractive error is called "manifest," since it is the amount of hyperopia for which the patient does not accommodate. It is in objective refraction (retinoscopy) and subjective refraction with the use of a cycloplegic agent or other means to relax accommodation that the latent hyperope's true refractive error becomes apparent.

The total refractive error of the hyperope, which includes both manifest and latent components, may not be prescribed right away because he or she is so accustomed to accommodating that the spectacle lens power would be overwhelming. In these instances, the professional judgment and experience of the prescribing doctor of optometry are important. If hyperopia were simply a name of a configuration of an optical system, full power would be the logical conclusion. Rather, it is a condition of a human being, and an individual's subjective response to correction is critical in its ultimate success. A gradual reduction of accommodative effort can often relieve the symptoms and detrimental behavior.

Binocular anomalies may accompany latent or undercorrected hyperopia. Accommodation and convergence are interrelated as coupled reflexes, each occurring when the other does. Excessive accommodative effort at near can cause excessive convergence at near. When the eyes "over cross," two images result, which the brain will not simultaneously perceive. Because the eyes cannot turn back out to the point at one image on demand without releasing accommodation and causing the eyes to lose focus on the near object, these two systems will battle in a no-win conflict. An easy solution is simply not to be confronted with the near demand. Another solution is to close one eye, thereby eliminating the conflicting image while retaining adequate accommodative power to clear the near object. Using either of these solutions, however, may result in Johnny's not wanting to read or may result in his developing amblyopia through nonuse of an eye.

Treatment for hyperopia is usually with convex, or plus, spectacle or contact lenses. Because they converge light rays before they enter the eye, plus lenses provide the power necessary to bring the focus point forward to the retina. Whereas myopes are frequently given their full minus prescription, hyperopes may not be given their full plus power for the reasons mentioned above (Figure 3-15).

Comparing the optical component of the nonaccommodating hyperopic eye with the average eye and its 60.00 D of power, the hyper-

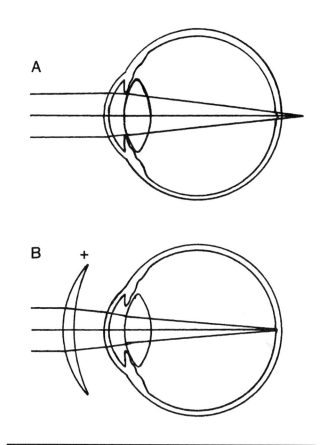

FIGURE 3-15—Use of plus lens to redirect light rays in hyperopia.

opic eye does not have enough power to focus light rays on the retina properly. If its optical power is 57.00 D, a +3.00 D lens would compensate for the difference. Again, this is an oversimplification, and again, the total power may not be prescribed initially.

Plus lenses magnify objects, so first-time wearers may remark that viewed objects seem bigger or closer. The curves of plus lenses may also produce a "pincushion" effect, in which straight lines appear caved-in. These are normal reactions, and patients become accustomed to them in time. Since their depth perception may be altered for a while, patients should be cautioned to walk carefully, particularly around curbs or steps.

Astigmatism

Astigmatism is defined as a refractive condition in which parallel light rays entering the eye do not focus at a single point but instead form two line images in different meridians, generally at right angles to each other.

In lay terms, astigmatism is often described by comparing a baseball or basketball with a football. The curves on the baseball's surface are all the same; they are round, or spherical. If the baseball's surface were a lens, light shining through it would focus at one point just as in spherical ophthalmic lenses used to correct simple myopia and hyperopia.

The football, on the other hand, has different curves throughout its surface. The extremes are represented by the minimum (weakest) curve from end to end and the maximum (strongest) curve around the middle. These two curves are designated as the two *principal meridians*, which are at right angles to each other, or 90 degrees apart. Because of the difference in curvature/power in these two principal meridians, light shining through a lens shaped like a football would form two lines in space. The football is analogous to the astigmatic cornea, and these types of curves are called *toric* or toroidal.

The distance between these two lines of focus is called the *interval of Sturm*. At the midpoint between these two lines, a circle is formed called the *circle of least confusion*. The closer the circle is to the retina, the less confused or blurred the vision will be. The smaller the difference between the curvatures of the two principal meridians, the smaller the interval of Sturm will be (Figure 3-16).

Astigmatism is measured as a function of corneal curvature and as a component of the total ocular optical system. Keratometry readings measure the curvature of the cornea in the two principal meridians. When the curvature differs with each meridian, the cornea is considered to be toric, and the amount and orientation of curvature in each meridian is recorded. During the refraction portion of the vision examination, astigmatism of the total optical system is measured, including the effects of corneal and lens or lenticular curvature. The difference between total ocular astigmatism and corneal astigmatism is called *residual astigmatism*.

In regular astigmatism, the two principal meridians are 90 degrees apart. *With-the-rule astigmatism* refers to steeper curvature in the vertical meridian, like the football lying on its side. *Against-the-rule astigmatism* refers to steeper curvature in the horizontal meridian, like the football standing on end. *Oblique astigmatism*

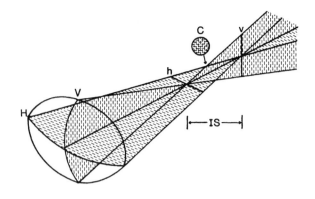

FIGURE 3-16—Astigmatism. Light rays from two different meridians, H and V, focus as two lines, h and v, between which are the interval of Sturm (IS), and the circle of least confusion, C.

occurs when the meridians are between 30 and 60 degrees and 120 and 150 degrees.

Irregular astigmatism is not common in nontraumatized eyes. It occurs when the principal meridians are not 90 degrees apart or when they are not uniformly positioned from point to point along a meridian. Corneal astigmatism may be induced postsurgically by sutures that are too tight or loose along the limbus, thus binding or buckling the cornea. This may be reversible, if detected quickly, by adjusting the tension on the sutures. Corneal curvature may also be affected by an encroaching pterygium, a fleshy growth on the conjunctiva, and it will most definitely be affected by keratoconus. In all of these cases, irregular keratometry readings are likely and are important components in the resultant diagnosis of irregular astigmatism.

Astigmatism is a refractive error caused by the cornea or the lens being toric or not spherical. (It is impossible for astigmatism to be axial, since an eyeball cannot be of two different lengths.) The three types of astigmatism are mixed, simple, and compound. In *mixed astigmatism*, one focal line is in front of the retina, and the other is behind the retina. In *simple astigmatism*, one line is on the retina, and the other is either in front of the retina (simple myopic astigmatism) or behind the retina (simple hyperopic astigmatism). In *compound astigmatism*, both lines are either in front of the retina (compound myopic astigmatism) or behind the retina (compound hyperopic astigmatism) (Figure 3-17).

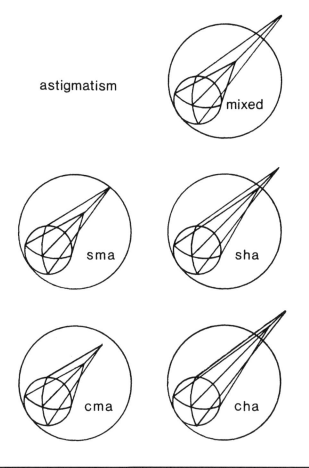

FIGURE 3-17—Classifications of astigmatism. Mixed astigmatism, simple myopic astigmatism (sma), simple hyperopic astigmatism (sha), compound myopic astigmatism (cma), and compound hyperopic astigmatism (cha).

Astigmatism with any substantial amount of refractive error may present symptoms such as blurred vision, headaches, eyestrain, and spatial disorientation. Signs may include squinting (to reduce the aperture size and thus reduce the size of the circle of least confusion in an attempt at clearer vision) and rubbing the eyes. Except for the mixed astigmat with low refractive error, astigmatism should be readily detected through visual acuity screening. Individuals with astigmatism confuse letters such as H and N; F, B, and E; and so forth.

Correction of astigmatism is usually with spectacle or contact lenses. Spectacle lenses incorporate curves to direct the incident light rays the appropriate amount in the appropriate direction to produce a point focus on the retina. The orientation of the lens before the eye is critical to proper positioning of the power in the two meridians. One meridian on the lens is designated as the *axis*, measured in degrees. Any lens prescribed for astigmatism must include the power *and* the axis orientation.

The simple astigmat needs power in only one meridian, since the other focus is on the retina. A lens with power in only one meridian is called a *cylinder*, or a cylindrical lens.

The lens used for compound or mixed astigmatism is a combination of a spherical lens, such as those used for simple myopia or hyperopia, and a cylindrical lens. It is called *spherocylinder*, and it has different power in each of its principal meridians.

Adaptation to astigmatic lenses might be similar to that of minus or plus lenses, depending on the prescription. It may also be complicated by the difference in power in the two meridians. Although the brain might not like what it sees, its inability to do anything about it in the case of uncorrected astigmatism forces it to accept and become accustomed to a slightly crooked world. When that world is "straightened out" by an astigmatic prescription, the initial response might be just the opposite, that it now appears slanted. This may also occur when the power or orientation of the prescription is modified significantly. These nominal reactions of the floor appearing slanted or "coming up toward" the patient are usually eliminated after a period of adaptation.

The use of contact lenses introduces additional considerations in the correction of astigmatism. A hard contact lens has a rigid spherical back surface that rests on the corneal tear film. The tear film fills in the spaces between the back of the lens and the change in curvature on the cornea. Since liquid acts as a refracting medium, most corneal astigmatism can be neutralized by the combined optical effect of the lens and the tear layer (Figure 3-18).

When residual astigmatism is significant, a toric contact lens is used to compensate for the amount and orientation of the residual astigmatism. Bitoric contact lenses, which have toric curves on both the front and back surfaces, are used in cases of combined significant residual astigmatism and corneal astigmatism.

A soft contact lens conforms more closely to the shape of the cornea. Although some spherical soft lenses may partially neutralize corneal astigmatism, they are usually not the lens of choice for higher amounts of corneal astigmatism. Toric soft

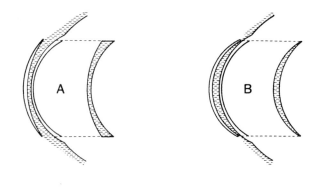

FIGURE 3-18—Tear layers fill in space between the back of a hard contact lens and the front of the cornea with a minus tear film "lens" A, or a plus tear "lens" B.

lenses may be prescribed to provide correction for many astigmatic refractive errors.

Patient education regarding astigmatism is very important. A common remark among patients is that they have "stigmatism." The part of the word that stands out in their minds is "stigma." Stigma as a Greek root means "spot." The prefix a- indicates a negative meaning. Therefore, astigmatism can be literally translated to mean simply that something (in this case, point light focus) does not hit the spot. Astigmatism can be simply explained to patients as a physical condition of out-of-roundness that is easily corrected with lenses. A matter-of-fact explanation should ease patient fears and misunderstanding.

Surgical Treatment of Myopia, Hyperopia, and Astigmatism

In recent years, treatment of myopia, hyperopia, and astigmatism has included surgery. To date, the most common surgical technique is called *radial keratotomy*, in which spoke-like incisions are made into the cornea. The placement and depth of the incisions determines the outcome, that is, reduction of myopia or astigmatism. Other techniques involve replacing part of the cornea to change the curvature in cases of high myopia, high hyperopia, and keratoconus. The "new" cornea may be from a donor, or it may be a reshaped section of the patient's own cornea. Laser surgery allows a section of the cornea to be removed. It is then frozen, reshaped by a lathe in much the same way as a contact lens is made and sutured back into place. The reason for the surgery, the technique, and the expertise of the surgeon are factors in determining the success of these procedures.

Presbyopia

Presbyopia is a reduction in the ability to accommodate that occurs normally with age. Physiologically, the ciliary muscles are no longer able to effect sufficient bulging of the crystalline lens (to create enough power) to focus for objects at the patient's near point. This may be a result of a reduction in lens elasticity or in the strength of the ciliary muscle (ciliary tonus).

The process generally occurs uniformly and bilaterally, although the timing and degree may vary among individuals due to several factors:

General health. Some systemic or ocular diseases affect visual function. Various medications, such as muscle relaxers, may inhibit proper functioning of the ciliary muscle. Certain conditions of the lens, such as cataracts, may also affect accommodation.

Age. Accommodative amplitude decreases with age to the point where near point tasks become increasingly uncomfortable, and, finally, clear focusing for near is impossible. This may first be manifested by difficulty in clearing objects at a distance after doing close work for a time. Often some symptoms begin to appear around age 40 years, sooner for some, later for others.

Visual demand. The type, distance, and duration of near point tasks will certainly affect any near point difficulty noticed. People who encounter more fine near point tasks in their occupation or hobbies may be more symptomatic than those who do not. The watchmaker may work at an average distance of 25 cm and may spend a great deal of time focusing at this distance. A sales clerk's near work may be at an average of 45 cm, and frequent distance viewing may allow breaks from the near demand. The watchmaker would require approximately 4.00 D of accommodative amplitude for long durations, whereas the sales clerk would require approximately 2.25 D from time to time. All other things being equal, the watchmaker may notice focusing difficulties before the sales clerk.

Ametropia. The 38-year-old myopic watchmaker may be able to remove his or her spectacles to achieve clear vision at his or her working distance. The 38-year-old hyperopic watchmaker may be beyond his or her accommodative capability.

Environmental conditions. One's ability to see clearly at near is also influenced by illumination and clarity of the target. Brighter illumination on the object of regard usually allows clearer vision due to decreased pupil size. The more clear or sharp the target, the easier it is to see. For example, type in a magazine may be easier to read than newsprint of the same size.

Stature. Shorter people with short arms will comfortably hold reading material closer than taller people with long arms. The 40-cm near point average assumes an average body size, whereas a 30-cm or a 50-cm near point may be more appropriate for a given individual.

Self-image. The reputation of presbyopia as an occurrence of old age, followed inevitably by gray hair, wrinkles, trembling fingers, retirement, and senility, is still in the minds of many. Admitting to difficulty seeing at near is tantamount to admitting defeat. An individual's ego may prevent his or her acknowledgment of near point problems, and a herculean effort may be made to see.

Most of the above considerations may be reviewed within the context of a case history with a patient. The case history taker can determine general health and any medications currently taken; age; occupational and avocational near point demands (not just where the patient works or what type of work is done, but also the distance, frequency, and duration of specific near point tasks); working environment, including illumination; and the patient's subjective assessment of the quality of near point vision. Since presbyopia may be manifested initially by a sluggishness in focusing ability from far to near or from near to far, questions to ascertain the presence of this phenomenon may be asked.

Techniques for measuring near visual acuity of an emerging or progressing presbyope may vary. If the routine or physically comfortable working distance has been established for the patient, testing may occur at that distance. Again, the standard 40-cm near point may not be appropriate for people of certain size and occupations. A typical action of uncorrected and undercorrected presbyopes is to "trombone" reading material, to move it toward and away from them until it is clear. The point at which they stop moving the material may be farther away than is appropriate. This point may also generally correspond with their accommodative amplitude.

Symptoms of presbyopia may be similar to those of hyperopia—for example, eyestrain when reading and blur at near—but they may be of a more recent and noticeable onset. The distinction between hyperopia and presbyopia is the reduction of accommodative amplitude. Unlike accommodative insufficiency, accommodative amplitude is at a normal level for the patient's age range. It is quantitatively measured during the vision examination.

Treatment for presbyopia is usually spectacle lenses that provide additional plus power for near. The amount of plus power will vary with the patient's needs (e.g., distance of task, ametropia, etc.), but it generally increases along with the patient's age. The emmetropic 40-year-old who has 5.00 D of accommodation and who needs 3.00 D to see at 33 cm has only 2.00 D in reserve. Since the reserve is 1.00 D less than the demand, he or she may be prescribed a +1.00 D lens for near work. By the time he or she reaches age 60 years and has no accommodation left, the full +3.00 may be prescribed.

The type of spectacle lenses used are usually single-vision reading glasses or bifocals. Whereas *reading glasses* may help one to see clearly for near tasks, they produce a blurry scene when viewing through them across a room. To understand the limitations of reading glasses, let's review focal distance relative to dioptric power of a lens. The focal length of a +1.00 D lens is 100 cm (1 m); of a +2.00 D lens, 50 cm; of a +3.00 D lens, 33 cm; and so on. This also represents the approximate maximum distance at which objects may be seen clearly through these lenses. An emmetropic presbyope who looks through a +2.00 D lens will be able to see clearly objects from his or her near point to approximately 50 cm. Objects farther away will appear blurry. Whereas the emmetrope can simply remove his or her glasses for distance vision, ametropes must remove their reading glasses and put on their distance prescription.

Although this problem undoubtedly perplexed many before him, Benjamin Franklin was the first person known to do anything about it. Franklin is credited with inventing what are now called *bifocals*.

Bifocals may be very convenient, as they provide distance and near vision in one lens. The wearer simply looks down into the segment for near work and straight ahead through the upper portion of the lens for distance vision. Their convenience may be tempered by the wearer's needs. In certain occupations, such as drafting and word processing, the near task is not down but straight ahead. Bifocals may be more of a hindrance than a help in these situations.

The far point limitation of the near add in the segment may also be a problem. For the patient who is not too steady on his or her feet, inability to see the ground when walking may be disconcerting and even dangerous.

Many more examples of the pros and cons of reading glasses versus bifocals could be cited. The point is that many considerations are incumbent in selecting the most appropriate type of lens for a patient. A good case history provides much useful information, and a psychological profile of a patient's potential acceptance of any type of lens is desirable.

The progression of presbyopia decreases accommodative amplitude. Although the near point is first to be affected, objects within an intermediate distance of between approximately 2 and 6 feet will eventually lose their clarity to the presbyopic eye. When clear, sharp vision is required within this intermediate range, lenses may be prescribed that incorporate corrections for distance, for this intermediate area, and for near. The three focal planes give these lenses their name, *trifocals*. Progressive addition lenses gradually change power from the distance prescription to the near prescription, affording clear vision in all ranges. Other special types of multifocal lenses are available for specific tasks, for example, having segments at the top of the lens for overhead near tasks.

Lens therapy for presbyopia may also involve the use of contact lenses. When contact lenses are used to correct distance vision, reading glasses or multifocals will still be needed for near work. Another method of prescribing contact lenses for presbyopia is called the *monovision technique*: One eye is corrected for distance vision (usually the dominant eye), and the other is corrected for near vision (usually the nondominant eye). Bifocal contact lenses are also available in rigid and soft materials in a number of designs.

Whatever type of lens therapy is chosen, proper instruction in the use and limitations of the lenses is very important. A positive and knowledgeable attitude on the part of the dispenser can be the key to patient acceptance, proper use, and the ultimate effectiveness of the lenses. The psychological welfare of the patient must always be highly regarded, so every attempt should be made to educate the patient as to the routine nature of presbyopia.

ASSOCIATED VISION ANOMALIES

Aphakia

Aphakia is the absence of the crystalline lens of the eye. The most frequent cause of surgical removal of the crystalline lens is a cataract. Many myths and fears are associated with cataracts.

A cataract is an opacity of the crystalline lens or its capsule. An opacity is a complete or partial loss of transparency. Lenticular opacification, or loss of lens transparency, usually results from changes in the tissues or fibers of the lens. These changes may be attributable to trauma; genetic or metabolic disorders; the effects of radiation, drugs, or infection; or most commonly, the aging process.

Traumatic cataracts result from some injury to the lens. Congenital and infantile cataracts are present at birth or appear in infancy, and they may accompany other genetic, metabolic, or systemic disorders. Prognosis for good vision after cataract surgery depends on the involvement of these other disorders. Cataracts may also occur with or immediately after certain intraocular or systemic pathologic processes, and there is some evidence that connects ultraviolet light with the formation of cataracts. There are more than 175 subdefinitions listed under "cataract" in the *Dictionary of Visual Science*. The major categories, however, include those discussed above and senile cataracts.

By far the most prevalent type of cataract is the senile cataract. Although this term merely refers to those cataracts that form as part of the natural aging process, the word "senile" is perhaps better not used when discussing cataracts with a patient. Many people associate cataracts with blindness. They regard a cataract as a growth or a tumor that will take over the eye.

The biochemical or biophysical changes in the lens as a result of trauma or associated pathology are usually easily explained to and accepted by patients. They understand scarring as a change in tissues following injury, and though cataracts are not scars, the analogy works.

Patient understanding and acceptance of senile cataracts relies on the presentation of the condition. Words or phrases such as "senile," "growth," "blindness," "progressive," and "it's not ready yet" should be avoided because of their negative connotations. The normalcy of cataracts should be emphasized, just as gray hair and "age spots" are conditions occurring normally with age. Whereas cataracts rarely regress, their extent may remain stable for a long time, or they may slowly progress.

The size and position of a cataract in the lens will dictate its effect on vision. A *nuclear cataract* may cause an increase in myopia (or decrease in hyperopia) because of an increase in the refractive index of the lens. Positioned on the visual axis, a nuclear cataract may also cause monocular double vision (diplopia) because of an image-splitting phenomenon. *Subcapsular cataracts* often appear at the posterior pole of the lens. They cause glare effects in bright illumination and reduced near acuity of greater proportion than that of distance acuity because of the position on the visual axis relative to accommodative light rays. Cortical cataracts, cataracts within the cortex itself, are often not noticed by a patient unless they are quite prominent. Small opacities in the periphery of the lens will generally remain undetected by a patient. A larger opacity in the periphery may be noticed under dim illumination when the pupil is dilated. Once a cortical cataract is of sufficient size and encroaches on the visual axis, a

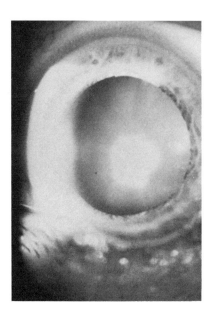

FIGURE 3-19—A cataract.

patient may complain of gradual visual loss and a haziness, fogginess, or film over the eyes that does not go away (Figure 3-19).

When a cataract does not interfere with vision, it may be left in place. When vision is substantially altered and further testing reveals ocular potential for better vision without the lens and its opacity, the decision may be made to remove the lens. The absence of possibly 18.00 D of power and of the entire accommodative capability of the eye creates another set of optical and psychological challenges for the practitioner whose patient desires normal vision again.

Treatment for aphakia employs one or a combination of three methods: spectacle lens correction, contact lenses, or IOL implant. The power of spectacle lenses necessitates that they be quite thick. In glass, they are quite heavy, so most are made of molded plastic. The front curve is usually aspheric, meaning that the curves become slightly flatter toward the periphery of the lens. This lens design compensates for the change in vertex distance (distance between the eye and the lens) between the center and periphery of the lens. Aphakic spectacle lenses are either full-field or lenticular. The full-field lens has power throughout the lens that decreases from center to edge. To reduce thickness and weight, the lenticular design confines

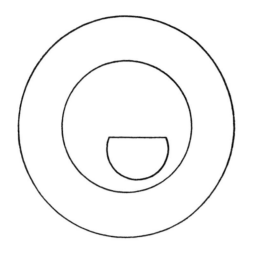

FIGURE 3-20—Aspheric lenticular ophthalmic lens.

power to a 38–40 mm "bowl" surrounded by a thin, nonoptical carrier (Figure 3-20).

Several drawbacks exist with aphakic spectacle lenses. Their high plus power, usually in the range of +10.00 to +16.00 D, creates significant magnification of objects viewed through them and of the eyes behind them. The field of vision is reduced due to the combined effects of magnification and placement of the lens before the eye. Orientation of the lens before the eye is critical. Improper vertex distance may result in changes in magnification and field. Incorrect position of optical centers of the lenses may cause discomfort, distortion, and diplopia. For a monocular aphake, satisfactory binocular correction with spectacle lenses is virtually impossible, as the difference between lens powers and magnification will create an unmanageable discrepancy in image size.

The second option for aphakic correction is contact lenses. Frequently hydrophilic (soft) contact lenses are chosen because they tend to be more comfortable than rigid or gas-permeable contact lenses. Contact lenses afford the patient a comfortable, nonmagnified, wide-field vision. Contact lenses have the capability of lens power modification. The major disadvantage of contact lenses is that they are not maintenance-free. They must be inserted, removed, recentered, cleaned, and disinfected. Daily-wear lenses seem to be giving way to extended-wear lenses for aphakes. Since aphakes cannot accommodate, they cannot see the contact lens they are trying to put in their eye. Many older people also lack the manual dexterity necessary for contact lens handling. Although extended-wear lenses offer freedom from the daily chore, the material is not highly durable. The patient is still required to remove them or have them removed for cleaning, which may present certain limitations. Frequent replacement lenses can avoid some of these maintenance problems. The incidence of decentered or lost lenses causes inconvenience. Contact lenses may even be contraindicated in the presence of certain ocular drug therapies.

IOLs are surgically placed in the eye after removal of the lens with cataract. They were first used in 1949, but overcoming various complications through refinement of design, sterilization, handling, and insertion techniques delayed their widespread use until the mid-1970s. Advantages of the use of IOLs include convenience and the potential of near-normal distance vision. Since they cannot be lost, scratched, or broken and since they need not be located first thing in the morning, IOLs ideally afford around-the-clock, maintenance-free vision. An experienced surgeon who specializes in lens implants can calculate the necessary power of the IOL fairly accurately. IOLs also do not cause the magnification or visual field reduction of spectacle lenses of the same power. The disadvantages of IOLs relate to unknowns. The power is calculated presurgery, and its accuracy cannot be verified until after the fact, so minor changes cannot be made. Another unknown is the long-term effects of an IOL on ocular health.

The choice of the treatment option to follow depends on many factors. They include ocular health, general health, the patient's physical and mental dexterity, the refractive status of the other eye, and the patient's informed preference. These are also not exclusive options. Patients for whom contact lenses are prescribed should be dispensed a back-up pair of spectacles with their full aphakic prescription. When an IOL does not fully correct distance vision, a contact lens or a spectacle lens may be worn over it. Glasses may also be worn over contact lenses to achieve more optimum vision. Monocular aphakes can benefit from either an IOL or a contact lens in the aphakic eye to equalize image size as much as possible.

There are cases, of course, in which both an IOL and a contact lens are contraindicated. For the binocular aphake, this presents the same drawbacks associated with aphakic spectacles. For the monocular aphake, the eye with the better corrected visual acuity is usually corrected, resulting in a necessary blur in the other eye.

The treatments discussed so far have only addressed distance vision. Since the accommodative capability of the eye is removed along with the lens, a prescription for near work will be required. Reading glasses or multifocals may be prescribed depending on the patient's near demand.

Lens therapy may provide optimum vision based on the altered condition of the visual system. It may not, however, satisfy the patient's expectations. Today's patient with cataracts has a much better prognosis than aphakes of the previous generation, but this may be little consolation in this age of "medical miracles." The best surgeon and the best optical correction can only do so much. The patient must adjust to a different way of seeing. The most difficult adjustments are experienced by those for whom spectacles are the only option, as their world is distorted, magnified, and narrowed. Fortunately, they are becoming the minority. For the others, it is a matter of offering assurance and support and instilling confidence in the benefits of their correction.

Anisometropia

Anisometropia is a condition of unequal refractive state of the two eyes. The definition becomes apparent when the word itself is dissected into its component parts: *an-* means not; *iso* means same; *metric* means measurement. Frequently, anisometropia refers to the results of unequal refractive error rather than the error itself.

The three types of anisometropia are simple, compound, and mixed. In *simple anisometropia,* one eye is emmetropic and the other is ametropic. *Compound anisometropia* refers to both eyes being myopic, hyperopic, or astigmatic, but in differing amounts. In *mixed anisometropia*, one eye is myopic and the other is hyperopic, and it is also referred to as *antimetropia* (anti = opposite).

Typical symptoms of anisometropia coincide with those of the ametropic condition. In addition, binocular anomalies may arise due to suppression of the more ametropic eye. One eye may feel more "pull" or eyestrain. It may tire or feel dry, and the patient may report that vision of one eye seems better than that of the other eye.

Treatment for anisometropia is with spectacle or contact lenses. *Refractive anisometropia,* which is attributed to a marked difference in corneal curvature of the two eyes or monocular aphakia, is best corrected with contact lenses. *Axial anisometropia* is attributed to difference in axial length between the two eyes along with fairly equal corneal curvature, which results in a marked difference in total refractive error. This type is best corrected with spectacle lenses. The lens type of choice, spectacles versus contact lenses, is based on the goal of achieving equal image sizes through the different-powered lenses.

In cases of refractive anisometropia, a contact lens will act as part of the optical refracting system, bringing the optical systems of the two eyes into closer alignment and thereby equalizing the sizes of the retinal images or reducing the discrepancy to an easily manageable level.

In axial anisometropia, the optical systems of the two eyes are already very similar, and the disparity is a result of different eyeball lengths. To apply contact lenses would create optical systems of two different powers, thereby inducing different image sizes on the retina. The curves of spectacle lenses may be used to alter magnification or minification of retinal image size in axial anisometropia.

Aniseikonia

Aniseikonia is a difference in size of the two retinal images. The two major subdivisions of aniseikonia are inherent and acquired. *Inherent aniseikonia* refers to different image sizes caused by the refractive condition of the two eyes. *Acquired aniseikonia* occurs as a result of the effects of corrective lenses. Both are related to anisometropia.

Clinical measurement of aniseikonia is with an instrument called an *eikonometer*. Eikonometry is performed with the eyes disassociated, either with polarized filters or with independently adjustable optical systems for each eye. The patient reports various information regarding the spatial orientation of viewed targets. Calculation tables accompanying the instrument provide the equivalent aniseikonic correction.

The symptoms and treatment of aniseikonia are basically the same as for anisometropia.

Many problems related to aniseikonia have been reduced with the increased use of contact lenses. The variable parameters of spectacle lenses are material, curvature, and thickness, all of which may be specified to provide certain refractive characteristics of the lenses. The vertex distance of lenses can also be adjusted to achieve appropriate magnification. Lenses specifically designed to alleviate aniseikonia are called *iseikonic lenses*.

Amblyopia

Amblyopia is reduced visual acuity with no apparent cause and not correctable by refractive means. It is more commonly referred to as "lazy eye."

Functional amblyopia is divided into three categories: strabismic, refractive, and stimulus depravation. The first two are the most commonly seen clinically.

Strabismic amblyopia is also called *amblyopia ex anopsia*. It is the result of abnormal binocularity. Conflicting images of the two eyes may result in the suppression of one. When one eye suppresses for a significant amount of time, it may tend to turn in or out, and it may maintain this position habitually. The incidence of amblyopia is somewhat higher among hyperopes than among myopes.

The most appropriate treatment for strabismic amblyopia depends on its extent, the goal of the treatment, and the availability of resources. Vision therapy can be successful in many cases, but it is time consuming and may require the special expertise and instrumentation of a qualified vision therapist. Surgery to align the eyes may be faster and cosmetically appealing sooner, but the prognosis for consistent binocular vision and the correction of amblyopia may depend on the referral to a vision therapist to secure and maintain binocular vision skills.

Refractive amblyopia is associated with uncorrected refractive errors. High refractive errors that remain uncorrected for a significant amount of time prevent normal visual stimulation, leading to a habitual state of reduced visual acuity. Refractive amblyopia may be reversible when it is not too deeply ingrained. The myope is less likely to become a refractive amblyope as a result of his or her ability to see up close. Although the myope's world may appear small, it can be clear. The earlier the onset of the refractive error, the greater its magnitude, and the longer it remains uncorrected, the more profound will be the amblyopia and the more resistant it may be to treatment. Visual stimulation may provide more "normal" vision for the refractive amblyope. It may be accomplished through lens therapy or a vision therapy program. Sometimes spectacle lenses cannot produce 20/20 visual acuity when contact lenses can.

Stimulus depravation results when sensory receptors do not receive input (i.e., the retina does not receive light) due to some factor, such as a congenital cataract. In the absence of stimuli, the receptors may not develop properly, and full visual capability may not be achieved. The duration of the depravation will be a factor in the severity of the problem and in the prognosis for success of treatment.

For additional information, refer to Chapters 2, 4, and 13.

SUGGESTED READING

Grosvenor T, Flom M. Refractive Anomalies: Research and Clinical Applications. Boston: Butterworth-Heinemann, 1990.

Milder B, Rubin M. The Fine Art of Prescribing Glasses Without Making a Spectacle of Yourself. Gainesville, FL: Triad Scientific Publishers, 1981.

4 / The Ophthalmic Prescription

Victoria B. Cipparrone and Rita M. Pierce

This chapter presents the basic concepts of light, lenses, and prisms and how these relate to the ophthalmic prescription.

CONCEPTS OF LIGHT AND LENSES

Optics, a complex subject, is greatly simplified for the purposes of this chapter. Several theories of light are used to explain how light responds when traveling through lenses and prisms. This chapter does not examine these theories individually, but it covers certain aspects of the theories to explain the relationship between light and lenses (see Chapter 3 for an in-depth discussion of the optics of light).

Light travels in a wave motion and moves in a specific direction. For the purpose of optics drawings, it is assumed that light waves move from left to right. Light waves are capable of producing vision in human beings by stimulating the retinal receptors known as rods and cones.

Light travels at a speed of 186,000 miles per second (mps) in air. This speed is much faster than the speed of sound. The speed of light in air is also much faster than in other transparent substances, such as glass or water, because these substances offer more resistance than air does to the light. When light enters a medium such as glass or water at any angle other than 90 degrees, the light is refracted or bent. The amount of resistance the medium offers, along with the curvature of the surface, helps determine how much and in which direction light rays will be bent.

A comparison, or ratio, of the speed of light in air to the speed of light in another medium is called the *index of refraction*. As an example, to find the index of refraction for water, compare the speed of light in water at 140,000 mps with the speed of light in air at 186,000 mps—186,000/140,000, which results in an index of refraction of 1.33 for water. This means that when light rays pass from air to water, they will be slowed down. This slowing down of the light rays results in the light rays being bent on entering the water, as water offers more resistance than air. This will happen to any light ray that strikes the surface at any angle other than 90 degrees.

Light rays striking a surface at 90 degrees will slow down, but the path of the light rays will not be changed. A simple experiment demonstrates this principle. Put a pencil in a glass of water. The pencil will appear displaced at the water line. This is the refraction, or bending of the light waves due to the difference in the refractive index. The indices of refraction for some common optical media are as follows:

- Air   1.00
- Water   1.33
- Polymethylacrylate (PMMA) plastic   1.49
- Ophthalmic crown glass   1.523
- Flint glass   1.616

The amount an ophthalmic lens refracts, or bends, light can be used to determine its power. The metric system is used for calculating

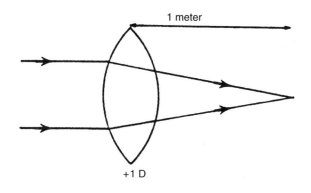

FIGURE 4-1—1.00 D lens with a 1.00 m focal length.

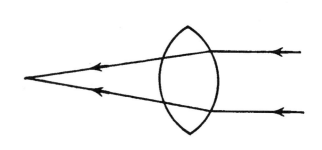

FIGURE 4-2—Parallel light rays traveling through a convex lens.

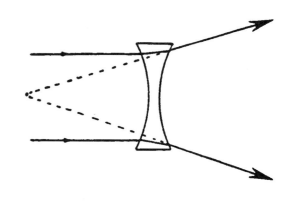

FIGURE 4-3—Parallel light rays traveling through a concave lens.

diopters, the unit of measurement of lens power. One meter is equal to 100 cm and to 1,000 mm. Therefore, the following formula can be used to calculate lens power in diopters:

$$\text{Diopters} = \frac{1 \text{ m}}{\text{focal length (m)}}$$
$$= \frac{100 \text{ cm}}{\text{focal length (cm)}}$$
$$= \frac{1,000 \text{ mm}}{\text{focal length (mm)}}$$

The focal length is the distance from the lens to the point where the parallel light rays come to focus. A 1.00 D lens is of such power that it will refract or bend parallel light rays to a focus 1 m from the lens (Figure 4-1). If the diopter power is known, it can be used to calculate the focal length for the lens using the following formula:

$$\text{Focal length} = \frac{1 \text{ m}}{\text{diopters}}$$
$$= \frac{100 \text{ cm}}{\text{diopters}}$$
$$= \frac{1,000 \text{ mm}}{\text{diopters}}$$

Very simply, the higher the lens power, the more the light rays will be bent or the shorter the focal length will be.

There are two basic types of ophthalmic lenses: plus and minus. *Plus lenses*, also called convex lenses, have several identifiable characteristics. These lenses are designed so that the center of the lens is thicker than the edges of the lens. Objects viewed through a convex lens will appear magnified, or larger. Parallel light rays passing through a plus lens will be converged, or brought together, to a real focus (Figure 4-2). *Minus lenses*, also called concave lenses, are designed so that the edges of the lens are thicker than the center of the lens. Objects viewed through a minus lens appear minified, or smaller. Parallel light rays passing through a concave lens will be diverged, or spread apart. A concave lens has a virtual, or imaginary, focus. This virtual focus is found by tracing the light rays back to where they appear to be coming from in front of the lens (Figure 4-3).

Prism power may also be incorporated in an ophthalmic prescription. A prism can be thought of as a triangle, which has nonparallel sides. The apex, or point, of the triangle is thinner than the base, the flat bottom. Light rays

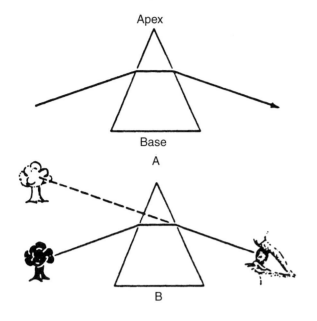

FIGURE 4-4—Light traveling through a prism. (Reprinted with permission from SS Bates. Fundamentals for Assisting in Primary Care Optometry. New York: Professional Press/Fairchild, 1983.)

passing through a prism will always be bent toward the base of the prism. A prism will neither converge nor diverge the light rays, only bend the light toward its base, thus displacing, or moving, the image of objects. Looking through a prism, objects will appear to be displaced toward the apex of the prism (Figure 4-4). A prism can be oriented in any direction in an ophthalmic prescription in order to get the light rays bent properly to correct a patient's visual problem (see Figure 4-4).

Because prism power is measured by *prism diopters*, which are different than the diopters for lens power, a different formula is used to calculate the power of a prism.

$$\text{A prism diopter } (\Delta) = \frac{\text{deviation of light ray (cm)}}{\text{distance from prism (m)}}$$

A 1Δ prism will deviate a ray of light or displace an image 1 cm for every meter of distance, measured on the tangent scale (Figure 4-5).

During the refraction, the doctor of optometry will determine either or both of the specific lens power and prism power needed by the patient for the light rays coming into the eye to be bent in such a way as to put a clear image on the retina.

LENS FORMS

There are two basic lens forms used for ophthalmic prescriptions: the spherical lens, which deviates rays of light in the same direction, and the cylindrical lens, which deviates rays of light in more than one direction. Various types of these two lens forms exist.

A *spherical lens* can be thought of as a portion of a round ball. It can be any of the following types:

Biconvex: Both of the lens surfaces are plus and converge light to one focal point (see Figure 4-2).

Plano convex: This lens has one plus surface and one surface that is plano or flat. This lens also converges light to a single focal point (Figure 4-6).

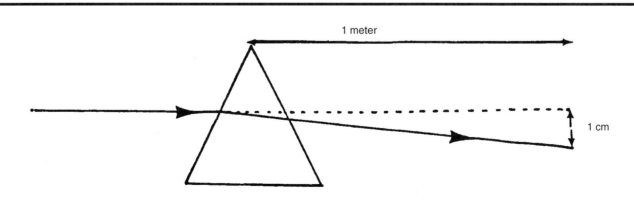

FIGURE 4-5—1.00Δ prism.

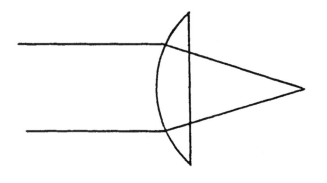

FIGURE 4-6—Light converges to a single focal point in a plano convex lens.

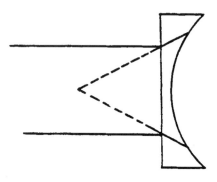

FIGURE 4-7—Light rays diverge as if the focal point was in front in a plano concave lens.

Biconcave: Both lens surfaces are concave or minus. They diverge light rays as if the focus was in front of the lens (see Figure 4-3).

Plano concave: This lens has one surface that is minus or concave and another surface that is plano or flat. It diverges light rays as if the focal point were in front of the lens (Figure 4-7).

Meniscus: This lens has one surface concave or minus and another surface convex or plus. It will either converge or diverge light rays, depending on which surface has more power (Figure 4-8). Most lenses used in ophthalmic prescriptions are meniscus lenses.

The second lens form is a *cylindrical lens*. A cylindrical lens deviates light in different directions. The simplest concept of a cylinder lens can be visualized by cutting a can in half (Figure 4-9). The front surface acts actually has two surfaces, one curved and the other flat. When rays of light strike the cylinder, the curved portion of the surface will converge light, acting like a convex sphere, and the flat portion of the surface will not bring the rays to a focus. Therefore, this cylinder has no power in one meridian and spherical plus power in the other meridian.

A *spherocylindrical lens*, which is common in ophthalmic prescriptions, has one power in one major meridian and a different power in the meridian 90 degrees away. A spherocylinder lens can be visualized by picturing a football (Figure 4-10). There is a spherical plus power along the length of the football and stronger plus power along the more curved width of the football. Spherocylinder lenses can be of a convex or plus nature, in which both meridians are convex, or a concave or minus nature, in which both meridians are concave.

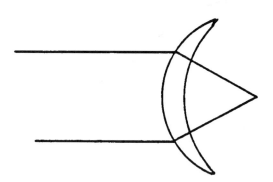

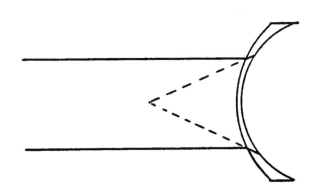

FIGURE 4-8—Meniscus lenses can either converge or diverge light rays.

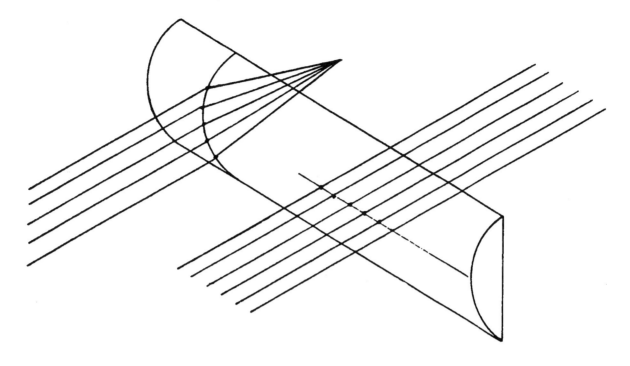

FIGURE 4-9—Light rays passing through a simple cylinder lens.

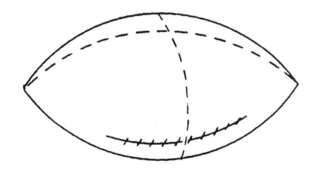

FIGURE 4-10—A spherocylinder lens pictured as a football.

THE OPTICAL CROSS

An optical cross is a diagram that denotes the dioptric power in the two *principal meridians* of a lens. The principal meridians are the meridians of greatest power and least power. The principal meridians are 90 degrees apart. The total optical cross for a lens is a combination of the front surface power and the back surface power. A spherical lens will have only one front curve in all meridians and only one back curve in all meridians.

A convex or plus spherical lens could be represented in the following manner:

```
   front           + back          = total
  ─┼─ +6.25       ─┼─ –5.00       ─┼─ +1.25
   +6.25           –5.00           +1.25
```

Combining the front and back surfaces in each meridian (+6.25 + –5.00), the total lens power is +1.25 D. If the lensometer were used to find the power of this lens, it would be +1.25 D.

A concave or minus spherical lens could be represented in the following manner:

```
   front           + back          = total
  ─┼─ +7.00       ─┼─ –8.75       ─┼─ –1.75
   +7.00           –8.75           –1.75
```

Again, combining the front and back surface powers in each meridian (+7.00 + –8.75) results in the total lens power, –1.75 D.

A spherocylindrical lens is a combination of a spherical surface and a cylindrical surface. The total cross will have a different curve or power in each of the two principal meridians. An example of a spherocylindrical lens is as follows:

```
  front           + back          = total
   |  +4.00         |  -6.00        |  -2.00
---+---          ---+---         ---+---
   |               |              |
 +4.00            0.00          +4.00
```

This total cross indicates –2.00 D of power in the horizontal meridian (+4.00 + –6.00) and +4.00 D of power in the vertical meridian (+4.00 + 0.00). The horizontal meridian is at 180 degrees, and the vertical meridian is at 90 degrees. The written prescription for this total cross would be +4.00 –6.00 x 090. A written prescription consists of three components: the sphere power, the cylinder power, and the axis of the cylinder. In this written prescription, the first number (+4.00) is the spherical power, the –6.00 is the cylinder power, and the 090 is the axis of the cylinder. This is a minus cylinder correction, since the cylinder portion of the correction is on the back surface of the lens instead of on the front surface. In a plus cylinder correction, the two different curves would be ground on the front surface of the lens. Doctors of optometry most often write prescriptions in minus cylinder form.

The total cross can be used to arrive at the written prescription in minus cylinder form. To begin, select the power that is the most plus (or the least minus). This becomes the spherical component in the prescription. In this example, it would be the +4.00 D. The meridian that the most plus power is located on becomes the axis of the cylinder for the written prescription. This means cylinder power is located 90 degrees away from the spherical power. The +4.00 D is located on the vertical meridian or on the 90-degree line, so the axis is recorded as 090. To find the total cylinder power, algebraically subtract the spherical power from the power in the meridian 90 degrees away from the spherical power. In the example then, +4.00 would be subtracted from –2.00, for a total of –6.00 D for the cylinder power. It is important to keep track of the plus and minus signs when adding and subtracting diopter powers. The final prescription would then be written as +4.00 –6.00 x 090. To relate this to the lensometer, the spherical power would be located first at +4.00 D on the lensometer power wheel. The power wheel would be turned toward the minus power until –2.00 D is reached, which is where the cylinder lines focus. This would be a total of 6.00 D that the power wheel was moved, and it was moved in the minus direction, for the –6.00 total. The axis indicator is on 090 degrees.

Here is another example of a spherocylinder lens:

```
  front           + back          = total
   |  +2.00         |  -3.00        |  -1.00
---+---          ---+---         ---+---
   |               |              |
 +2.00            -5.00         -3.00
```

To write the prescription for this total cross, first find the sphere power, which is the most plus or the least minus power on the total cross. In this example, it would be the –1.00. The –1.00 is located on the 180-degree meridian, so the axis of the cylinder becomes 180 in the written prescription. To find the total cylinder power, algebraically subtract the –1.00 (the sphere power) from –3.00 (the power in the meridian 90 degrees away from the sphere power). The result is a –2.00 D for the cylinder power. Again, watch the plus and minus signs on the diopter powers. This prescription then would be written at –1.00 –2.00 x 180. This is also a minus cylinder form lens because the two different curves are ground on the back of the lens. Understanding the optical cross should provide a better understanding of the ophthalmic prescription.

TRANSPOSITION

Ophthalmic prescriptions written by doctors of optometry will usually be in minus cylinder form, for example, +2.00 –1.00 x 080. Occasionally, the office might receive a prescription written in plus cylinder form, for example, +2.00 + 1.00 x 080. This prescription form is commonly used by ophthalmologists. The following is a step-by-step procedure for transposing plus cylinder prescriptions into minus cylinder form.

Example A: +2.00 +1.00 x 080

1. Combine the sphere and cylinder power mathematically to achieve the new sphere power: +2.00 + (+1.00) = +3.00.

2. Change the sign of the cylinder so that +1.00 becomes −1.00.
3. Change the axis so that it is 090 degrees away by either adding or subtracting 90 to the existing axis so as not to make the new axis greater than 180 degrees: 080 degrees + 090 degrees = 170 degrees.
4. The transposed prescription will now read +3.00 − 1.00 x 170.

Example B: −1.00 + 3.00 x 045

1. Combine the sphere and cylinder power mathematically to achieve the new sphere power: −1.00 + (+3.00) = +2.00 sphere.
2. Change the sign of the cylinder from plus (+) to minus (−) so that +3.00 cylinder becomes −3.00.
3. Change the axis by adding 090 degrees: 045 + 090 = 135 degrees.
4. The transposed prescription would now read +2.00 −3.00 x 135.

Example C: −4.00 +0.75 x 105

1. Combine the sphere and cylinder power mathematically to achieve the new sphere power: −4.00 + (+0.75) = −3.25 sphere.
2. Change the sign of the cylinder from plus (+) to minus (−) so that +0.75 cylinder becomes −0.75.
3. Change the axis by subtracting 090 degrees: 105 degrees − 090 degrees = 015 degrees.
4. The transposed prescription would now read −3.25 −0.75 x 015.

SPHERE EQUIVALENT

A sphere equivalent of an ophthalmic prescription is used for a patient's prescription when the doctor of optometry desires to prescribe less than full cylinder power. Most of the time the optometrist will provide the sphere equivalent for the paraoptometric, but an understanding of how it is determined is helpful.

Assume that the prescription for a patient is +2.00 −1.00 x 090 in the right eye. The optometrist does not want the patient to have the cylinder power but wants the patient to see clearly. To achieve the sphere equivalent of this prescription, divide the cylinder power in half and algebraically combine it with the sphere power. The sphere equivalent of the above prescription is +1.50 because half of −1.00 (the cylinder power) is −0.50, and it is combined with the sphere power so that +2.00 + (−0.50) = +1.50 D.

The sphere equivalent for +3.00 −2.00 x 080 is +2.00 D, which is found by taking half of −2.00 (the cylinder power) and adding it to +3.00 (the sphere power).

The following is an example of finding sphere equivalent of −2.50 −0.75 x 015. Begin by taking half of −0.75 (the cylinder power), which is −0.37. Algebraically combine −0.37 with the sphere power of −2.50 for a sphere equivalent for this prescription of −2.87 D.

PRISM

The doctor of optometry may prescribe prism when the two eyes do not align properly. If the optometrist prescribes prism in a spherical ophthalmic prescription, the written prescription may look like this:

OD −2.00 D.S. ◯ 1∆ BI

OS −1.00 D.S. ◯ 1∆ BI

(D.S. stands for diopter sphere.) Not only does the prescription need to show the amount of prism in each lens, but it also needs to show the direction of the base. The base direction can be up, down, in, or out, abbreviated BU, BD, BI, or BO, respectively.

If the optometrist prescribes prism in a spherocylinder ophthalmic prescription, the written prescription may look like this:

OD −3.00 −0.75 x 180 2½∆ BO

OS −2.50 −1.00 x 165 ½∆ BU

Most prescription lenses are made so that the optical center (the spot in the lens with no prism power) is placed at the patient's interpupillary distance (PD) (Figure 4-11). There will be induced prism in the lenses if the laboratory does not position the optical centers at the same distance as the patient's PD. Prentice's rule is used to calculate induced prism. The rule states

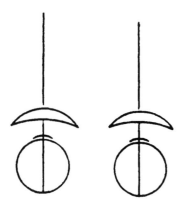

FIGURE 4-11—The optical centers at these convex meniscus lenses are placed at the patient's interpupillary distance.

that induced prism is equal to the lens power multiplied by the displacement in centimeters of the lens optical centers from the patient's PD.

To avoid induced prism, *decentration* is done. The formula for calculating decentration is the frame PD (eye size plus bridge size) minus the patient's distance PD divided by 2. For example, if the patient's PD measures 60 mm and the frame PD measures 64 mm, in order for the laboratory to match the optical centers to the patient's PD, the laboratory would need to decenter each lens 2 mm inward. Decentration is inward when the frame PD is larger than the patient's PD and outward when the frame PD is smaller than the patient's PD.

MULTIFOCALS

Multifocals were designed to meet the visual requirements people have at different distances. A spectacle wearer who has a correction for distance may require more plus power to be able to see clearly at near.

The terms *add power* or *near addition* are used when referring to multifocal segments because the segment is plus power that is added to the distance power. To calculate the proper multifocal power, the optometrist must determine how much power the patient needs at distance and how much power the patient needs at near.

Example A

If a patient requires a distance power of +2.00 D and needs a total of +3.00 D to see clearly at near, the bifocal or segment power would then be +1.00. (Segment power is always in plus power.) The formula used is as follows:

$$\frac{\text{distance}}{\text{power}} + \frac{\text{segment}}{\text{power}} = \text{total near power}$$

Example B

The patient's distance prescription is −2.00 −1.00 x 080, and the segment power is +1.00. The total near power is −1.00 −1.00 x 080, found by combining the distance spherical correction of −2.00 and the segment power of +1.00 for the total near spherical power of −1.00. The cylinder power, if there is any in the distance prescription, is always included in the total near power.

When ordering a prescription, indicate the segment power, not the total near power. Some spectacle wearers require three lens powers: a correction for distance, a correction for near (usually calculated for a working distance of 16 inches), and a different correction for intermediate distances. Multifocals used to correct three working distances are called *trifocals*.

The *intermediate power* is commonly half the near add power, for example, distance +2.00 D, near add +1.00 D. Half the near add power would be +0.50 D. In this prescription, the total near power would be +3.00 D because the distance and the near power are added together. The total intermediate power would be +2.50 D, which is the distance power added to the intermediate power.

When ordering a trifocal lens, the intermediate power, when not specified, will always be made half the near add power. It is possible to special order intermediate powers other than half the near add power if necessary.

SUGGESTED READING

Fannin T, Grosvenor T. Clinical Optics (2nd ed). Boston: Butterworth-Heinemann, 1996.
Grosvenor T, Flom M. Refractive Anomalies Research and Clinical Applications. Boston: Butterworth-Heinemann, 1990.
Milder B, Rubin M. The Fine Art of Prescribing Glasses Without Making a Spectacle of Yourself. Gainesville, FL: Triad Scientific Publishers, 1981.

5 / Ophthalmic Lenses

Marian C. Welling and Lynn E. Konkel

Ophthalmic lenses are an intrinsic part of daily life for millions of people. The lenses are used for a variety of reasons, the most common being the correction of faulty vision. Choosing the correct lens for a patient can be a complex task. The patient's prescription must be considered, along with the lens design, material, and treatments that will best meet his or her lifestyle needs.

The ophthalmic lens industry is continually making advances in design and style to serve the visual needs of patients better. This chapter provides an overview of the most commonly used ophthalmic lenses and their uses. This is essential information for all optometric assistants and technicians.

OPHTHALMIC LENS MATERIALS

The principal types of lens materials used today are glass, CR-39 (standard ophthalmic plastic), and polycarbonate. Each has its own unique qualities, uses, advantages, and disadvantages. A listing of various lens materials is shown in Table 5-1.

There are three characteristics that must be considered when designing an ophthalmic lens: thickness, chromatic aberration, and weight. The thickness of a lens can be reduced by using materials made with a higher index of refraction (see Chapter 3). Likewise, chromatic aberration (typically a colored fringe around an image) may be reduced by using a material of higher Abbé number, which describes the dispensive power of the material. Finally, the weight of the lens may be reduced by using a material of lower specific gravity. The American National Standards Institute (ANSI) has established and published standards for the manufacturing of lenses for ophthalmic use.

Glass

Crown glass is the name given to the ophthalmic quality of glass most commonly used. It is a soda-lime-silica glass similar in composition to the best grades of plate glass. It has a refractive index of 1.5230, Abbé value of 58.5, and specific gravity of 2.54. Crown glass is the lens material that has been used the longest. It has the superior optical qualities that newer lens materials try to match, particularly the Abbé value for chromatic aberrations. It has a hard surface that makes it naturally scratch-resistant; however, in order to meet ANSI standards for impact resistance, the lens must be either heat-tempered or chemically tempered. Patients should be made aware that scratches in the surface of lenses reduce the impact resistance of the lens. Also, due to the relatively high specific gravity of crown glass, the lenses are heavy, which may be uncomfortable.

CR-39

Standard ophthalmic plastic lenses are made from a material called CR-39, a hard resin. Plastic lenses were first introduced in the United States shortly after World War II. Since then, due to constant advances in technology, they comprise 72% of the ophthalmic lens mar-

TABLE 5-1. Lens materials

Nominal index	Actual index	Abbé number	Trade name (manufacturer)
Glass materials			
1.523	1.523	58.6	Ophthalmic crown (several manufacturers)
1.60	1.601	40.7	1.60 crown (Schott, Duryea, PA)
1.70	1.706	31	High-Lite (Schott, Duryea, PA)
1.80	1.805	25.4	1.80 High Index (Schott, Duryea, PA)
Plastic materials			
1.50	1.498	58	CR-39 (PPG Industries, Pittsburgh, PA)
1.54	1.537	47	Spectralite (Sola, Petaluma, CA)
1.55	1.549	38	Easylite (Younger, Los Angeles, CA)
1.56	1.556	37.7	HiRi (PPG Industries, Pittsburgh, PA)
1.58	1.577	37.5	Cristyl Hi Index 1.58 (Titmus, Petersburg, VA)
1.59	1.586	31	Polycarbonate (several manufacturers)
1.60	1.595	36	Thin & Lite (Essilor, St. Petersburg, FL)
1.66	1.660	32	Hyperindex 166 (Optima, Stratford, CT)

Note: The *higher* the nominal index number and the actual index number, the *thinner* the lens for equal power. (Polycarbonate may be surfaced to 1.5 center thickness [CT], and both polycarbonate and high-index 1.6 plastic are available in finished at 1.5 CT: This reduced CT further reduces edge thickness in minus-powered lenses.) The *lower* the number, the *greater* the image distortion away from the center of the lens (chromatic aberration). In other words, because *all* powered lenses have this property, the lower the number, the closer to the center of the lens noticeable distortion will occur. Moreover, the higher the power, the more noticeable this becomes. The *higher* the number, the *heavier* the material. (NOTE: Because higher index materials use flatter base curves to achieve equal powers, they will be thinner and therefore contain less material. Even if the specific gravity of two lenses were equal, for equal powers, the lens with the higher index of refraction would weigh less.) Ultraviolet radiation is recognized by the American National Standards Institute to be radiation of up to 380 nm. This figure shows the relative effect of various lenses on blocking ultravoilet rays. The *lower* the number, the more effective the lens material.

ket. CR-39 has an index of refraction of 1.498, Abbé value of 57.8, and a specific gravity of 1.32. When these values are compared with that of crown glass, a lens in CR-39 is thicker, produces almost the same amount of chromatic aberration, and is significantly lighter in weight (approximately 50% lighter).

The advantages of CR-39 lenses are many. They do not have to be treated in any way to meet the standards for impact resistance. Plastic lenses are comfortable to wear due to their light weight. They have less tendency to fog than glass lenses when going from a cold to warm environment. They have uniform color density when tinted because the dye used to color the lenses is absorbed directly into the lens surfaces after the lens is made. This process of color manipulation is easy. Colors can be added, changed, or removed in the office. Plastic lenses produce less glare than glass lenses and give rise to relatively few internal reflections. Plastic lenses transmit slightly more light than glass, thereby tending to improve visual performance.

The major disadvantage of CR-39 lenses is that they scratch more easily than glass lenses. Most CR-39 lenses dispensed today include a scratch-resistant coating; however, this does not mean the lenses will not scratch. Patients should be instructed on how to clean their lenses and to store them in a case when they are not being worn. The proper cleaning method is to rinse them with warm tap water; apply a cleaning solution if desired; and then pat them dry with a soft, lint-free cloth or tissue.

Another disadvantage of CR-39 lenses is that they are thicker than glass lenses due to the lower index of refraction. Also, CR-39 lenses are more prone to warp than glass lenses. Warpage results from the tension put on the lens by the eyewire of a frame. If the lens is forced into a frame, the pressure exerted on the lens will cause it to warp. This problem is avoided by making sure that the lenses are cut to the proper size before being placed in a frame.

Polycarbonate

This material is another form of plastic, an ophthalmic grade of lexan. It is a highly impact-resistant material, first used for bulletproof windows and windshields in the early 1960s. A polycarbonate lens has an index of refraction of 1.586, which makes it 10% thinner than crown glass and 15% thinner than CR-39 lenses. Polycarbonate lenses are also light in weight. These lenses also provide patients with ultraviolet (UV) light protection without the added expense of applying a coating. This material filters 99% of the UV rays naturally. A disadvantage of these lenses is the low Abbé value, causing chromatic aberration. Some patients will notice a rainbow effect in the periphery of the lens.

Polycarbonate lenses are available in single-vision, multifocal, and some progressive addition lens designs. The material is also available in several aspheric designs, offering thinner, ultra-lightweight lenses in high plus and minus powers. Polycarbonate has the same tinting characteristics as CR-39. Polycarbonate lenses should be recommended for all patients when protection and safety are major factors. Athletes, children, and monocular patients are generally good candidates for lenses made of this material.

High-Index Plastic

Lenses made of polyurethane are often called *high-index plastic*. The index of refraction will vary with the manufacturer, but will range from 1.58 to 1.61. Therefore, lenses made of this material are the thinnest, most distortion-free lenses. High-index material will begin to make a difference in lens thickness beginning at –2.00 D; a significant difference in lens thickness will be found starting at –4.00 D. The main disadvantage of high-index plastic is that it is less impact-resistant than polycarbonate, although it is slightly more impact-resistant than CR-39 plastic. This lens is quickly becoming the lens of choice for patients with powers over –3.00 D in low-risk environments where the lack of strength is not a problem. High-index lenses are available in single-vision, multifocal, and some progressive addition lens designs. They are also available in aspheric designs. Depending on the manufacturer, they are available with scratch-resistant and antireflective coatings. Most brands of this lens also tint very well.

HOW TO DISPENSE THE THINNEST LENS POSSIBLE

When a patient desires the thinnest lens possible, there is more to the process than simply selecting the appropriate lens material. Frame size, aspheric design, and center thickness must also be considered.

Frame size: The smaller the frame, the thinner the lens. Try to match the distance between centers, which is the distance between the two geometric centers of the lenses (eye size plus bridge size), to the patient's interpupillary distance (PD). This will minimize the amount of movement necessary to adjust to the lens blank's optical center. Also, try to select a frame that places the patient's eye slightly above the vertical center of the frame.

Lens material: The thinnest materials are polycarbonate or high-index plastic. Remember to recommend polycarbonate when maximum impact protection is desired.

Aspheric design: A lens that decreases in power toward the periphery of the lens creates a thinner lens. This lens is very effective for high plus powers. Aspheric lens design will reduce the bulge and magnification of plus lenses. The patient may notice a decrease in peripheral visual acuity with this design, however.

Center thickness: Order lenses as thin as possible. Polycarbonate can be made with a 1.0–1.5 center thickness.

IMPACT RESISTANCE

All lenses used in ophthalmic eyeglasses and sunglasses must meet federal standards for impact resistance. There are two categories of impact-resistant lenses: dress eyewear and occupational protective lenses.

Dress Eyewear

Dress eyewear must have lenses that are impact-resistant to the degree that they will withstand the impact of a ⅝-inch steel ball dropped from a height of 50 inches, commonly called *drop-ball testing*.

CR-39, polycarbonate, and high-index plastic lenses, by design, are more impact-resistant. These lenses offer protection from breakage and potential injury and are available in both dress and occupational styles. The materials have been proven strong enough that each individual lens does not have to be drop-ball tested by a local laboratory. Random drop-ball testing is done by the manufacturer of the lens blanks. These materials are less likely to break than the safest glass lens.

Glass lenses must be treated in one of two ways to meet the impact-resistance standards and pass the drop-ball test. The first method is *heat tempering*. After a lens is cut and edged to its desired shape and size, it is placed in a vacuum and brought close to its melting point. Then the lens is rapidly cooled so that tension is created between the inner and outer molecular layers of the glass. This process results is some lens surface distortion.

The second method is called *chemical tempering*. Lenses are placed in a very hot chemical bath where an ion exchange takes place in the surface of the glass. The lenses are left in the bath for 15–17 hours so that the ion exchange goes deeply into the lens.

Patients wearing glass lenses that have been treated by either method should be told that the impact-resistant properties will be compromised if the lens surface is scratched. Patients should not be led to believe that any lens material is unbreakable; all lenses are impact-resistant, with some materials being stronger than others.

Occupational Lenses

These lenses are commonly known as *industrial safety lenses*. Safety lenses must also pass a drop-ball test; however, the steel ball used here is 1 inch in diameter. Along with the drop-ball test, safety lenses must have a minimum thickness (the center for minus lenses and the edge for plus lenses) of 3.0 mm. The only exception to this is high plus lenses. For these lenses, the minimum thickness must be 2.5 mm.

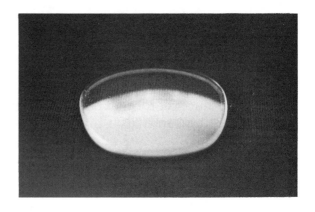

FIGURE 5-1—A single-vision lens has only one point of focus.

LENS DESIGNS

Single-Vision Lenses

Single-vision lenses have one optical center that will correct vision at a given distance (Figure 5-1). There are three designs of single-vision lenses: spherical, planocylindrical, and spherocylindrical.

A *spherical lens* has the same power in all meridians. This lens is used to correct simple myopia or hyperopia.

A *planocylindrical lens* has no power in one meridian, and the meridian 90 degrees away has the most power. All other meridians have powers that vary from that of the least to the greatest power. This lens is used to correct astigmatism.

A *spherocylindrical lens* has a spherical component throughout the lens, and this spherical component is the exclusive power in the axis meridian. The cylindrical power varies in all meridians, with the maximum cylindrical power being 90 degrees from the axis meridian. This lens is used to correct a combination of myopia or hyperopia with astigmatism. Lenses can be ground in either plus or minus cylinder form. A plus cylinder lens has the cylinder ground on the front surface of the lens. A minus cylinder lens has the cylinder ground on the back surface. Most lenses used today are in the minus cylinder form.

Multifocal Lenses

A multifocal lens is a single lens with more than one point of focus (Figures 5-2 and 5-3). There are several types of multifocal lenses, and patients are usually not familiar with all of their

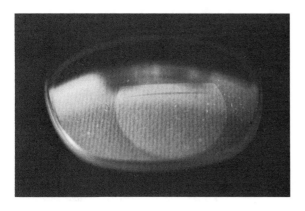

FIGURE 5-2—A bifocal lens has a point of focus in the distance portion and also in the near segment.

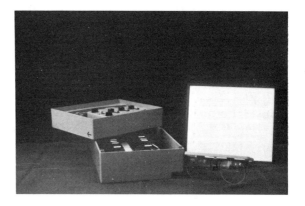

FIGURE 5-4—A multifocal demonstration kit allows a patient to try progressive addition lenses and compare them to traditional multifocal styles.

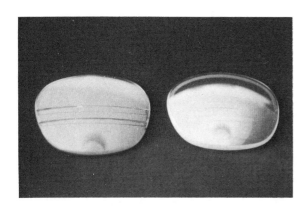

FIGURE 5-3—A trifocal lens has three points of focus: one in the distance, one in the intermediate, and one in the near segment.

choices. It is your professional responsibility to educate them by explaining and demonstrating their lens options. There are a variety of products available to help you, such as kits of sample lenses, diagrams, sample eyewear, and multifocal demonstration kits (Figure 5-4).

Progressive Addition Multifocal Lenses

One type of multifocal is the progressive addition lens. These lenses have the distance prescription in the upper portion of the lens, with this power progressively changing to the near prescription in the lower portion of the lens. This allows the wearer clear vision and a smooth, comfortable transition as he or she moves his or her eyes for all working distances without the interference of lines and with the added cosmetic advantage of no visible lines.

For many practitioners, progressive addition lenses are the multifocal of first choice for their patients. Fitting success rates are high, even for current flat-top bifocal and trifocal wearers.

In all progressive addition lenses, there is an area where the add power increases. This area is the cause of the peripheral distortion the patient notices. There are three major designs of progressive addition lenses. The first is the *hard design*. In the hard design, the area of add power change is small. This gives the patient a wide reading area and good distance viewing. This lens will produce peripheral distortion caused by unwanted cylinder power, however. The difference between the various brands of hard design lenses is where the manufacturer chooses to locate this unwanted cylinder power. Hard design lenses are recommended for patients who need a wide reading area or who are hyperopic.

Soft design progressive addition lenses have a wider transition zone, spreading out the unwanted cylinder power. This type of lens has a long intermediate corridor and softer optics. Since the soft design is easier to adapt to, it is recommended for emerging presbyopes and those whom the paraoptometric suspect may have adaptation problems.

The final type of progressive addition lens design is the *multidesign*. This lens uses characteristics of soft design in the lower add powers, gradually creating a lens that is harder in design in the higher add powers. Work with your doctor and laboratory representatives to learn all you can about the progressive addition lenses used in your office.

FITTING PROGRESSIVE ADDITION LENSES

There are five steps involved in successful fitting of progressive addition lenses:

1. *Adjust the frame.* The frame must be in proper adjustment before the height of the progressive power is measured (see Chapter 6). Make certain the vertex distance, pantoscopic angle, and bridge are properly adjusted. This step is crucial to the success of the lenses.
2. *Measure the height of the progressive power.* Measure the height from the deepest part of the frame to the center of the pupil. Make sure the patient is looking straight ahead and that you are eye level with the patient. Having the patient move around and then rechecking the measurement is desirable. The use of seg height gauges is highly recommended for this procedure. The minimum fitting height is 24 mm for progressive addition lenses to work properly. If the height is less than 24 mm, a different frame must be selected. At this time, you can use a lens cut-out chart provided by the lens manufacturer to make certain the lens will cut out in the frame.
3. *Measure monocular distance PD.* The quickest, simplest, and most accurate method of doing monocular PD measurements is with a corneal reflex pupillometer.
4. *Verify the lenses.* Once the lenses arrive from the laboratory, verify the prescription accuracy (see Chapter 6). Leave the markings on the lenses so that you may use these for the final frame adjustment. The cross on the lens should be directly over the center of the pupil when the patient is looking straight ahead.
5. *Demonstrate the lenses.* Demonstrate the proper head movements for using the lenses. Remind the patients to keep their chins up and drop their eyes.

Straight-Top Bifocals

Straight-top bifocals are also known as *flat-tops* and *D-segs*. They are available in one-piece plastic and fused glass (Figures 5-5 and 5-6). They are produced by all major manufacturers and are the most widely prescribed bifocal in the world.

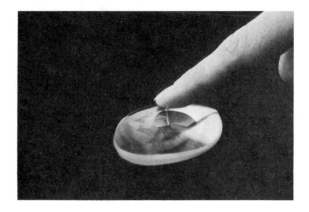

FIGURE 5-5—The segment line can be felt in a one-piece bifocal design. The segment line can be seen but not felt in a fused design segment.

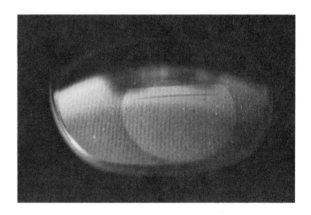

FIGURE 5-6—The straight-top bifocal is the most frequently prescribed multifocal design.

Straight-top bifocals are available in a variety of widths: 25, 28, 35, and 40 mm. The optical center of a straight-top bifocal is located closer to the segment line. Therefore, there is less image jump with this lens than that of a round bifocal. As a rule of thumb, the width of the bifocal should increase proportionately to the amount of near work a patient does. Generally, the straight-top bifocal height is measured from the deepest part of the frame's eyewire to the wearer's lower lash line. They are designated by using the initials *ST, FT,* or *D* for "straight-top," "flat-top," and "D-seg," respectively, along with the width of the desired segment.

Round Bifocals

Round bifocals are also available in both one-piece and fused types. The most commonly used

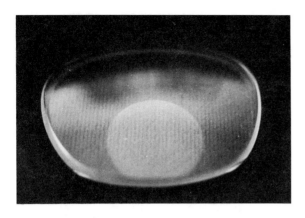

FIGURE 5-7—A round bifocal is less visible in a lens than a straight-top bifocal.

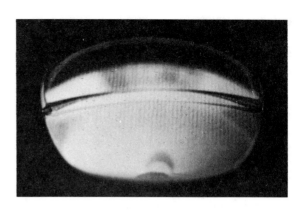

FIGURE 5-8—The full-width bifocal is commonly called an Executive and gives a wide field of near view.

round bifocal has a diameter of 22 mm (Figure 5-7). The major advantage to the round style bifocal is that it is less visible than a straight-top. Its major disadvantage is that it creates more image jump than a straight-top due to the lower placement of the segment optical center. The small diameter of the segment can also cause problems for a wearer with a lot of near-point demand.

A *kryptok bifocal* is a glass lens with a 22-mm round fused segment of flint glass. Because of the chromatic aberration associated with flint glass, the lens is not widely prescribed. The advantage of the kryptok bifocal is that it is less expensive than the round style mentioned above.

When fitting round style bifocals, the fitting height is measured from the deepest part of the frame's eyewire to the wearer's lower lash line.

Full-Width Bifocals

Full-width bifocal lenses are often called *executive* or *Franklin bifocals*. They are available in both glass and plastic and are always made with one-piece construction. They are easily identified by a large ridge that runs across the entire width of the lens (Figure 5-8). The major advantage of this lens is the wide field of near vision that it affords the patient. There is almost no image jump with this lens because the optical center of the segment is located on the segment line. There are some mechanical difficulties with this lens that have limited its use in recent times, however. The lens thickness, curves, and ledge result in a less secure fit of the lenses in the frame eyewire. Also, this lens has a more limited availability of blank sizes, so it often cannot be used with large eyesize frames. Another major disadvantage of this lens is its lack of cosmetic appeal. The construction of this lens makes it thicker and heavier than a straight-top or round style bifocal. The fitting height of these lenses is generally positioned at the wearer's lower lash line.

Trifocals

Most trifocals are manufactured with an intermediate power that is 50% of the near power. Any other percentage requires a special-order lens. Trifocals are available in straight-top and Executive styles. They are specified not only by style name and width of the segment, but also by the height of the intermediate portion of the segment. Therefore, "ST 7/25" designates a straight-top segment that is 25 mm wide, with an intermediate segment that is 7 mm high (Figure 5-9).

The intermediate area of the trifocal is designed to give the patient clear vision at arm's length. The use of trifocals is gradually diminishing as progressive addition lenses, with clear viewing at all possible distances, continue to gain in popularity.

When fitting a trifocal, the top line of the segment is generally positioned at the lower pupil edge when the wearer is looking straight ahead in normal room illumination.

Occupational Segments

There are a variety of lens designs available for special occupational needs. The most common is

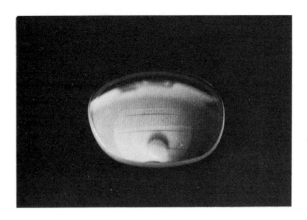

FIGURE 5-9—A straight-top 7/25 trifocal gives clear vision at arm's length as well as distance and near.

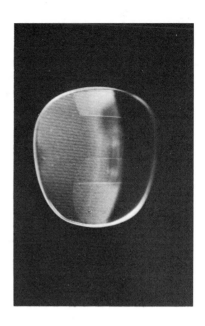

FIGURE 5-11—A quadrifocal lens gives a patient four points of clear vision.

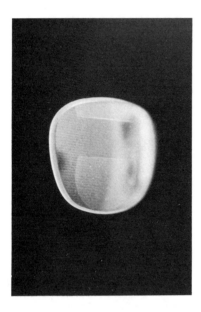

FIGURE 5-10—A double bifocal segment is used to provide a clear near field in the upper field as well as in the lower field.

the *double segment bifocal*, which has a segment at the top and the usual segment on the bottom of the lens (Figure 5-10). It is available in straight-top, round, and full-width styles. These lenses are designed with a 13- to 15-mm separation between the upper and lower segments. Distance vision is limited to this separation area.

Another commonly prescribed occupational lens is called a *quadrifocal*. It has a straight-top trifocal as its bottom segment and a straight-top bifocal as its top segment (Figure 5-11). It is available in widths of 22, 25, and 28 mm. The intermediate heights can be 6, 7, 8, or 10 mm high. A progressive addition lens called the *Overview* is designed to be used for patients currently wearing a progressive lens who have overhead near viewing demands occupationally. The Overview uses an upper semicircular segment over a traditional progressive lens.

The *E/D style occupational lens* is designed for patients requiring a greater intermediate viewing area, such as computer terminal users and accountants. It looks like an Executive bifocal with a straight-top segment inside it. Actually, the Executive portion of the lens is the intermediate power and the straight-top segment is the near power. The top of the lens is the distance power.

American Optical Corporation manufactures the *Technica* progressive addition lens specifically designed for computer users. It progresses from an intermediate power when the patient is looking straight ahead, to the near power as they look down. Approximately 12 mm above the pupil center there is a window of distance vision in the lens.

SPECIAL LENS DESIGNS
Aspheric Lens Designs

Aspheric lens designs have been used previously in the manufacture of lenticular lenses designed for the aphakic patient as well as progressive addition lenses. Aspheric lenses are gaining popularity in single-vision and traditional multifocal designs, however, especially when used in conjunction with high index lens materials. Aspheric lenses are designed using a series of curves on the front surface rather than the one simple (spherical) curve, making the surface more elliptical than spherical. The result of the aspheric design is a thinner lens with less distortion. Also, in plus powers there is less magnification and in minus powers less minification.

Aphakic Lenses

The need for aphakic lenses has greatly decreased in recent years due to the increase in the use of intraocular lens implants in aphakic patients during cataract surgery. A patient who has not been fit with an intraocular lens, however, will require either contact lens or spectacle correction. The multiple-drop aspheric lens is the lens of choice for this patient. This aspheric lens is designed so there is a drop in power that begins several millimeters from the center of the lens and continues to the periphery. This 3.00 D to 4.00 D drop in power varies from manufacturer to manufacturer.

This lens is cosmetically more appealing than other aphakic designs. The drop in power toward the periphery of the lens lessens the distortion and image jump an aphakic lens wearer experiences. This also gives the patient a more normal visual field. These lenses are available in single-vision and multifocal designs.

For the most efficient use of these bifocals, the manufacturers recommend that they be set 1 mm below the patient's pupil. The lenses should also be used in a frame with an eyesize no larger than 50 mm.

Myodisc Lenses

A myodisc lens is a high minus lens with a lenticular design. The front surface of the lens is plano (perfectly flat). The lenticular bowl is on the back surface of the lens and is usually 30 mm in diameter. This bowl consists of a deep concave depression in the back of the lens. The portion of the lens surrounding the bowl on the back surface is plano like the front surface

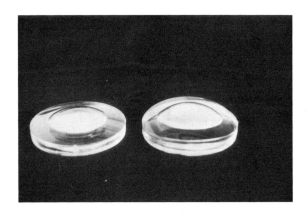

FIGURE 5-12—A lenticular lens can have either a round or an oval field.

(Figure 5-12). These lenses are available in single-vision, fused, and one-piece bifocal designs.

Balance Lenses

A balance lens is ordered for a monocular patient to balance the eyewear cosmetically. The laboratory uses an available lens of similar design and power as the specified prescription lens for the patient's good eye.

Fresnel Membrane Press-On Lenses

The Fresnel Press-On membrane is a thin plastic sheet approximately 1 mm thick that is placed on the ocular surface of an existing lens. It is available in prism powers, plus and minus powers, and a precut plus power straight-top bifocal style. Application is quick and simple. Water is the only substance needed to hold the membrane in place.

Fresnel membranes are often used in vision therapy and postsurgical temporary lenses for aphakes, as well as permanent treatment for a hemianopsia. Although these membranes have many applications, their use is limited because they are cosmetically unappealing and may result in reduced visual acuity.

LABORATORY CONSIDERATIONS: LENS BASE CURVE

The definition of the base curve of a lens has changed over the years as the design of lenses has changed. Today, ophthalmic laboratory technicians consider the base curve of a single-vision spherical lens as the front surface curve. The base curve of a spherocylinder lens is the flattest front surface curve, and since plus cylinder ground lenses (where the cylinder is ground on the front surface) are essentially obsolete, the flattest curve is most often the only front surface curve.

The base curve of a multifocal lens is the curve of the distance portion on the segment side. Since segments are almost exclusively on the front surface, so is the base curve. The cylinder is always ground on the side opposite to the segment.

Every major lens manufacturer distributes corrected curve lenses having specific base curves that are designed to eliminate aberrations. All quality laboratories have trained technicians who can determine what curves will give the best optical and cosmetic effect for a given prescription. Often, calculation for the optimum base curve is computerized.

In special situations, paraoptometrics may specify the base curve on a laboratory lens order. These situations may include the following: when the lens powers are very different for each eye, high-diopter power corrections, and prescriptions for patients who have shown a sensitivity to base curve changes.

It is wise to record the base curve of eyewear when it is received from the laboratory for future reference. Such information is helpful when pinpointing possible sources of problems with lens adaptation.

LENS ENHANCEMENTS

Scratch-Resistant Coatings

Plastic (CR-39) lens surfaces are not as hard as glass lens surfaces, making them more susceptible to scratching. Scratch-resistant coatings are a layer of resin that protects the lens from many surface scratches. This coating is so popular today that it is often considered part of the lens rather than an "add-on" option. Many large laboratories automatically use scratch-resistant plastic to fill their orders for plastic lenses.

The best scratch-resistant coatings are factory applied. The lenses are actually molded and cured with the hard-coated surface. Thus, scratch resistance is truly part of the lens rather than a coating applied to the finished lens blank. These lenses are available with the scratch resistance on both sides of a finished lens blank or on the front surface of a semifinished blank. Scratch-resistant coatings usually carry a manufacturer's warranty against scratching from normal wear for 12–24 months. They do not interfere with the tinting process and will not peel or crack off the lens. Some laboratories also coat the back surface of a lens.

Antireflective Coatings

Antireflective coatings offer improvements in both a patient's vision and the cosmetic appeal of the lenses. They increase the light transmission of a clear lens from 92% to approximately 99%. Antireflective coatings improve vision by increasing the amount of light entering the eye, eliminating ghost images and light reflection in the lenses. This makes them particularly useful for night driving, for playing sports, for using a computer, and in reducing glare from television studio lighting. The cosmetic value of the lens is improved by making the lens itself less visible. This makes the minifying or magnifying distortions of high-powered lenses much less visible, as the eye itself becomes more visible through the lenses. The patient will also notice a reduction in the annoying back surface reflections of the wearer's eyes and eyelashes.

Antireflective coatings are applied by coating companies or by the lens manufacturer. They cannot be applied in the office or by your local laboratory. The coatings consist of many microscopically thin layers of various metallic oxides that are applied in a vacuum under highly controlled conditions. Antireflective coatings are available on all lens materials.

New versions of the multilayer antireflective coating offer a more smudge-resistant surface. This smudge resistance is achieved by the addition of a layer of silicone to the lens surface. They are easier to clean than the conventional antireflective coatings; hot water and a soft, lint-free cloth will usually suffice.

Ultraviolet Coatings

UV coatings are designed to filter out UV light up to 400 nm, even in a clear lens. This coating protects the eye from potentially damaging UV light in both indoor and outdoor settings. Scientific studies have found a correlation between exposure to UV light and increased cataract development. People who spend a great deal of time outdoors; aphakes; and women using birth control medication, which increases the eye's sensitivity to light, will especially benefit from UV coating. The UV coatings are added to plastic lenses in a tinting unit. This can be done in the optical laboratory or in the office. Glass UV coatings must be applied by a coating company. As previously stated, polycarbonate lenses do not need special treatment, as their surfaces are already UV-absorbing.

The UV absorption properties of some brands of UV coatings can lessen over time. When this happens, the protective coating may be reapplied to the same lens.

Mirror Coatings

Prescription sunglass wearers may request that a mirror coating be applied to the front surface of the lens. Mirror coatings reflect some of the light striking the lens and increases the density of the lens. A mirror coating can also improve contrast and visual acuity without darkening the lens. Mirror coatings are usually applied over a lens that has been sunglass tinted.

Sports Coatings

Sport enthusiasts may want to wear special lens coatings designed to improve contrast sensitivity and reduce glare. The sport coatings currently available are the following:

Snowscreen for skiers. This coating is designed to function in white-on-white light.

Seascreen for water sports. This coating is designed to function best in blue-green light.

Landscreen for land-based sporting activities. This coating is designed to reduce visible light, not reflective light.

These coatings are applied as a series of coatings that begin with a yellow-brown coating applied to the concave side of the lens. On the convex side is a double-gradient filter designed to reduce glare from above and below. The third layer is a reflection-reducing coating applied to the concave side. These lens coatings eliminate 100% of UV light, 80% of infrared (IR) light, and 90% of distracting blue light.

Lens Tints

There are four general categories of colored lenses: glass lenses with absorptive tints, glass lenses coated with color, plastic lenses colored in a dye bath, and photochromic glass or plastic lenses that change color when exposed to sunlight.

Lens tints are often graded by the percent of light transmission, with a #1 being the lightest (greatest amount of transmission) and #3 being the darkest (least amount of transmission). These classifications are slightly subjective, but a generally accepted definition of the grades is as follows:

#1 tint—light transmission of 65–80%

#2 tint—light transmission of 45–60%

#3 tint—light transmission of 15–40%

As a point of reference, keep in mind that a clear spectacle lens has a light transmission of 92%.

Absorptive Glass Tints

Absorptive glass tints are produced by adding color to the glass during the manufacturing process, while the glass is in its liquid state. Oxides of the following elements are used to tint the glass to the corresponding colors:

- Cobalt—blue
- Manganese—violet, gold, red
- Uranium—yellow
- Didymium—pink
- Cerium—brown
- Iron—green
- Nickel, iron, cobalt—gray

The amount of the element that is added to the glass determines the darkness or lightness of the tint. It is important to note that the color of an absorptive tint cannot be altered, and absorptive glass lenses are not available with gradient-style tints. Also, absorptive tints in glass lenses are **not** uniform in density. A minus lens with a thinner center than edge will produce a tint that is lighter in the center and darker at the edges. A plus lens with a thicker center than edge will produce a tint that is darker in the center and lighter at the edges.

Each color tint has its own absorptive properties and uses. Charts of absorption curves are readily available from lens manufacturers.

Pink-tinted lenses are used for partial absorption of UV light. They are frequently used when a patient complains of photophobia, especially when working under fluorescent lighting. They transmit the visible spectrum evenly through the lenses, thereby preserving the natural color values. Their flesh color blends easily with the skin and gives the face a warm tone.

Gray-tinted glass lenses reduce the intensity of all transmitted wavelengths evenly, so colors are seen in their normal relationship. They are used primarily when absorption of UV and IR rays is needed. They make excellent sun lenses.

Green-tinted lenses provide absorption of UV and partial absorption of IR rays. They are used primarily for industrial uses. This tint alters color values slightly.

Brown-tinted lenses absorb UV and some IR rays. They are used to reduce blue haze and fog. They greatly alter color values. They have achieved a great deal of popularity recently as "blue blockers."

Yellow-tinted lenses are used on dark, foggy days to brighten the background. This tint absorbs UV light but has a high transmission of IR light. They have become popular as shooting glasses and for downhill skiing on cloudy days. Some claim visual acuity is increased on foggy or cloudy days and in the early-morning hours. Theoretically, they cut through haze to render distant objects more visible.

Glass Color Coatings

Another method of obtaining a colored glass lens is through coating a clear lens. This is done by applying a metallic oxide to the lens front surface in a vacuum.

A major advantage to these coatings is that they are of uniform density, regardless of the power of the lens. Another plus is that any lens design can be coated. Color coating also makes gradient tinting available in glass.

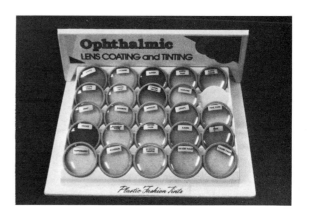

FIGURE 5-13—Plastic lens tints are available in a rainbow of colors and are often used to enhance the frame color to create a fashionable look.

A drawback of color-coated glass lenses is that they have a slight metallic reflection that some people find objectionable. Another disadvantage is that coated lenses tend to attract dust, lint, and grease, making it more difficult to keep the lenses clean.

Plastic Lens Dye-Bath Tinting

Plastic lenses are tinted by dipping them in a liquid dye bath. CR-39, polycarbonate, and most high-index plastic lenses can be tinted this way. The dye is heated in a double-boiler–type system. The dye penetrates the lens surfaces evenly so uniform density of color is achieved regardless of lens powers. The longer the lens remains in the dye, the darker the tint will be. This lens coloring method allows for gradient shades and also multiple colors in one lens. It also makes possible countless different colors of lenses because dyes can be mixed. Offices will have a sample tint selection to assist the patient in selecting the appropriate tint. Since plastic lens tints will fade over time, it is recommended that dyed plastic lenses be redyed yearly (Figure 5-13).

Lens colors can be changed, darkened, lightened, or removed should the patient find the initial tint undesirable.

Photochromic Lens Tints

Photochromic lenses change color when exposed to radiant energy, primarily, but not exclusively, the near UV rays. Photochromic lenses are available in glass or plastic (CR-39) lens materials.

PROPERTIES OF GLASS PHOTOCHROMIC LENSES

The color-changing performance of glass photochromic lenses is permanent. It will not fatigue or deteriorate over time. PhotoGrey Extra and PhotoBrown Extra, the most popular glass photochromic lenses, will darken in 60 seconds. They will also lighten over 75% of their range in 10 minutes. The main darkening force of photochromic lenses is UV light, but they will also react slightly to visible light. This means they will darken to some degree in brightly lit rooms and when flash photographs are being taken.

All photochromic lenses require a break-in period. It takes several exposures to the sun for the lenses to achieve their full darkness. This process usually takes approximately 2 weeks.

Photochromic lenses absorb UV light but do not absorb IR light. The tint in these lenses is not uniform in density; the color varies with the thickness of the lens. Photochromic glass lenses are available in a full range of prescription powers and lens designs. All batches of photochromic glass do not react exactly the same. A pair of lenses should always come from the same batch. Ordering single lens replacements could result in uneven tints between the two lenses. The lens is available in single-vision, straight-top, and progressive addition lens designs.

FORCES AFFECTING TRANSMITTANCE OF PHOTOCHROMIC GLASS

There is constant competition between the darkening and fading forces in photochromic glass. If the darkening forces outweigh the fading forces, the lenses are dark. If the fading forces dominate, the lenses are light.

Darkening forces	*Fading forces*
UV light energy	Visible red or IR light energy
More recent exposure	Less recent exposure
Colder	Warmer
Thicker	Thinner
Heat tempering	Chemical tempering

1. *Wavelengths of light*: The nature of the wavelengths of light affects transmission. UV light is the main darkening force.
2. *Recent exposure*: Photochromic lenses have an exposure memory. Lenses that have had more recent exposure to sunlight will darken faster than those with a less recent exposure history.
3. *Temperature*: For a given sunlight exposure, the colder the temperature, the darker the lens will get.
4. *Thickness*: The thicker the lens, the darker it will get for a given sunlight exposure.
5. *Tempering*: Chemical tempering is recommended for optical performance of all photochromic glass lenses. Chemical tempering causes a slight increase in the darkened transmission.

PLASTIC PHOTOCHROMIC LENS TINTS

The ophthalmic world has long awaited a plastic photochromic lens. There have been several attempts to market plastic photochromics, albeit mostly unsuccessful, because they just did not work well.

In March 1989, Rodenstock introduced to the United States the *Colormatic* plastic photochromic lens. The Colormatic lens is a light tan indoors with approximately 80% light transmission. With exposure to UV light, it changes to a medium gray tint that has an approximate transmission of 50%. Temperature is a factor in the color-changing performance—the colder the temperature, the darker the lens will get. This lens is not designed as a sun lens but rather as a comfort lens—a fashion tint that changes color and provides protection in bright glare producing situations.

Photocolors is another plastic photochromic lens with changeable tints in fashion colors. The colors are aquamarine, amethyst, and emerald. These lenses are almost clear indoors with approximately 86% light transmission. They darken to approximately 45% light transmission when exposed to UV energy. Similar to the Colormatic lens, they are also sensitive to temperature.

The color changing performance of these lenses does slowly wear out but will easily last for the normal life expectancy of a pair of lenses.

In January 1991, the *Transitions* photochromic plastic lens became available in single-vision, straight-top 28, and progressive addition lens designs. It was updated in November 1992 with the release of the *Transition Plus* lens. The Plus lens becomes darker outside and is less sensitive to temperature than its predecessor. The lens always returns fully to its light tan indoor color. The lens is marketed as a tint that will reduce glare and provide visual comfort in bright light situations. Transition lenses possess the following properties:

- Lightweight plastic
- Scratch resistance
- 100% UV absorption
- Medium to dark gray tint outdoors
- Light blush color indoors
- Automatic adjustment to light
- No darkening for flash photography
- Always fully lighten indoors and darken quickly when exposed to UV light

Transition lenses are a great general-use lens for patients who are wearing plastic lenses and would enjoy the added feature of a changeable tint.

As with all photochromic tints, Transition lenses react to UV light and temperature. In a temperature of 72°F, the lens reacts similarly to a PhotoGrey Extra glass photochromic. The colder the air temperature becomes, the more the lens will darken. In high-temperature situations, the lens will be slightly lighter. For example, at 95°F, the lens will darken to approximately 48% light transmission. The lens turns gray when exposed to UV light.

These lenses are lightweight, UV light absorbing to 380 nm, tintable, and scratch-resistant coated. Transition lenses lighten and darken uniformly, regardless of the lens power. This is because of the way the lenses are made. It is a process whereby a photochromic material is injected deeply within the front surface of a plastic lens. The color changing performance lasts for the life of the lens without noticeable differences in the color-changing capability.

Polarized Sun Lenses

The polarized lens is designed to eliminate glare reflected from flat surfaces. Some polarized sun lenses are made of films of polarizing material: mitrocellulose packed with ultramicroscopic crystals of herapathite, with optic axes parallel to each other. This material is laminated between clear or lightly tinted lenses. Other polarized lenses are made with the polarizing material molded in them. The polarized filter transmits approximately 37% of the incident light. When combined with a sun tint, the transmission drops to approximately 15%. The lens reduces glare from horizontal surfaces, such as highways, car bumpers, water, and snow.

Polarized lenses are available in glass and plastic, in shades of gray, green, and brown.

SUGGESTED READING

Brooks CW, Borish IM. System for Ophthalmic Dispensing (2nd ed). Boston: Butterworth-Heinemann, 1996.

6 / Neutralization and Verification

Gregory L. Stephens

One of the more important tasks commonly assigned to the paraoptometric is that of working with optical laboratories, which provide spectacle frames and lenses to the optometrist. All spectacles must be ordered properly, with the order written in such a manner that it is easily understood by laboratory personnel. In addition, all spectacles received from the optical laboratory should be examined (verified) for manufacturing accuracy. All lens powers must be within acceptable error tolerances. Frames, lens materials, multifocal types, and tints must match what was ordered. Although laboratory personnel usually check all spectacles before sending them to the optometrist, errors can occur, and in-office verification will prevent improperly made spectacles from reaching the patient. This chapter describes both the procedures to be followed when ordering spectacles and the procedures to be used when verifying spectacles made by the optical laboratory.

ORDERING FROM THE OPTICAL LABORATORY

Most optometrists order spectacles for their patients from local optical laboratories. Although many laboratories accept orders given by telephone, it is more common for the lens and frame parameters to be written on order forms that are then mailed or faxed to the laboratory. Each laboratory will have its own order form design, and individual forms are labeled with an invoice number that the laboratory uses to follow the order as it passes through the various manufacturing processes. In addition, the optometrist's name and address will usually be printed on the form. Most order forms are designed so that multiple copies are made when the order is written. One copy should always be kept at the optometrist's office for future reference.

Figure 6-1 illustrates a completed order for a pair of spectacles containing bifocal lenses. The order form is that of Benedict Optical of Lewisville, Texas, but it is representative of forms supplied by most optical laboratories. The following points should be noted when writing an order:

1. Writing must be legible, with all information printed in large, bold letters. It is best to use a ballpoint pen when writing the order so that all copies are readable.
2. Lens powers should usually be written in minus cylinder form, the standard used by optometrists to specify lens powers. Some laboratories prefer that plus cylinder form spectacle prescriptions be transposed to minus cylinder form before being written on the order form.
3. All lens powers should be written with two digits after the decimal point, and the sign must be included for both minus and plus powers. Lens powers between −1.00 and +1.00 diopters (D) should be written with a zero to the left of the decimal point (e.g., −0.25). The word plano or its abbreviation, pl., should be used rather than "0.00" to specify a lens with zero sphere power.
4. An order that includes prism must specify both the amount of prism in prism diopters (Δ) and the prism base direction.

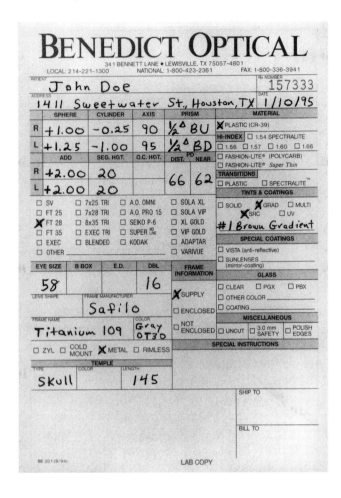

FIGURE 6-1—Completed order for a bifocal spectacle prescription. The laboratory supplies both the frame and lenses.

5. Both the distance and near interpupillary distances (PDs) must be included when ordering most multifocals. The exception is the progressive addition lens (PAL), which requires only split (monocular) distance PDs. Some order forms will not have a space for split PD information. In this case, write the split PDs in the PD box on the order form or in the special instructions section.

Some order forms require that the distance PD and the segment (seg) inset be provided, rather than the distance and near PDs, when ordering multifocals. Seg inset for each lens is equal to the following:

$$\frac{(\text{Distance PD} - \text{near PD})}{2}$$

For the example used in Figure 6-1, the seg inset for each lens is

$$\frac{(66 - 62)}{2} = 2 \text{ mm}$$

Only the distance PD is needed when ordering most single-vision (nonmultifocal) spectacles. The near PD is used by itself only when ordering single-vision reading glasses.

6. A number of other parameters must also be specified when ordering a multifocal lens. These include segment type (a D-28 bifocal), segment height (20 mm), and add power (+2.00 D for each lens). PALs are usually ordered by trade name (e.g., Sola XL [Sola Optical USA, Inc., Petaluma, CA], Varilux Comfort [Varilux Corp. Oldsmar, FL]). The fitting height (bottom of box to center of pupil) information for a PAL may be placed in the seg height box.

7. The lens material (glass, plastic, or high index plastic of specific index of refraction or trade name) and any lens tint or coating must be included. Most plastic lens tints require two specifications: the color of the tint and a measure of the tint transmittance (#1, #2, #3, or #4). A gradient tint is one that lightens toward the bottom of the lens. Many order forms use the terms "clear" or "white" if a lens is to be ordered without a tint.

8. Special impact resistance or thickness requirements can be included if needed. All spectacle lenses manufactured for everyday use (dress lenses) must meet impact resistance requirements as required by the U.S. Food and Drug Administration (FDA). Specifically, a lens must be able to withstand the impact of a ⅝-inch steel ball dropped 50 inches onto its front surface (the drop-ball test). Most lenses must be approximately 2 mm thick to meet this standard, although the FDA has no specific thickness requirement. Polycarbonate and some of the high-index plastics can be made with center thicknesses as low as 1 mm in minus powers and still meet impact resistance requirements.

Spectacle lenses used for industrial or occupational eye protection must meet a more stringent impact resistance test (a 1-inch steel ball dropped 50 inches onto the lens front surface), as required by the U.S. Occupational Safety and Health Administration (OSHA). OSHA also requires that industrial lenses have a minimum thickness of 3 mm. (High plus power lenses may have a minimum thickness of 2.5 mm.)

Most order forms contain a section for specifying impact-resistance requirements. Often, the form lists impact resistance as either "2 mm" or "3 mm." Circling or checking 2 mm implies that the lenses are for everyday (dress) use, although the lenses will not necessarily be 2 mm thick. Circling or checking 3 mm implies that the lenses are to meet the more rigorous standards for industrial eye protection. The term *dress* or *industrial* may also be used on some forms. Center thickness information can be written in the "special instructions" section of the form. The form shown in Figure 6-1 has a box only for 3-mm thick (industrial) lenses. If this box is not checked, the laboratory assumes that the lenses will be for everyday use, and the lenses will meet the FDA dress requirements.

9. When a spectacle frame is to be part of the order, both the frame name and manufacturer must be included. This is done to prevent confusion, since the same frame name may be used by a number of manufacturers.
10. It is common in today's marketplace for the optometrist to buy spectacle frames directly from the manufacturer, then ship the frame to the optical laboratory. To prevent confusion, the type of order should be indicated on the order form. Terms commonly found on order forms to describe the order include *frame enclosed*, *frame to come*, *supply frame*, *lenses only*, and *frame only*.

The order shown in Figure 6-2 is for a pair of temples only. The most important point to note is that no unnecessary information has been supplied. Lens powers are not needed to order a pair of temples, nor is frame eyesize or bridge size needed. The order has also been clearly marked so that laboratory personnel will know that only temples are being ordered. By providing just the needed information, it is less likely that an error will occur when the order is filled.

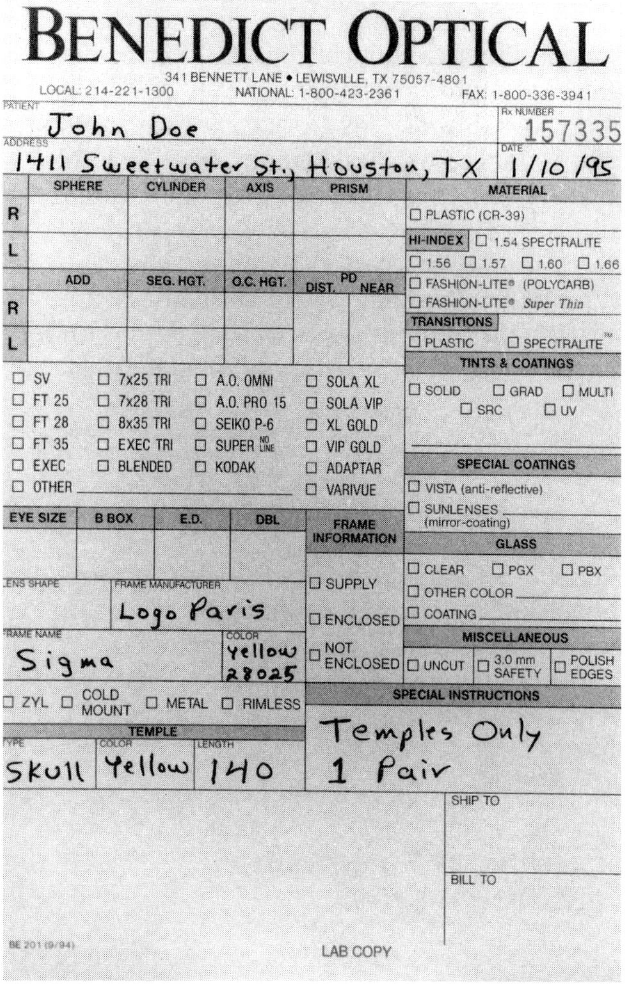
BENEDICT OPTICAL
341 BENNETT LANE • LEWISVILLE, TX 75057-4801
LOCAL: 214-221-1300 NATIONAL: 1-800-423-2361 FAX: 1-800-336-3941
PATIENT: John Doe
Rx NUMBER: 157335
ADDRESS: 1411 Sweetwater St., Houston, TX
DATE: 1/10/95
SPHERE | CYLINDER | AXIS | PRISM
R
L
ADD | SEG. HGT. | O.C. HGT. | PD DIST. NEAR
R
L
MATERIAL
☐ PLASTIC (CR-39)
HI-INDEX ☐ 1.54 SPECTRALITE
☐ 1.56 ☐ 1.57 ☐ 1.60 ☐ 1.66
☐ FASHION-LITE® (POLYCARB)
☐ FASHION-LITE® Super Thin
TRANSITIONS
☐ PLASTIC ☐ SPECTRALITE™
TINTS & COATINGS
☐ SOLID ☐ GRAD ☐ MULTI
☐ SRC ☐ UV
☐ SV ☐ 7x25 TRI ☐ A.O. OMNI ☐ SOLA XL
☐ FT 25 ☐ 7x28 TRI ☐ A.O. PRO 15 ☐ SOLA VIP
☐ FT 28 ☐ 8x35 TRI ☐ SEIKO P-6 ☐ XL GOLD
☐ FT 35 ☐ EXEC TRI ☐ SUPER NO LINE ☐ VIP GOLD
☐ EXEC ☐ BLENDED ☐ KODAK ☐ ADAPTAR
☐ OTHER ☐ VARIVUE
SPECIAL COATINGS
☐ VISTA (anti-reflective)
☐ SUNLENSES (mirror-coating)
EYE SIZE | B BOX | E.D. | DBL
FRAME INFORMATION
☐ SUPPLY
☐ ENCLOSED
☐ NOT ENCLOSED
GLASS
☐ CLEAR ☐ PGX ☐ PBX
☐ OTHER COLOR
☐ COATING
LENS SHAPE
FRAME MANUFACTURER: Logo Paris
FRAME NAME: Sigma
COLOR: Yellow 28025
MISCELLANEOUS
☐ UNCUT ☐ 3.0 mm SAFETY ☐ POLISH EDGES
☐ ZYL ☐ COLD MOUNT ☐ METAL ☐ RIMLESS
SPECIAL INSTRUCTIONS: Temples Only 1 Pair
TEMPLE
TYPE: Skull COLOR: Yellow LENGTH: 140
SHIP TO
BILL TO
BE 201 (9/94)
LAB COPY

FIGURE 6-2—Completed order for a pair of temples.

PRINCIPLES OF LENSOMETRY

The instrument used to measure the power of spectacle lenses is the *lensometer*, or *focimeter*. This instrument measures the sphere power, cylinder power, and cylinder axis of a lens, the amount of prism in a lens and the orientation (base direction) of that prism, the location of the prism reference point of a lens, and the powers of multifocal adds. *Focimeter* is actually the most general term for an instrument that measures lens power, but *lensometer* will be used throughout this chapter because it is the more commonly accepted terminology. Trade names for lensometers include Lensometer (American Optical Corp., Southbridge, MA), Lensmeter

(Marco Ophthalmic, Inc., Jacksonville, FL; Topcon America Corp., Paramus, NJ), Vertometer (Reichert Ophthalmic Instruments, a Division of Leica, Inc., Buffalo, NY), Vertexometer (Nikon, Inc., Torrance, CA), and Lens Analyzer (Humphrey Instruments, Inc., San Leandro, CA). Rather than discuss each type of lensometer separately, the operation of a "generic" lensometer will be described in detail. Where differences among instruments are important for proper understanding, these differences will be described and illustrated.

Parts of a Lensometer

Figure 6-3 illustrates the parts common to most lensometers. In the following discussion, a number in parentheses will be included when a specific lensometer part is mentioned for the first time. This number can be matched to the numbered parts in the figure.

Lensometer Focus and Calibration Check

1. Turn the power switch (1) on. A pilot light (2) will indicate that the lensometer has power.
2. Focus the eyepiece (3). Look into the eyepiece and blur the reticle (the set of black rings, as shown in Figure 6-4) by turning the eyepiece end counterclockwise. It may be easier to see the reticle lines if a piece of white paper is held in front of the lens stop (4). The lens holder (5) can be moved out of the way if necessary.

    Next, slowly turn the eyepiece clockwise until the reticle lines are just sharply focused. Do not turn past the point at which a sharp focus is first obtained. The eyepiece is now properly focused.

    An eyepiece focus position scale (6) is found on most lensometers. If the position of this scale is noted when the eyepiece is first focused (Figure 6-5), the scale can be returned to this position after someone has changed the eyepiece focus, and it will not be necessary to repeat the eyepiece focusing procedure.

    Focusing the eyepiece is an important step and must always be performed when first using a lensometer or when using a lensometer after someone else has used it. If the eyepiece is not properly focused, significant measurement errors can occur. In addition, if the eyepiece is focused improperly (turned past the point at which a sharp reticle focus is first obtained), accommodation will be required to keep the reticle clear, and this can be tiring when the lensometer is used for long periods of time.
3. Check the power calibration. Rotate the power wheel (7) into the plus, to approximately +4.00 D on the scale. (The power wheel of most lensometers is a large wheel labeled with power in diopters. Black numbers usually indicate plus power and red numbers minus power. Some lensometers may also have an internal power scale. This scale is viewed by looking into the eyepiece.) Next, while looking through the eyepiece at the lensometer target, slowly rotate the power wheel back toward the zero power position until the target is just sharply in focus (Figure 6-6). (Do not oscillate the power wheel back and forth on each side of the focus to find the best position of focus. This could cause measurement errors.) If the lensometer is in proper calibration and the eyepiece has been properly focused, the power scale should now read zero.

    If the power wheel does not read zero when the target is sharply focused, repeat the eyepiece-focusing procedure. Then perform the power calibration procedure again. If the power wheel still does not read zero when the target lines are in focus, the instrument is out of calibration and future power readings must be corrected for this error. For example, if the target lines focus at +0.25 D on the power wheel scale when the calibration procedure is performed, 0.25 D must be subtracted from all future lens power readings to correct for this calibration error. A lens power reading of –2.50 D would thus be corrected to –2.75 D.

    The lensometer calibration procedure should be performed periodically to insure that the instrument stays in calibration. Loss of calibration is uncommon.

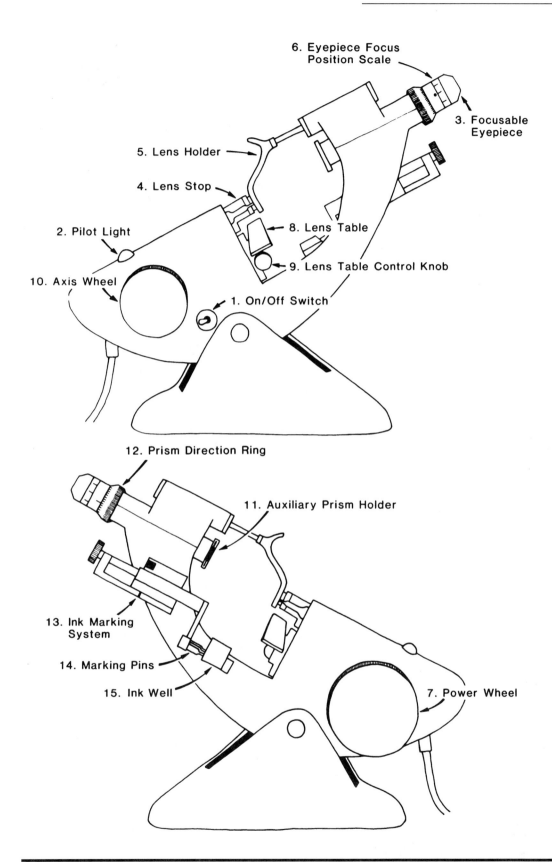

FIGURE 6-3—Two views of a generic lensometer. Part numbers correspond to those used in the text.

110 Chapter 6

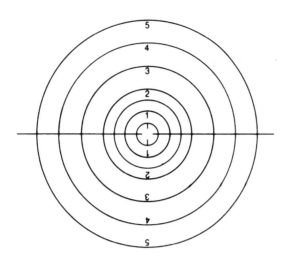

FIGURE 6-4—A typical eyepiece reticle.

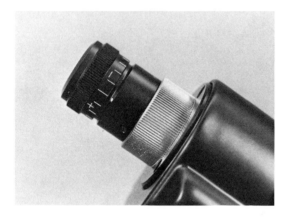

FIGURE 6-5—Eyepiece focus position scale. Consider the long line to be the zero position of the eyepiece and each short line a step of ±1 unit. Record the eyepiece position relative to the small white dot.

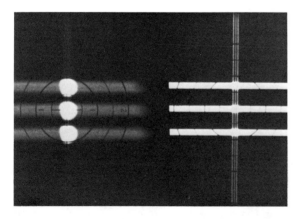

FIGURE 6-6—Left. Out-of-focus lensometer target. Right. Target in sharp focus.

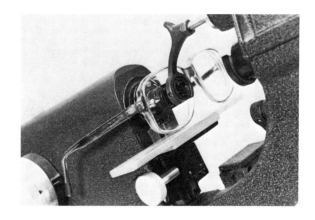

FIGURE 6-7—Proper positioning of spectacles on the lens stop.

Measuring the Distance Power of Single-Vision and Multifocal Lenses

1. Position the spectacles on the lens stop. Place the back (concave) surface of the lens to be measured against the stop (temples pointed away from the eyepiece). Move the lens table up or down using its control lever or knob (8 and 9), until the lens is approximately centered on the lens stop and the bottoms of both eyewires are touching the lens table. Lower the lens holder gently against the lens to hold the lens in position. Figure 6-7 illustrates proper positioning.

   Note: If the lens is a bifocal or trifocal, the uppermost portion of the lens (the portion used for distance vision) should be in front of the lens stop. Stay away from the segments (add portions) for the time being.

2. Attempt to focus the target. Turn the power wheel into the plus (more plus than the power of the lens), then slowly rotate the wheel back toward the minus until the lensometer target begins to come into focus. If necessary, lift the lens holder slightly off the lens and move the lens around on the lens stop to center the target on the reticle (see Figure 6-6B). Always remember to move the lens table back against the bottoms of the frame eyewires.

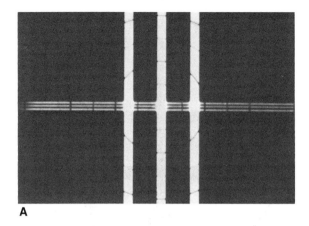
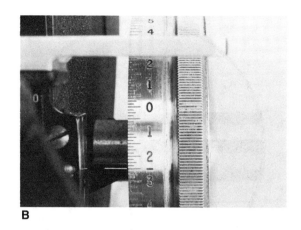

FIGURE 6-8—Power measurement for a sphere lens. A. The two sets of target lines are both sharply focused. B. The power wheel reading at the scale pointer is –2.50 D.

If both sets of lines making up the target (the closely spaced set and the widely spaced set) sharply focus at the same time, the lens is a spherical power (sphere) lens. If both sets of target lines cannot be focused at the same time, the lens is a spherocylinder. The two types of lenses are measured using slightly different methods.

3. When a lens is a sphere, both the closely spaced set and the widely spaced set of target lines will focus at the same time. The power of the lens is the power wheel reading when the entire target is in focus. (The lens has no cylinder power, so the axis wheel can be ignored.) Figure 6-8 provides an example. Both sets of target lines are sharply focused at –2.50 on the scale. The lens power is recorded as –2.50, –2.50 sph., or –2.50 D.S. As previously mentioned, power is recorded with two digits after the decimal point, and the sign is always included, "–" for minus powers, "+" for plus powers. The abbreviation D.S. (diopter sphere) or sph. (sphere) indicates that the lens is spherical, not a spherocylinder.

The power wheel scale shown in Figure 6-8 is graduated in steps of ⅛ D for powers between ±3.00 D and in steps of ¼ D for higher powers. Power should always be measured to the nearest ⅛ D (0.12 D), however. For example, the scale gradations between –2.00 D and –3.00 D correspond to the following power readings:

```
_____ –2.00
    _____ –2.12
_____ –2.25
    _____ –2.37
_____ –2.50
    _____ –2.62
    _____ –2.75
    _____ –2.87
_____ –3.00
```

The numbers to the right of the decimal point are standard for specifying lens powers in steps of ⅛ D. No other numbers should be used. If the power wheel scale reads zero, power should be recorded as "plano," or its abbreviation, pl.

4. The two sets of target lines cannot be focused at the same time when measuring the power of a spherocylinder. It is therefore necessary to focus first one set of lines, then the other; however, the lines must be focused in a specific order. The more closely spaced set of target lines will be termed the *sphere lines*, and the more widely spaced set will be the *cylinder lines*. Figure 6-9 illustrates targets for the most commonly used lensometers, with the sphere and cylinder lines labeled.

Rotate the power wheel into the plus (more plus than the lens power), then slowly

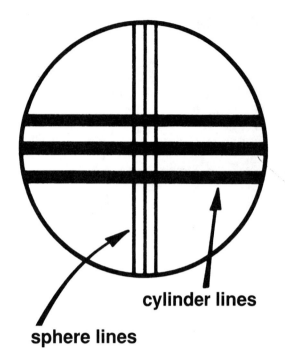
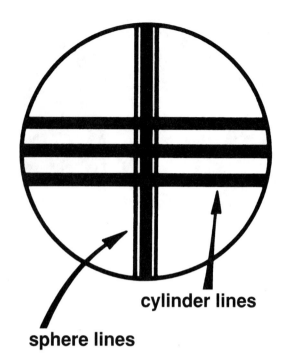

FIGURE 6-9—Target lines for some of the more commonly used lensometers. The three closely spaced lines are the sphere lines. The three more widely spaced lines are the cylinder lines. The target on the left is found in the Reichert Vertometer, some Nikon Vertexometers, and the Marco Lensmeter. The target on the right is that of the American Optical Lensometer.

decrease the power until one set of target lines starts to focus. If the lines appear broken (Figure 6-10) or if the cylinder lines are in focus, rotate the cylinder axis wheel (10) until the sphere lines (the more closely spaced set of lines) are in focus and appear unbroken (Figure 6-11). The sphere power of the lens will be the power reading at which the sphere lines focus. Measure to the nearest ⅛ D.

Continue to rotate the power wheel in the minus power direction until the cylinder lines focus sharply (Figure 6-12). (DO NOT move the axis wheel.) The algebraic difference between the power wheel reading with the sphere lines in focus and the power wheel reading with the cylinder lines in focus is the amount of cylinder power. This difference is given a minus sign, so lens power is always written in minus cylinder form.

Read the cylinder axis from the axis wheel.

A key point: The cylinder lines must focus at a more minus power reading than the sphere lines. If the cylinder lines are the first (more plus) focus, rotate the cylinder axis wheel by 90 degrees. The sphere lines will then become the more plus focus.

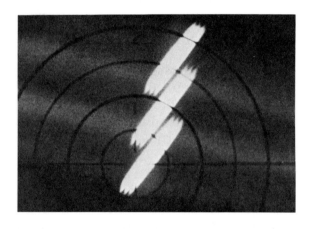

FIGURE 6-10—When measuring the power of a spherocylinder lens, both sets of target lines will not focus sharply at the same time. Here, the sphere lines are in focus, but the target lines appear broken because the cylinder axis is not set correctly.

Example 1 (see Figures 6-11 and 6-12)

When measuring the power of a right lens, the target sphere lines focus at +3.25 D, with the cylinder axis wheel at 90 degrees. The cylinder

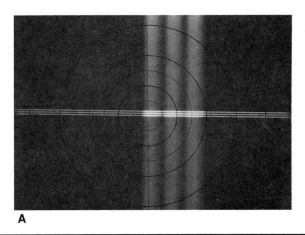 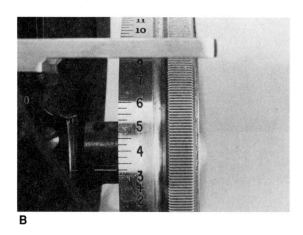

FIGURE 6-11—A. Sphere lines are in proper focus and appear unbroken because the cylinder axis wheel has been positioned correctly. B. Power wheel reading +3.25 D, at which the sphere lines focus. This is the lens sphere power.

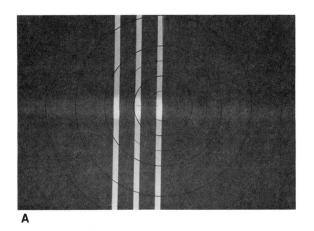 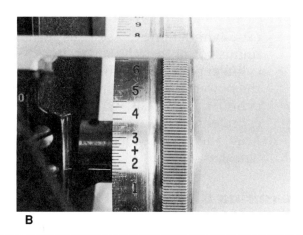

FIGURE 6-12—A. Cylinder lines are unbroken and in sharp focus. B. Power wheel reading +1.75 D, at which the lines focus. The lens cylinder power is the difference between the power wheel readings at which the sphere and cylinder lines focus.

lines focus at +1.75 D (without changing the cylinder axis). The difference of the two readings is 1.50. The lens power (using the standard method of recording in minus cylinder form) is

O.D. +3.25 −1.50 x 090

The first number is the lens sphere power, the second the cylinder power, and the last the cylinder axis. The lowercase "x" is the abbreviation for axis.

To summarize, the following steps are used to measure the power of a lens in minus cylinder form:

1. Focus the eyepiece and check the power calibration.
2. Mount the lens with its back surface against the lens stop. Hold the lens in position with the lens holder and lens table.
3. Turn the power wheel into the plus, then decrease the power until either the entire target or one set of target lines focuses.
4. If both sets of target lines focus at the same time, the lens is a sphere. Read the lens power from the power scale.
5. If both sets of target lines cannot be focused at the same time, the lens is a spherocylinder.
   a. Turn the power wheel into the plus, then decrease power until the target begins to focus.
   b. Rotate the cylinder axis until the sphere lines are unbroken and are the more plus focus. The sphere power will be the power at which the sphere lines focus.
   c. Continue to rotate the power wheel into the minus until the cylinder lines focus.

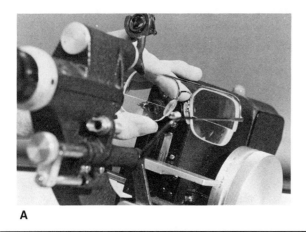 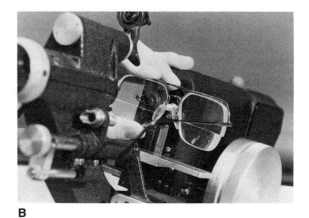

FIGURE 6-13—Measurement of bifocal add power. The lens front surface must be against the lens stop. A. Lens position for first power measurement, above the bifocal line. B. Lens position for second power measurement, below the bifocal line.

(The cylinder lines must focus at a more minus power than the sphere lines.) The cylinder power is the difference between the powers for the sphere line focus and cylinder line focus, written in minus cylinder form.

d. Read the cylinder axis from the axis wheel.

Measuring Bifocal Add Powers

A bifocal lens has two areas of different power, the major (upper) portion of the lens, usually used for distance vision, and the segment in the lower part of the lens, usually used for near vision. The power of the distance portion is measured as was previously described. The power of the segment is expressed as an addition or "add" over the distance portion power and is measured using a different procedure.

1. Turn the spectacles around so that the front (convex) surface of the lens is against the lens stop. Position the lens so that its distance portion is in front of the stop (Figure 6-13A). Hold the lens in position with the lens holder and lens table.
2. Focus one set of target lines and note the power wheel reading at which the lines focus. (It is generally recommended that the more vertical target lines be the ones focused.) The target lines must be unbroken. Rotate the cylinder axis wheel, if necessary, to obtain unbroken target lines.
3. Move the lens upward so the bifocal segment is in front of the lens stop (Figure 6-13B) and hold the lens in position with the lens holder. Turn the power wheel toward the plus, and focus the **same** set of target lines that was focused in the previous step. Note the power wheel reading that focuses the lines.
4. The bifocal add power is the difference of the two power readings. Record to the nearest ⅛ D, with two digits after the decimal point. Be sure to include the plus sign. (The add will always be a plus power.)

Example 2

The distance portion power of a right bifocal lens (measured with the lens back surface against the lens stop) is +5.00 –0.75 x 090. The spectacles are then turned around, with the front surface against the lens stop, for measurement of add power. With the distance portion of the lens in front of the lens stop, the more vertical lines focus at +4.75 D. With the segment (the lower portion of the lens) in front of the lens stop, the same set of target lines focuses at +7.12 D. The difference of the two readings is 2.37 D. The lens power is

O.D. +5.00 –0.75 x 090

+2.37 Add

Measuring Trifocal Add and Intermediate Powers

A trifocal lens has three areas of different power: (1) the distance portion, which is usually the

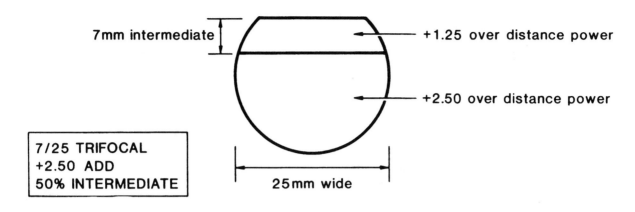

FIGURE 6-14—Measurement of trifocal add and intermediate powers. The add power of each segment is measured as for a bifocal. The lens add power, however, is considered to be the add power of the lower segment (+2.50 D). The add power of the intermediate (+1.25 D) is expressed as a percentage (50%) of the lower segment add power.

upper largest part of the lens; (2) the near portion, the lower of the two segments and which has the most plus power; and (3) the intermediate portion, which is usually a segment just above the near portion and which has a power between that of the distance and near portions. The distance portion power is measured with the back surface of the lens against the lens stop, as usual, and its power is written in minus cylinder form. The add powers of the near and intermediate portions are measured in the same manner as for a bifocal. First, turn the spectacles around so the lens front surface is against the lens stop. Next, focus the more vertical target lines through the lens distance portion and then through each segment. The near add power is the difference of the distance focus and the near focus. The intermediate add power is the difference of the distance focus and the intermediate focus. The add power of the intermediate segment is not recorded directly, however. Instead, the intermediate portion add power is expressed as a percentage of the near add power.

Example 3

The add powers of a trifocal lens are to be determined. The lens is turned around on the lensometer so that the lens front surface is against the lens stop. With the distance portion in front of the lens stop, the more vertical target lines focus at +1.00 D. Through the intermediate portion, the same set of lines focuses at +2.25 D. With the near portion in front of the lens stop, the same set focuses at +3.50 D. The add power is +2.50 D (the difference of the distance and add). The intermediate add power is +1.25 D. Since this value is one-half (50%) of the near add of +2.50 D, the lens is said to have a 50% intermediate. Figure 6-14 illustrates this example.

Measuring Aphakic (Cataract) Lenses

The procedures that have been described for measuring the powers of single-vision and bifocal lenses are also used to measure the powers of aphakic or cataract lenses, the high plus power spectacle lenses worn by some patients after cataract surgery. The powers of aphakic lenses can be more accurately measured if a little extra care is used in making measurements. First, all power measurements made through the distance portion should be made with the targets close to the center of the reticle. Move the lens around as necessary to center the targets. Second, power measurements made through the segment should be made as close to the top of the segment as possible. This decreases prism that might otherwise deflect the targets out of the field of view and require the use of auxiliary prism. Third, the lens must be absolutely flat against the lens stop whenever a power measurement is made. If the lens tilts, large power measurement errors can occur.

Because of prismatic effects in these lenses, however, it is often very difficult to find and focus the target lines when the segment is positioned in front of the lens stop. In fact, because of the prismatic effects, the target may not be visible at all. When this occurs, the tar-

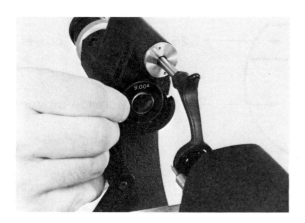

FIGURE 6-15—Placement of a 9Δ auxiliary prism in its holder behind the eyepiece. Prism base direction is changed by rotating the prism in the holder.

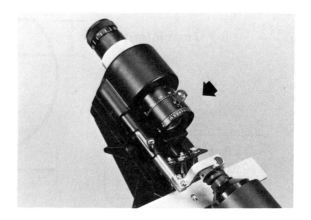

FIGURE 6-16—Permanent Risley auxiliary prism (arrow) behind the eyepiece. Prism is added or removed by rotating the knob. Prism base direction is varied by changing the orientation of the knob.

get must be moved back into view using auxiliary prism.

Auxiliary prism is available in two forms. Loose auxiliary prisms of various powers are supplied with many lensometers. These prisms, in round holders, fit into a slot just behind the eyepiece (Figure 6-15, and see Figure 6-3, number 11). Risley auxiliary prisms are an option for other lensometers. A Risley prism is a variable power prism permanently mounted on the back of the eyepiece (Figure 6-16).

Auxiliary prisms are used if the target cannot be found while measuring the add power of an aphakic lens. If the lensometer does not have a Risley prism, select a loose auxiliary prism of about 6Δ, and place it in its holder on the eyepiece. Rotate the prism in its holder while attempting to focus the target lines. As the prism is rotated, the target will move closer to the reticle center, and when this happens, the target lines can be focused. If the auxiliary prism chosen does not deflect the targets close enough to the reticle center, a prism of different power should be tried. It is not necessary to record the power of the auxiliary prism used.

To use Risley prism when measuring aphakic lens add powers, add prism power by rotating the knob on the Risley prism until the target lines are centered on the reticle. (Vary the direction of the prism added, if necessary, by changing the orientation of the knob.) The target lines can then be easily focused. With practice it should be possible to quickly add prism of the proper amount and direction and center targets that were completely out of the field of view.

Power Measurement with Other Lensometers

A few lensometers have targets differing significantly from those previously described. Some of these targets are shown in Figures 6-17, 6-18, and 6-19. The targets of Figures 6-17 and 6-18 can be used as previously described if the shorter lines are considered to be the sphere lines (the more plus focus) and the longer set the cylinder lines (the more minus focus).

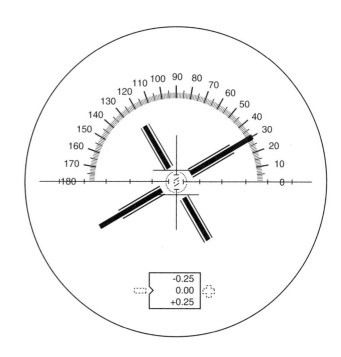

FIGURE 6-17—The target of one model of Nikon Vertexometer. The shorter set of lines (oriented at 120 degrees in the figure) are the sphere lines and must be the more plus focus. The longer set of lines, the cylinder lines, must be the more minus focus. (Courtesy of Nikon, Inc., Torrance, CA.)

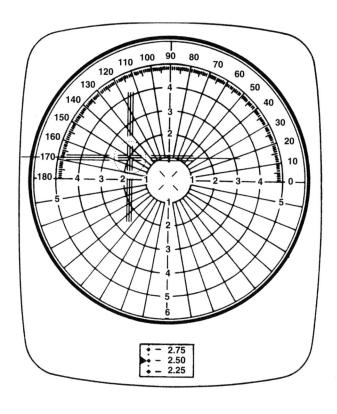

FIGURE 6-18—The target of a Nikon Projection Vertexometer. The sphere lines are the shorter set of lines and must be the more plus focus. The cylinder lines, the more minus focus, are the longer set (the set with the long middle line). (Courtesy of Nikon, Inc., Torrance, CA.)

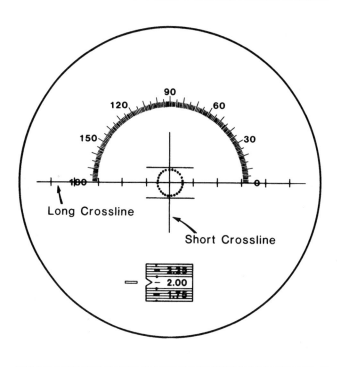

FIGURE 6-19—An example of a corona-and-crossline target. The circle of dots is focused by the power wheel. The short and long crosslines are part of the reticle.

The target of Figure 6-19 is a ring of dots. (This target is often termed a *corona-and-crossline target*.) When a spherical power lens is measured, the target will focus as a ring of dots. When a spherocylinder lens is measured, the dots elongate to form a series of lines. The more plus focus will be the lens sphere power. At the more minus focus, the lines will orient 90 degrees from their first focus. As usual, the difference of the two focus values is the cylinder power.

Measurement of cylinder axis requires the use of the long crossline, which is part of the reticle. At the more minus focus, the long crossline is rotated until it is parallel to the focused target lines. Cylinder axis can then be read from the scale inside the eyepiece. This type of lensometer does not have an axis wheel.

Power Measurement with Automatic Lensometers

An automatic lensometer measures the power of a lens at the touch of a button, with no need to focus a target. All the operator must do is properly position the lens. Automatic lensometers measure powers quickly, and operator measurement errors are minimized. Automatic lensometers, however, tend to be much more expensive than standard lensometers, which has somewhat limited their use.

Lens positioning for an automatic lensometer is similar to that of a standard lensometer (Figure 6-20). The back (concave) surface of the lens is placed against the lens stop. It is usually not necessary to put the lens front surface against the lens stop for add power measurements, however. Some automatic lensometers also record lens positioning as the shift is made from the right to the left lens so that PD measurements are automatically calculated.

Most automatic lensometers can print the results of measurements (Figure 6-21). Care must be exercised when interpreting prism readings, since the amount of prism measured will vary with position on the lens. This topic is discussed more fully in the section on measuring prism.

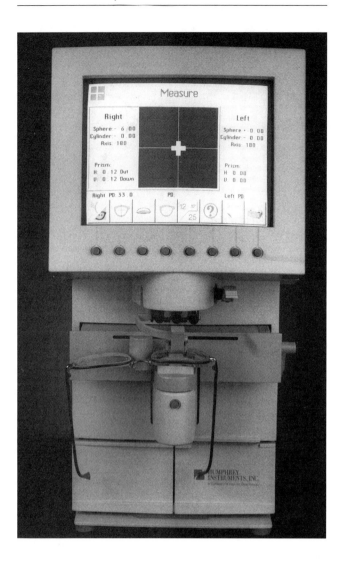

```
           HUMPHREY INSTRUMENTS
           LA  360      SEQ    02

Name _____

Date _____

RIGHT SPH  :   - 0.50
        CYL :   - 1.50    X   112°
        ADD :   + 1.50
   PSM HOR :     0.00     IN
        VER :     0.00    UP

LEFT SPH   :   - 0.50
        CYL :   - 1.50    X   82°
        ADD :   + 1.50
   PSM HOR :     0.00     OUT
        VER :     0.00    UP

NET PSM H  :     0.00
         V :     0.00

PD: 58.0

      (R  30.5   +   L  27.5)
```

FIGURE 6-21—Humphrey Lens Analyzer lens power printout.

FIGURE 6-20—Proper positioning of spectacles in a Humphrey Lens Analyzer, a type of automatic lensometer.

Automatic lensometers are simpler to use than nonautomated versions, but some operator skill is still required. Most important, if the spectacle lens to be measured is not flat against the lens stop, the tilt can create measurement errors. Holding the lens in position with the lens holder helps to avoid this error. High-index lens materials can cause problems because the color aberrations of these materials affect measurement accuracy. Many of the newer automatic lensometers can correct for this error if the operator indicates the index of refraction of the material being measured. Tinted lenses may also cause measurement difficulties. It may not be possible to measure dark sunglass lenses with some automatic lensometers.

Measuring Prism

Once lens powers have been measured, the accuracy of the positioning of the lenses in the frame, or the amount of prism in each lens, can be determined. Measurement of prism is more difficult than measurement of power. The amount of prism is different at different points on a lens, and usually only one point on a lens will have no prism (the optical center). In addition, the patient's PD must be taken into account when measuring prism.

Prism is specified by its magnitude or amount in prism diopters and also by its direction. The direction of a prism is given by the orientation of its base, either base in (BI), base

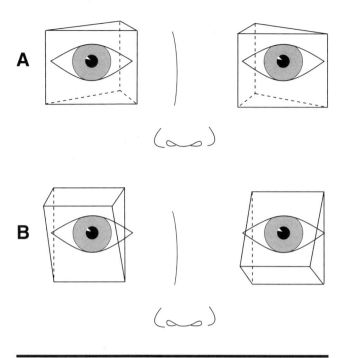

FIGURE 6-22—Prism base directions are specified relative to the eye. A. Base-in prism is present in front of both the right and the left eye. B. The prism for the right eye is base up, whereas that for the left eye is base down.

out (BO), base up (BU), or base down (BD). These directions are specified relative to the eye, with base in and base out referring to prisms having their bases oriented nasally and temporally, respectively. For the example shown in Figure 6-22A, the prism in front of each eye is base in, since the base of each prism is oriented toward the patient's nose. The prism of Figure 6-22B is base up in front of the right eye and base down in front of the left.

The amount of prism in a lens is measured using the lensometer reticle, with the lens back surface against the lens stop. Prism deflects the lensometer target away from the center of the reticle, and the reticle rings measure the amount of deflection in units of prism diopters. One reticle design is illustrated in Figure 6-23. For this design, the innermost ring marks 0.5∆ of deflection from the reticle center, the outermost ring 5∆. The ring progression is thus (from innermost to outermost) 0.5, 1, 1.5, 2, 3, 4, and 5∆.

The long horizontal line (crossline) of the reticle can be rotated to different positions

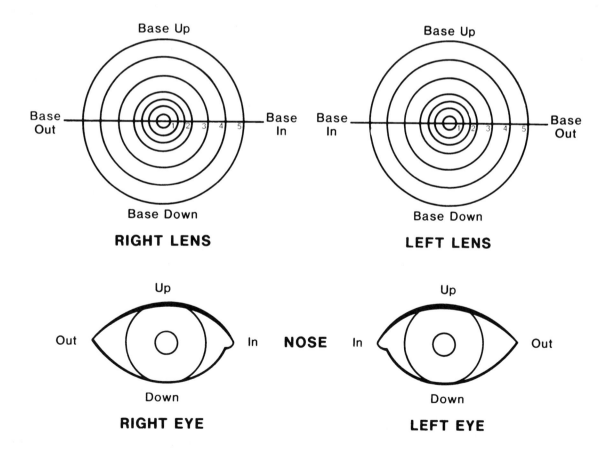

FIGURE 6-23—Specification of prism orientation in the lensometer. Prism deflects the target in the direction of the prism base, and base direction is specified relative to the eye.

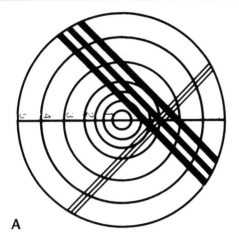 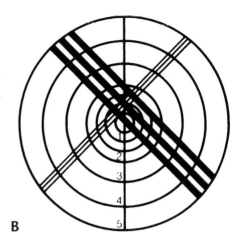

FIGURE 6-24—Examples of prismatic deflection, assuming that a right lens is being measured. A. 2Δ base in. B. 1Δ base up.

using the prism direction ring (see Figure 6-3, number 12) on the outside of the eyepiece. The angular position of this crossline is indicated by a scale either on the outside of the eyepiece or on the reticle itself.

Prism deflects the target of all lensometers in the direction of the prism base. The base direction, at least for horizontal prism, depends on whether a right or a left lens is being measured (see Figure 6-23). For example, if a right lens is being measured, target deflection toward the left side of the reticle (toward the temporal or outer portion of the lens as it is mounted on the lens stop) means that base-out prism is being measured. If a left lens is being measured and the target is deflected to the left side of the reticle, the prism direction is base in, toward the nasal or inner part of the lens. Base-up prism deflects the targets upward; base-down prism deflects the targets downward on the reticle, regardless of whether a right or left lens is being measured.

Figure 6-24 presents examples of prism measurement. Assuming that a right lens is being measured and that the lens is properly positioned on the lens stop, the target of Figure 6-24A has been deflected to the 2Δ BI position. The center of the lensometer target (where the middle sphere line crosses the middle cylinder line) is at the 2Δ ring, and the deflection is to the right, which is nasally or inward for a right lens. Figure 6-24B illustrates the target position when 1Δ of base-up prism is present. Note that the reticle crossline has been rotated to a vertical position to make the measurement of vertical prism easier.

At times, it may be necessary to measure prism when the target is deflected both vertically and horizontally. The preferred method of measurement is to resolve the two prisms into their vertical and horizontal components. Figure 6-25 provides an example. Assuming this drawing to be the lensometer view for a right lens, the target is deflected both upward and nasally—that is, a combination of base-up and base-in prism is present. The amounts of each component are determined by projecting the center of the lensometer target (dropping perpendiculars) to the horizontal and vertical, as shown by the dotted lines in the figure. The deflections along the horizontal and vertical are measured to the nearest ¼ or ⅓Δ. For this example, the target deflection is a combination of 2.5Δ BU and 3.5Δ BI. The prism would be recorded as follows:

O.D. 2.5Δ BU ◯ 3.5Δ BI.

(◯ means "combined with.")

A spectacle prescription is usually designed so that each prism reference point (PRP) (also termed *major reference point*, or MRP) is centered laterally on the patient's pupil. The patient will then be looking through the proper amount of horizontal prism (base in or base out) when looking straight ahead. Lateral PRP positions are

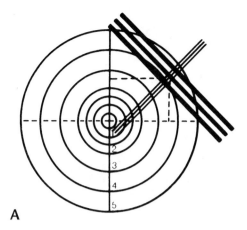
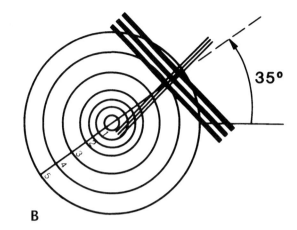

FIGURE 6-25—Prism measurement when both vertical and horizontal prism are present. A. The target deflection is resolved into its horizontal and vertical components. Assuming that a right lens is being measured, the deflection is 3.5Δ base in, 2.5Δ base up. B. Target deflection is specified as an amount in an angular direction. Assuming a right lens is being measured, the deflection is 4.25Δ base up and base in at 35 degrees.

specified on the order form by the patient's PD. If no prism is prescribed (the usual case), the optical center, the point with no prism, will be the PRP. The optical centers of the two lenses will then be separated by the patient's PD if the spectacles are correctly made.

Vertical PRP positions are not commonly specified when writing orders for spectacle lenses. In most cases the laboratory will place the PRP or optical center at the same height in both lenses. When a specific vertical PRP position is desired, it is given on the order form as a "level PRP" or "optical center height." The *level PRP* is the vertical distance from the lowest part of the lens bevel at the bottom of the lens (the bottom of the boxing system box, as described in the next section) to the PRP position. The optometrist or paraoptometric, when measuring a level PRP, usually tries to position each PRP 3–5 mm below the center of the pupil.

THE BOXING SYSTEM

Adopted in 1962 as a voluntary standard by the optical manufacturing industry, the boxing system is used for specifying the sizes of most spectacle lenses and frames made today. A brief description of the boxing system is presented here.

All boxing system measurements are made to the tips of the lens bevel (the bevel apex) or to

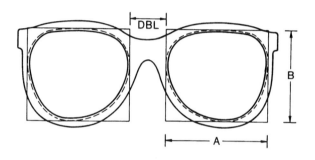

FIGURE 6-26—The boxing dimensions of a frame or of lenses mounted in a frame. The dashed lines surrounding each lens opening represent the tips of the lens bevels. The bevel tips usually extend approximately 0.5 mm into the frame.

the tips of the groove on the inside of the frame eyewire (Figure 6-26). The "A" dimension of a frame or lens, or the *frame eyesize*, is the largest horizontal distance across the lens or eyewire opening as measured between the two vertical tangents to the lens bevel tips (or the eyewire groove tips). The "B" dimension is the largest vertical dimension as measured between the two horizontal tangents to the bevel tips. The A and B dimensions therefore correspond to the horizontal and vertical dimensions of the smallest rectangular box into which a lens just fits; hence, the term *boxing system*. Other spectacle lens measurements, such as bifocal segment height or level prism reference point (PRP) (optical center height or level PRP), are specified using the bottom edge of the box as the reference point.

The separation of the two lenses in a frame is given by the boxing measurement termed *distance between lenses* (DBL). This measurement, also known as the *bridge size*, is the minimum horizontal separation of the two nasal lens bevel tips or the minimum separation of the two boxes surrounding the lenses.

VERIFICATION OF SPECTACLE LENSES

Any spectacle prescription made by an optical laboratory must be verified for accuracy before being dispensed to a patient. All lens and frame parameters must match what was ordered. The spectacles should always be verified against the original order, which will usually be a copy of the order form sent to the laboratory. A copy made by laboratory personnel should not be used because errors may occur when information is transferred at the laboratory. The following is a discussion of the various lens and frame parameters that must be verified and the procedures used to verify them. The American National Standards Institute (ANSI) accuracy standards for ophthalmic lens manufacture are also presented. These standards provide the error tolerances that are acceptable when a lens parameter does not exactly match the ordered value.

Power

Ophthalmic lens power, both the distance portion power and the powers of any multifocal segments, is verified using the lensometer as previously described.

Lens Centration and Prism

Prism and lens positioning are most easily verified when both the patient's PD and the level PRP are specified on the order form. The following is a recommended procedure for verifying these lens parameters:

1. Check the original order form for the amounts of either or both vertical and horizontal prism (if any) that were ordered for each lens.
2. Mount the right lens of the spectacles in the lensometer (lens back surface against

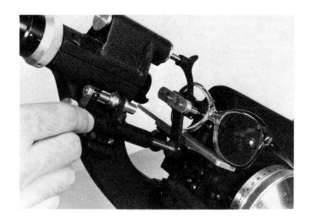

FIGURE 6-27—Use of the lensometer ink marking system to dot a lens at its prism reference point.

the lens stop). Move the lens around on the lens stop until the target lines are positioned on the reticle at the prism value specified on the order form. Hold the lens at this position using the lens holder and lens table. For example, in most cases no prism will be ordered for either lens. The lensometer target should then be positioned at the zero prism position, the center of the reticle. As a second example, if 1Δ BU vertical prism is ordered for the right lens, the target should be positioned at the 1Δ BU position on the reticle.

3. Use the lensometer ink marking system (see Figure 6-3, numbers 13, 14, and 15) to dot the lens. Dip the three pins of the marking device into the ink well, then move the pins into position over the lens. (The center pin will be centered on the lens stop and lens holder.) Press the pins against the lens surface (Figure 6-27), then lift them away. Three dots will now be on the lens. The middle dot marks the lens PRP, the point on the lens having the amount of prism prescribed. The side dots can be ignored.
4. Repeat the above procedure for the left lens. A set of three dots will now be on each lens.
5. Measure the separation of the two center dots with a PD rule (Figure 6-28). If the laboratory has made the spectacles correctly, the separation of the dots should match the patient's PD as specified on the order form. If split (monocular) PDs were specified on the order form, the distance from

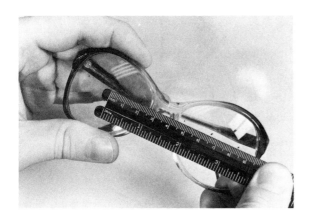

FIGURE 6-28—Measurement of the horizontal separation of the lenses' prism reference points. The separation of the two center dots (65 mm) should match the interpupillary distance ordered.

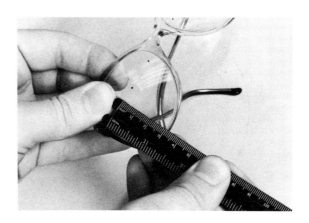

FIGURE 6-29—Measurement of level prism reference point. The level prism reference point (31.5 mm) is the vertical distance from the dots to the bottom of the box (the lowest part of the bevel along the bottom of the lens).

each center dot to the center of the frame bridge should match the split PD ordered.

6. Measure the distance from each PRP dot to the lowest part of the lens bevel (the bottom of the boxing system box), as shown in Figure 6-29. This measurement should match the level PRP ordered.

If level PRPs or optical center heights are not specified on the order form, it is still necessary to verify vertical lens positioning or to measure the amount of vertical prism in the spectacles. This requires that a somewhat different procedure be used.

1. Determine which lens of the spectacles has the more power (larger number or larger absolute value) in its vertical meridian. For example, if the right lens of a pair of spectacles has a power of –2.00 –1.50 x 180 and the left lens a power of –4.00 –2.00 x 180, the left lens has 6.00 D of power in its vertical meridian and the right lens 3.50 D of power. The left lens therefore has more power in its vertical meridian.
2. Place the lens with more power in its vertical meridian on the lens stop, back surface against the stop, as usual. If the difference in powers of the two lenses is small, it does not matter which lens is placed on the lens stop first. Large measurement errors can occur, however, if the lens powers are very different and the lower power lens is positioned on the lens stop first.
3. Center the target on the reticle (the zero prism position) by moving the lens around on the lens stop, and move the lens table so it is against the bottom of the frame.
4. Move the other lens in front of the lens stop. The bottom of the frame must be against the lens table. DO NOT move the lens table up or down.
5. Focus the target lines and eliminate any horizontal prism by moving the lens sideways on the lens stop. Any remaining vertical target deflection from the reticle center is the amount of vertical prism in the spectacles. The amount measured should match the total amount of vertical prism ordered for the spectacles.

Figure 6-30 provides an example of this method of measuring vertical prism. The right lens has more power in its vertical meridian than the left. Therefore, the target is centered on the reticle for the right lens, and the lens table is moved against the bottom of the frame. Next, the left lens is moved in front of the lens stop, without moving the lens table up or down. The spectacles are then moved sideways until no horizontal prism is present. (The target is only deflected up, with no left or right deflection.) The target ends up at the position shown in the right illustration of Figure 6-30; 1Δ BU prism is present in the left lens.

The 1Δ BU prism in the left lens of Figure 6-30 may also be written as 1Δ BD in the right lens. Vertical prism in one direction for one lens

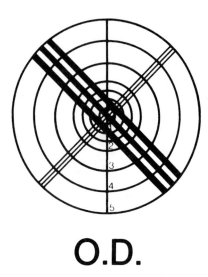 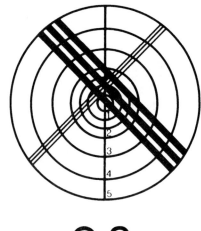

O.D.   O.S.

FIGURE 6-30—One commonly used method for measuring the amount of vertical prism in a pair of spectacles.

is equivalent to vertical prism in the opposite direction for the other.

The method of measuring vertical prism just described measures only the total amount of vertical prism in a pair of spectacles, not the amount present in each lens. The 1Δ BU vertical prism measured for the left lens in the example could have been distributed as ½Δ BD right lens and ½Δ BU left lens or as ¾Δ BD right lens and ¼Δ BU left lens (or any number of other possible combinations). It is not possible to determine how vertical prism is actually distributed unless level PRPs are provided on the order form. Optometrists usually need to know only the total prism in a pair of spectacles, however, not the amount in each lens, so this method of measuring prism is usually adequate.

A third, less commonly used method for verifying vertical lens positioning, is also available, as follows:

1. Check the order form for the amount of prism prescribed for each lens. Use the ink marking system to dot each lens at the prism amount prescribed.
2. Measure the distance from the bottom of the box (the lowest part of the lens bevel) to the center dot of each lens. The distances should be equal to each other if the spectacles were made correctly. This method is simple and quick to perform, but it is useful only for lower power lenses (below about ±2.00 D). It will be inaccurate for higher power lenses and must be used with caution.

Prism Measurement with Automatic Lensometers

The same procedures used to measure prism with a standard lensometer are also used with an automatic lensometer. Many automatic lensometers will calculate the horizontal separation of the PRPs if power is measured at the PRP point for each lens. Some will also calculate the separation of the optical centers, even if power measurements are not made at these points. Vertical prism measurements require that the lens with the more power in its vertical meridian be measured first. It is not a good idea to just measure prism at one arbitrary point on each lens, then add or subtract the values for the two lenses to obtain the total prism. These measurements can be considerably in error, especially if the two lenses are of very different power.

A Power Measurement Routine

The procedures just described can easily be incorporated into a standard routine for completely verifying lens power and prism for a pair of spectacles. One commonly used routine is as follows:

1. Starting with the right lens of the spectacles, measure the power of the lens (or measure the power of the distance portion of a multifocal lens) with the lens back surface against the lens stop.

2. If prism was prescribed, move the lens around on the lens stop until the targets are positioned at the prescribed prism position. If no prism was prescribed, position the targets at the center of the reticle. Dot the lens at this position using the ink-marking system.
3. Repeat steps 1 and 2 for the left lens.
4. Remove the spectacles from the lensometer and measure the separation of the two PRP dots (which should match the patient's PD). The dots should also be equidistant from the bottom of each lens.
5. Turn the spectacles around so the lens front surface is against the lens stop and measure the add powers for each lens.
6. All measurements should match what was ordered. If measurements do not match, ANSI standards must be consulted to determine if the spectacles should be sent back to the laboratory to be remade.

Measuring a Patient's Spectacles

When a patient arrives for an eye examination, the powers of the spectacles he or she is wearing must be measured. This is a job commonly assigned to the paraoptometric, and the procedures are similar to those used for verifying spectacles received from the optical laboratory. For these reasons, measurement procedures are dicussed here.

Powers of single-vision and multifocal lenses are measured with the lensometer as previously described.

Vertical prism can be measured using only the second of the three measurement procedures previously described, since level PRP information will not be available. Start by centering the target on the reticle for one lens (the lens with more power in its vertical meridian). Move the lens table up against the bottom of the spectacles. Then move the other lens in front of the lens stop without moving the spectacles up or down. Move the lens sideways to eliminate horizontal prism. Any remaining vertical prism will be the total amount of vertical prism in the patient's spectacles.

Horizontal prism measurement for a patient's spectacles is essentially the reverse of the method previously described, as follows:

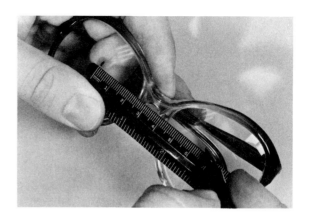

FIGURE 6-31—Marking lenses for measurement of horizontal prism. Given a patient's interpupillary distance of 65 mm, two marks have been placed on the lenses 65 mm apart. (The 32.5-mm position on the PD rule is centered on the frame bridge.)

1. Measure the patient's distance PD using a PD rule.
2. Use the PD rule and a felt-tipped pen to place two marks on the lenses, with the marks separated by the patient's PD (Figure 6-31). The marks should be placed symmetrically relative to the center of the frame bridge. For example, if the patient has a PD of 65 mm, place the 32.5 mm position of the PD rule at the center of the frame bridge, then put a mark at the 0 and 65 mm positions of the PD rule.

   Steps 1 and 2 can be combined, if desired. Instead of measuring the patient's PD, place the spectacles on the patient, and place a mark on each lens directly in front of the patient's pupil.
3. Center the mark for the right lens on the lens stop of the lensometer (Figure 6-32).
4. Focus the lensometer target. Move the lens up or down until any vertical prism is eliminated. DO NOT move the lens sideways. Any remaining horizontal prism is the amount present in that lens.
5. Repeat steps 3 and 4 for the left lens.

Lens Materials

Ophthalmic lenses may be manufactured from either glass or plastic, although most lenses made today are of plastic materials. Each material has its advantages and disadvantages, and it is important when examining a spectacle prescription to verify that the lens material matches what was

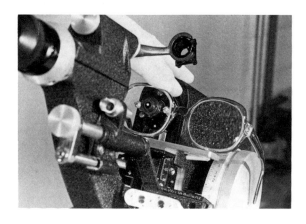

FIGURE 6-32—Mark centered on the lens stop for measurement of horizontal prism. The mark was placed on the lens as shown in Figure 6-31. The mark is centered horizontally on the lens stop, but it can be moved up or down to eliminate any vertical prism.

ordered. It is usually a fairly simple task to distinguish glass lenses from plastic lenses, but it can be difficult to differentiate one type of glass from another or one type of plastic from another.

Glass lenses are most easily distinguished from plastic lenses at high powers, as a plastic lens will be much lighter than a glass lens of the same power. At low powers, the weight difference between glass and plastic lenses will be small, so other methods must be used. Probably the most commonly used technique is to tap the lens with a fingernail. The sound made when a glass lens is tapped will be "sharper" than the dull sound of a plastic lens. It requires considerable practice, however, to be able to use this technique with any accuracy. Another method of differentiating glass and plastic is to touch the lens to the cheek. Plastic lenses feel warmer than glass. It may also be possible to distinguish a glass lens from a plastic lens using the polariscope, since a plastic lens may show characteristic stress patterns. Often, however, the only foolproof way to distinguish glass from plastic is to remove the lens from the frame and drop it gently a short distance onto a hard surface. Glass lenses will have a characteristic ringing sound, plastic lenses, a dull click.

It is sometimes easier to distinguish glass from plastic when the lens is a multifocal. A plastic "D" or flat-top bifocal has a ledge at the top of the segment that sticks out from the front of the lens. A glass D segment has no ledge. A plastic round 22 segment forms a small bump on the front of the lens, but no bump is present for a glass round 22 bifocal. Both glass and plastic Executive-style multifocals will have a ledge at the top of the bifocal. Neither glass nor plastic PALs will have a ledge. The presence or absence of a ledge cannot be used to identify the lens material for these two multifocal types.

It is more difficult to distinguish the high-index plastics from each other and from CR-39 plastic. Most of the high-index plastics sound similar to CR-39 when dropped onto a table top. Polycarbonate has a fairly characteristic sound when dropped, somewhat similar to the sound of a dropped poker chip; however, some of the other high-index plastics make a similar sound. Some high-index plastics have an inherent light tint, but this cannot be reliably used to identify the material. Optical laboratories must use extreme care when processing lenses so that lens materials are not accidentally switched. It is usually necessary to rely on the laboratory's statement that lenses are of the proper material. Some manufacturers have now begun to put markings on their lenses (similar to the markings of PALs) that allow a lens to be identified by index or material. This should be encouraged. At present, however, there is no reliable method available for identifying plastic lenses by material or index.

High-index glass materials are also difficult to differentiate from each other. These lens materials are no longer commonly used, so the identification problem is less of an issue than it is for plastic high-index materials.

Lens Design, Base Curve, and Warpage

Most spectacle lenses are of meniscus design, meaning that the front surface is of plus power and the back surface of minus power. The sum of the front and back surface powers will be approximately equal to the power of the lens. The lens prescribed in Figure 6-33 has a power of +5.00 D in its vertical (90-degree) meridian and a power of +4.00 D in its horizontal meridian. This power can be written as +5.00 –1.00 x 090 (or +4.00 +1.00 x 180, if transposed to plus cylinder form). Note that the lens power was obtained with a spherical front surface (+8.00 D) and a toric or cylindrical back surface (–4.00 D and –3.00 D) on the lens. Such a lens, with its

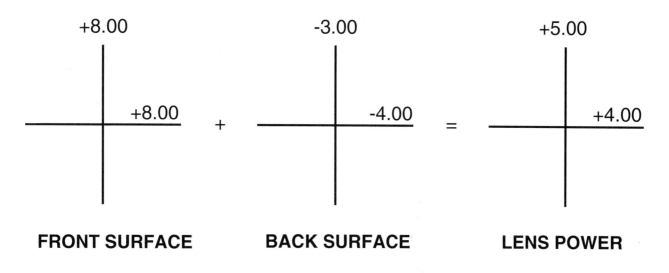

FIGURE 6-33—The power of a lens is approximately the sum of its front and back surface powers.

back surface toric, is termed a *minus cylinder design lens*. The vast majority of spectacle lenses made today, whether single vision or multifocal, are of minus cylinder design. Plus cylinder design lenses, with the cylinder on the lens front surface, are very rarely used.

The method of writing a spectacle prescription, in either plus or minus cylinder form, has nothing to do with the method by which a lens is manufactured. Almost all lenses are made with the cylinder on the back surface (minus cylinder design), yet optometrists and ophthalmologists may write their prescriptions in either plus cylinder or minus cylinder form and transpose from one form to the other.

The base curve of a single-vision lens is defined for most purposes as the front surface power as measured with a lens clock. The base curve of a multifocal lens is defined as the power of the front surface in the upper (distance) portion of the lens, again as measured with a lens clock. For the example used in Figure 6-33, the base curve is +8.00 D.

The Lens Clock

The surface powers and base curve of a lens are measured using a lens clock (Figure 6-34). The lens clock pegs are placed gently against the surface to be measured, with the lens clock perpendicular (normal) to the lens surface, and surface power is read from the lens clock scale. The black (plus) scale is used when making a measurement on the convex front surface of a

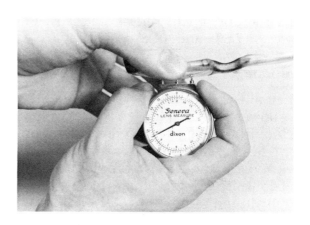

FIGURE 6-34—A lens clock is used to measure the surface powers of a lens. For this convex (plus) lens front surface, the inner (black) number scale is used. The power in the meridian being measured is +5.25 D.

lens, and the red (minus) scale is used when measuring the concave back surface of a lens. Measurements should be made to the nearest ⅛ D (0.12 D).

Since a toric surface has two principal meridians with different powers, the lens clock must be rotated to determine the powers of this type of surface. As the lens clock is rotated, the reading will reach a minimum value, then a maximum value. The maximum and minimum values are the principal meridian values and are the powers of the surface.

Extreme care must be used when measuring the power of a plastic lens with a lens clock, since the lens clock pegs can dent or scratch the lens. Older lens clocks designed for use on glass lenses have very sharp pegs and should never be used on plastic lenses. The rounded pegs of newer lens clocks are less damaging but should still be used with care. Be very careful not to scratch the lens surface when rotating the lens clock to measure principal meridian powers.

Lens Clock Calibration

A lens clock is a delicate instrument. Rough handling can cause loss of calibration, so the calibration should be checked occasionally. A good calibration surface is a plate glass window. When the lens clock pegs are placed against the window glass, the lens clock should read zero. If the lens clock is out of calibration, lens surface power readings must be corrected by the error. For example, if a lens clock reads +0.25 D when placed against a flat piece of glass, and it reads +7.50 D when placed against a lens surface, the lens surface power is +7.50 minus 0.25, or +7.25 D.

Warpage

When a lens clock is used to measure the surface powers of a lens, the lens will occasionally be found to have two different curves on its front surface and two different curves on its back surface. This lens is warped. The lens was probably inserted into a frame that was slightly too small, and the pressure of the frame caused the lens to flex or warp. The amount of warpage is the amount of cylinder on the lens front surface, that is, the difference of the front surface maximum and minimum readings. Since warpage affects both lens surfaces, it will not alter the lens power and warpage cannot be measured with the lensometer. Warpage, however, can cause a patient to have difficulty adapting to new lenses. It is always worthwhile to check for warpage when verifying spectacles received from the optical laboratory. Tolerances for warpage will be discussed in the section on ANSI standards.

The base curve and design of a lens are not commonly specified on the order form by most optometrists. Almost all lenses are made in minus cylinder design, and the base curve is standard for a given lens power. When base curve and lens design are specified on the order form, these parameters should be verified as being correct. It is good practice to always check plastic lenses for warpage.

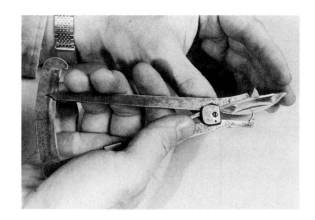

FIGURE 6-35—Measurement of lens thickness with a thickness caliper. Lens thickness at the position where the jaws touch the lens is 4.5 mm.

Center Thickness

The center thickness of a lens is the thickness at its optical center or PRP. Optometrists do not generally specify this parameter on an order form since thickness is usually determined at the optical laboratory. The laboratory's objective is to make a lens as thin as possible (to decrease weight and to improve cosmetic appearance) yet still safe to wear. When a center thickness is ordered, it is necessary to verify that the thickness of the lens received is correct. Thickness must be measured at a number of points on the lens, since center thickness will usually be the point of maximum thickness for a plus power lens and the point of minimum thickness for a minus power lens.

As previously mentioned, all industrial eyewear must have a minimum thickness of 3 mm. Minus lenses must have a minimum center thickness of 3 mm, and plus lenses must have a minimum edge thickness of 3 mm. (High plus power lenses may have a minimum thickness of 2.5 mm.) It will be necessary to measure the thickness at a number of points on the lens to determine the point of minimum edge thickness. All industrial eyewear should be checked to be sure that it meets thickness requirements.

The two instruments most commonly used to measure lens thickness are the thickness caliper and the dial-thickness gauge. A thickness caliper is shown in Figure 6-35. As with other instruments, it must first be calibrated. With the tips of the jaws touching, the pointer should point to zero on the scale. If it does not, then lens thickness measurements must be corrected

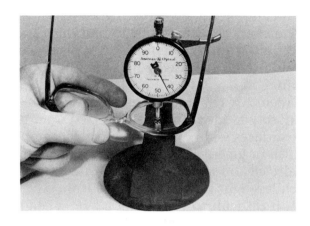

FIGURE 6-36—Measurement of lens thickness using a dial-thickness gauge. The metal arm at the upper right raises and lowers the gauge's upper jaw. The small knurled knob locks the dial scale in position. Lens thickness at the point measured is 4.3 mm.

for the error. Next, the lens to be measured is placed between the jaws of the caliper and the jaws released gently onto the lens surface. (Use care not to scratch the lens. Lift the jaws away from the lens before moving the caliper.) The lens thickness where the jaws touch the lens can be read from the scale.

The second instrument commonly used to measure lens thickness, the dial-thickness gauge, is shown in Figure 6-36. To check its calibration, the two rounded ends of the jaws are placed in contact. The dial scale should then read zero. If it does not, the error can be corrected by loosening the small knob on the top of the instrument that holds the dial scale in place. The entire scale is then rotated to align the scale zero mark with the needle. Lens thickness is measured by placing the lens between the gauge jaws and reading thickness from the dial scale. (The top jaw is raised and lowered using the arm at the top of the gauge.) The scale is graduated in 0.1 mm steps, but the labels can be confusing. A scale reading of 10 is a thickness of 1 mm, and a scale reading of 25 is a thickness of 2.5 mm. Thickness should be measured to the nearest 0.1 mm.

Lens Tempering

All spectacle lenses made of glass are treated by the optical laboratory to make the lenses more impact-resistant. (NOTE: This treatment does not make the lenses unbreakable, and patients should never be told that their lenses are unbreakable or shatterproof.) Two different processes are used. The first is air tempering or heat tempering. To heat temper a glass lens, the lens is heated almost to its melting point, then rapidly cooled. The second process, now much more commonly used, is chemical tempering. To chemically temper a lens, it is immersed in a molten potassium salt solution, usually for 16 hours.

Plastic lenses are not treated to increase impact resistance. Plastic lenses are almost as impact-resistant as any treated glass lens, and polycarbonate plastic lenses can be much more impact-resistant than any other lens type.

It is difficult to verify that a glass lens has been tempered. The instrument most commonly available for this purpose is a *polariscope* or *colmascope*. The polariscope consists of a light source and two polarizing filters with their axes of polarization 90 degrees apart. When a heat-tempered glass lens is placed between the polarizers, a light and dark pattern is observed, sometimes in the shape of a cross surrounded by a dark band or ring (Figure 6-37A). When a chemically tempered or untempered glass lens is placed in the instrument, the lens appears uniformly dark (Figure 6-37B). Therefore, it is not usually possible to verify that a glass lens received from the optical laboratory has been chemically tempered. Since most laboratories chemically temper their lenses, the usefulness of the polariscope is limited.

When a plastic lens is held in a polariscope, a light and dark pattern may occasionally be observed (Figure 6-37C). The lens has not been tempered. Instead, the pattern is an indication that the lens is under stress, often because the lens is slightly too large for the frame. A small amount of stress is probably not harmful, but large amounts of stress may cause plastic lenses to warp and may also weaken some plastic frame materials. A highly stressed lens should always be checked for warpage. If the optical laboratory is routinely providing highly stressed lenses, it may be necessary to contact the laboratory and suggest that edging and lens insertion procedures be modified.

Tints and Coatings

Verification of tints and coatings is straightforward for most lens types. The color of dyed plas-

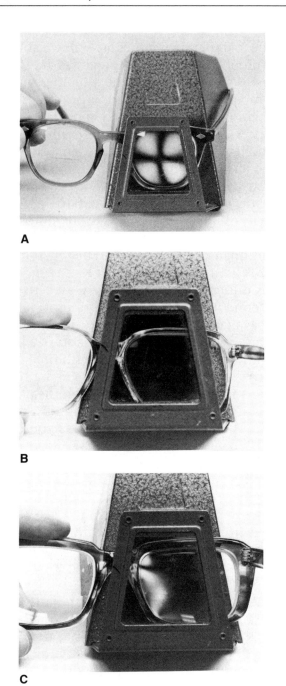

FIGURE 6-37—A. The cross-and-ring pattern visible when a heat-tempered lens is held in the polariscope. The pattern need not have a perfect cross shape. Any alternating light and dark pattern for a glass lens indicates a heat-tempered lens. B. When a chemically tempered or untempered glass lens is held in a polariscope, the lens appears uniformly dark. C. Light and dark pattern formed by a plastic lens under stress.

should also be correct. Coated glass lenses will have a characteristic purplish, bluish, or gold reflection from the lens back surface. This should not be confused with an antireflective coating.

A lens with an antireflective coating is relatively easy to identify. Light reflected from the lens surfaces will be colored, most commonly reddish or greenish, although the lens itself is usually clear. In addition, the lens will reflect much less light than an uncoated lens.

It is difficult to verify that a lens is coated with a scratch-resistant coating. A coated lens will appear identical to an uncoated lens, and reflections from the lens surfaces will not be colored. It is usually necessary to rely on the laboratory's statement that the lens has been coated.

Photochromic lenses are available in both glass and plastic materials. The best-known glass photochromic lens is PhotoGray Extra, from Corning, Inc. (Corning, NY). A new PhotoGray Extra lens received from the optical laboratory will have a characteristic light green tint that identifies the lens. The green color will disappear after the patient wears the lenses for a few days. The best-known plastic photochromic lens is Transitions (Transitions, Pinellas Park, FL), which is light gray in color. A simple method for identifying the lens as photochromic is to expose the lens to sunlight or to an ultraviolet (UV) radiation source (a "black" light) for a few minutes. The lens will darken when exposed to these light sources.

Ultraviolet Protection

An important concern with all spectacle lenses is the protection provided from UV radiation. Long-term, chronic exposure to UV radiation from the sun, especially to the UV-B radiation between 290 and 315 nm, is associated with the development of some types of cataracts. In addition, chronic exposure to solar UV-A radiation (315–380 nm) may be associated with retinal damage. Transmittance curves for representative clear (untinted) spectacle lens materials for the UV and a portion of the visible spectrum are shown in Figure 6-38. Polycarbonate and the high-index plastics absorb all UV radiation below 380 nm, and CR-39 treated with a UV-protective dye absorbs all UV radiation below 400 nm. All three of these lens types

tic lenses should be matched against demonstration lenses shown to the patient in the dispensary. The tint transmittance (usually specified as a number, i.e., #1, #2, #3, or #4)

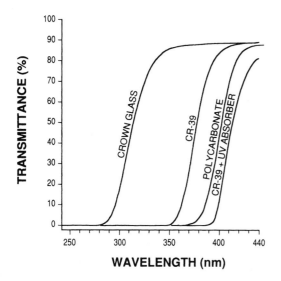

FIGURE 6-38—Transmittance curves for clear (untinted) spectacle lens materials. (Reprinted with permission from GL Stephens, JK Davis. Spectacle Lenses. In W Tasman, EA Jaeger [eds], Duane's Clinical Ophthalmology [Vol 1]. Philadelphia: Lippincott, 1993;55.)

Transmittance curves for some sunglass tints used with prescription CR-39 plastic and crown glass lenses are shown in Figure 6-39. The CR-39 plastic lens tints provide good protection against UV radiation, absorbing all UV below approximately 360 nm and most of the UV between 360 and 400 nm. The glass lens tints show more variability, with the gray and green tints allowing higher transmittance levels in the UV-A. Transmittance in the visible spectrum depends on the color of the lens. A green tint transmits more light in the green portion of the spectrum and less in the blue and red. A gray tint transmits all wavelengths of visible light almost equally. A brown tint transmits more of the longer wavelengths and less of the blue end of the spectrum.

Inexpensive transmittance meters that measure the UV transmittance of a lens are available (Figure 6-40), but these meters tend to overestimate UV transmittance. For example, a lens with an actual UV transmittance of 20% might read 50% when measured by a UV meter. Only when the meter reading is low will the reading be relatively accurate. If a meter reads less than about 5% transmittance when measuring a lens, then the lens probably transmits little UV radiation.

A more accurate but also more expensive instrument for measuring the UV transmittance

are considered to provide excellent protection against UV radiation. On the other hand, CR-39 plastic without a UV-protective dye and clear crown glass do not provide complete protection against UV radiation, with crown glass providing essentially no protection.

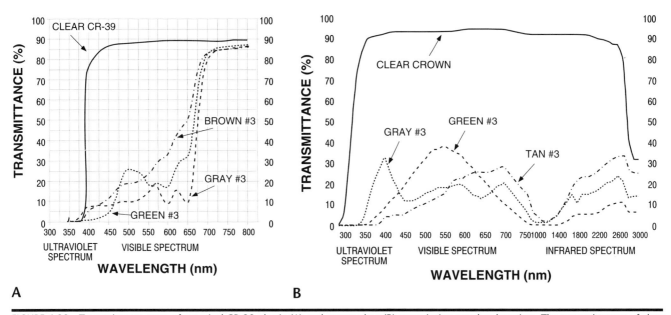

FIGURE 6-39—Transmittance curves for typical CR-39 plastic (A) and crown glass (B) prescription sunglass lens tints. The transmittances of clear CR-39 plastic and clear crown glass are included for comparison. (Reprinted with permission from GL Stephens, JK Davis. Spectacle Lenses. In W Tasman, EA Jaeger [eds], Duane's Clinical Ophthalmology [Vol 1]. Philadelphia: Lippincott, 1993.)

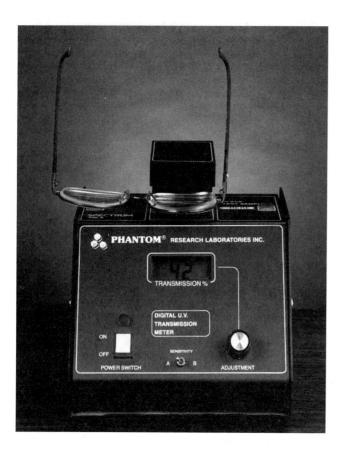

FIGURE 6-40—An ultraviolet transmittance meter.

of a spectacle lens is the Spexan spectrometer, an attachment for the Humphrey Lens Analyzer (an automatic lensometer). This instrument provides a graph of both the UV and visible transmittance of the lens, along with UV-B, UV-A, and visible light transmittance values (Figure 6-41).

Multifocals

In addition to multifocal add power, a number of other multifocal segment parameters must be checked when verifying a spectacle prescription. These include the segment type, segment height, segment width, segment alignment, and segment positioning relative to the patient's near PD. If any of these parameters are not correct, the patient may not be able to use the lenses properly, or the lenses may not have a good cosmetic appearance.

Segment Type

The type of multifocal segment in a pair of spectacles can be verified either by comparison with

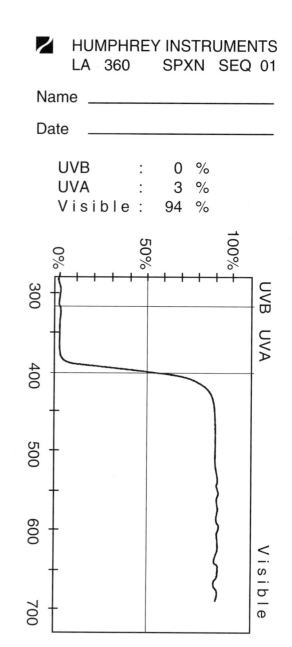

FIGURE 6-41—Transmittance curve for a polycarbonate lens as measured by the Spexan attachment of the Humphrey Lens Analyzer.

known samples or by reference to manufacturers' literature, although with experience the different types will be easily committed to memory. Commonly available multifocal types are described in Chapter 5.

Segment Height

Bifocal segment height is the distance from the bottom of the boxing system box surrounding a lens (the lowest part of the lens bevel) to the top of the segment. Trifocal height is the distance from the bottom of the box to the top of the intermediate segment (also the top of the segment). Figure 6-42A illustrates the proper method of making these measurements.

Segment Width

Bifocal or trifocal width is defined as the widest horizontal dimension of the segment (Figure 6-42B). If the edge of the segment has been removed during the edging process, it may not be possible to measure segment width accurately. It is also not possible to measure the width of an Executive-style multifocal.

Trifocal intermediate width is the vertical height of the intermediate portion of the segment (as shown by the small arrows in Figure 6-42B). This width is standard for most trifocal types and may not always be specified on the order form. D-shaped trifocals are available with several different intermediate and segment widths, however, and the type received must be verified. Standard terminology for specifying D-shaped trifocal size on an order form is as follows:

$$7/25D \text{ trifocal}$$

The number to the left of the slash is the vertical intermediate width in millimeters. The number to the right of the slash is the maximum horizontal segment width.

Segment Alignment

The top edges of segments that have flat tops (D-shaped segments and Executive-style segments) must be level with the horizontal. This is best verified by laying a PD rule across both lenses and attempting to align the edge of the rule parallel with the top edges of the two segments (Figure 6-42C). (If the two bifocal segments are not at the same height, it should still be possible to align the PD rule parallel to both segment lines, although one segment line may be closer to the rule edge than the other.) If the segment edges cannot be aligned, one or both lenses is either rotated in the eyewire or improperly made. It may be possible to correct this problem by turning the lens in the eyewire using lens-twisting pliers. If the rotation creates an error in the cylinder axis or distorts the frame shape, however, the lens will need to be remade.

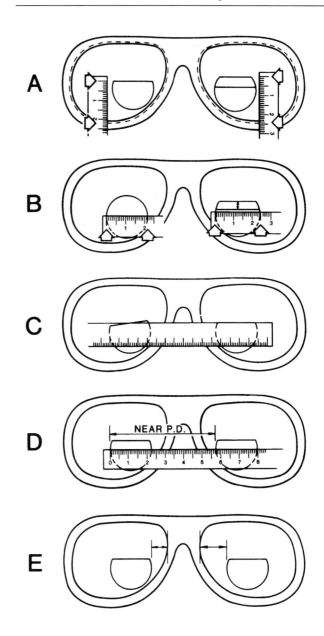

FIGURE 6-42—Multifocal verification. A. Segment height is the distance from the top of the segment to the lowest part of the lens bevel, 22 mm for the bifocal lens, 24.5 mm for the trifocal lens. B. Segment width is the largest horizontal dimension of the segment. The round segment is 22 mm wide. The D segment is 25 mm wide. Intermediate width for the trifocal is indicated by the small arrows. C. An example of improper segment alignment. The tops of both segments should be parallel to the interpupillary rule. D. The near interpupillary distance is the distance from the temporal edge of one segment to the nasal edge of the other. E. An example of asymmetric segment positioning. One segment is closer to the nasal eyewire than the other.

Near Interpupillary Distance

For a patient to view through the centers of the multifocal segments when looking at a near object, the segment optical centers must be separated by the patient's near PD. Segment optical

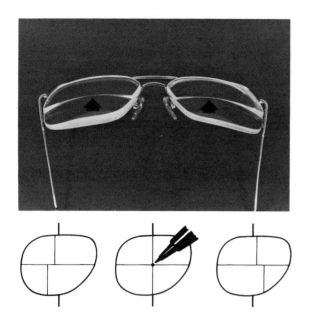

FIGURE 6-43—Verification of the near interpupillary distance of an Executive-style bifocal. Top. Each lens is dotted at the thinnest point on the bifocal ledge (arrows). The separation of the dots should match the near interpupillary distance ordered. Bottom. Each lens is dotted at the point where a line viewed through the lens appears unbroken. The separation of the two dots should match the near interpupillary distance ordered.

center separation is best verified by measuring the distance from the temporal edge of one segment to the nasal edge of the other (Figure 6-42D). This distance should match the near PD ordered.

While segment positioning is verified, the symmetry of the segment placement in the lenses should also be checked. The two segments should be equidistant from the nasal sides of the eyewires. An example of an asymmetric segment placement is shown in Figure 6-42E. Although the near PD may be correct, the spectacles may not be optically or cosmetically acceptable to the patient, and it may be necessary to return the spectacles to the laboratory to be remade.

The near PD of an executive-style bifocal cannot be measured using the method described above. Instead, the actual segment optical centers must be found and their separation measured. There are two ways to do this. The first is shown in the upper illustration of Figure 6-43. Holding the spectacles so the bifocal ledges are viewed from below, each lens is marked with a felt-tipped pen at the position where the ledge is thinnest (arrows). The near PD will be the separation of the marks as measured with a PD rule. The second method requires that a straight edge or line be viewed through the lens (see Figure 6-43, bottom). As the lens is moved back and forth, one point will be found where the line viewed through the distance portion and the line viewed through the near portion are aligned. This point of alignment should be marked on each lens with a felt-tipped pen. The near PD will then be the horizontal separation of the two marks. The same two methods can also be used to verify the near PD of executive-style trifocals.

Lens Bevel

When a lens blank is edged to the proper shape and size to fit into a spectacle frame, the lens edge can be finished in any one of a number of different shapes, termed *bevels*. The most commonly used of these are illustrated in Figure 6-44. The *standard bevel*, or *V bevel* (Figure 6-44A), is used for most low power lenses edged to fit into plastic and metal frames. The two surfaces of the bevel come together at an angle of approximately 115 degrees, and the sharp corners of the bevel are removed with what is termed a *safety bevel* or *pin bevel* (Figure 6-44B).

The *hide-a-bevel* (Figure 6-44C) is used with high minus power lenses to decrease the visibility of reflections from the lens bevel. The distance of the bevel apex from the lens front surface can also be specified. Positioning the bevel apex forward on the bevel edge can hide the thick edge of a high minus lens in a frame so that the edge is more cosmetically acceptable.

The *rimless bevel* (Figure 6-44D) is used for lenses to be mounted in some rimless and semi-rimless frames. This bevel is normally roughened so that it has a whitish appearance, but it can be polished to a smooth finish. It is also possible to round the sharp edge of the bevel, a process termed *roll-and-polish*. The *nylon suspension grooved bevel* (Figure 6-44E) is used for lenses that are held in a frame by nylon line. A groove is cut entirely around the edge of a rimless bevel, and the nylon line fits into this groove.

When verifying the bevels of a pair of spectacles, it is first necessary to verify that the type of bevel matches that ordered. A specific bevel type is usually ordered only for special designs

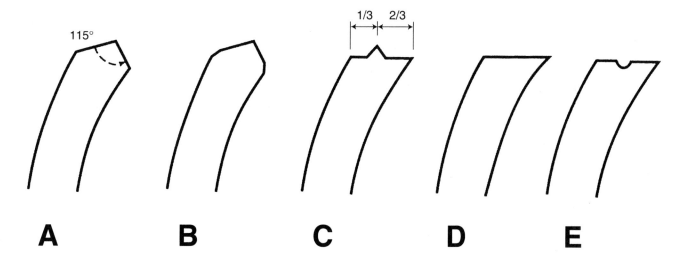

FIGURE 6-44—Lens bevel types as viewed in cross section. A. Standard or V bevel. B. Standard bevel with safety bevels. C. 1/3–2/3 hide-a-bevel. D. Rimless bevel. E. Rimless bevel with nylon suspension groove.

(e.g., polished edges, roll-and-polish). If a bevel type is not specified on the order form, the laboratory will usually provide a V bevel for low power lenses, a hide-a-bevel for high minus lenses, and a rimless bevel for rimless and semi-rimless frame designs. If the bevel apex position is specified on the order form, this should also be verified. For example, if a 1/3–2/3 hide-a-bevel is ordered, the laboratory should place the bevel apex one-third of the total edge thickness behind the front surface edge (as shown in Figure 6-44C). Finally, the quality of all bevels should be checked. The edges of a bevel should be safety beveled, and the bevel edges should not be chipped.

Optical Quality

Both the condition of the lens surfaces and the optical quality of the lenses should be examined for all spectacles received from the optical laboratory. Some lens defects are very difficult to see and may be missed at the final laboratory inspection, yet these defects may decrease the impact resistance of a lens or affect a patient's vision.

Lens surface defects are best found by examining the lens under bright lighting with the lens held in front of a dark background. Both the front and the back surfaces should be examined. Any scratches, pits, or dents are cause for rejection. The segment ledge of a multifocal should also be inspected for chips. This is a fairly common defect and is cause for return of the lens to the laboratory.

When verifying lens optical quality, the primary defect to search for is a localized area of poor optics. A high-contrast, well-lit grid pattern, such as a set of venetian blinds or the grating over a large fluorescent light fixture, makes a good test target. The pattern should be viewed through the lens while the lens is moved back and forth. Areas of localized waviness or distortion of the pattern, especially near the center of the lens, are cause for rejection. These areas should be circled with a felt-tipped pen or a wax pencil so that the defect can be confirmed by laboratory personnel. Note that there will always be some normal increase in distortion toward the periphery of any lens. This will cause straight lines viewed through the lens periphery to appear curved. This is not cause for rejection as long as the increase in distortion occurs gradually.

Other Lens Types

Moderate-Power Aspheric Lens Designs

Aspheric surface curves have long been in use for high plus power aphakic (cataract) lenses. Recent improvements in spectacle lens technology have allowed aspheric curves to be used for lower-power lenses, and this lens design has a much improved cosmetic appearance relative to nonaspheric lenses. Representative trade names for these moderate power aspheric lenses include the Cosmolit from Rodenstock USA Inc., Lens Division (Danbury, CT), the Profile from Gentex Optics (Dudley, MA), the ASL from Sola, and the Hyperal from Silor Optical, Division of Essilor of America Inc. (St. Petersburg, FL).

Moderate-power aspheric lenses have aspheric front surfaces—that is, the front surface of the lens steepens or flattens toward the edge or periphery of the lens. The lens back surface is spherical or toric. The main reason for using an aspheric curve is to improve the cosmetic appearance of a plus power spectacle lens. A hyperope wearing spectacles is often very self-conscious about his or her appearance. The eyes appear magnified behind the lenses; the lenses are thick and relatively heavy, even when made of plastic; and the lenses appear to bulge out of the front of the frame. Aspheric curves greatly decrease these effects. The lenses are much thinner, lighter, and flatter, and the eyes are less magnified. In addition, some aspheric lenses are available in high-index materials, further decreasing thickness, weight, and magnification.

Moderate-power aspheric lenses may also be used for the myope. These minus power lenses will have a decreased edge thickness relative to a nonaspheric design.

It is difficult to differentiate aspheric lenses from standard nonaspheric designs. It might be expected that the lens clock could be used, since different powers would be measured at the center and edge of the lens. The power difference is so small, however, that the procedure is not reliable. Aspheric lenses are appreciably thinner than nonaspheric lenses and the lens curves appear flatter, but it requires some experience to judge the differences reliably. It is usually necessary to rely on the laboratory's statement that the lenses are of an aspheric design.

Moderate-power aspheric lenses are often fit using split PD and level PRP measurements. Always be sure to verify that these measurements are correct when receiving new spectacles from the optical laboratory.

High-Power Lenses

Verification of high plus and high minus power lenses is generally the same as for other lens

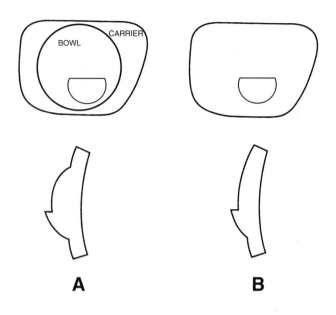

FIGURE 6-45—High plus (aphakic) spectacle lenses. A. Plus lenticular lens. B. Full-field lens.

types. Powers, prism, and lens positioning are measured as has already been described. Some high power lenses are made in a lenticular design in an attempt to decrease the thickness of the lens, however. A lenticular lens has a central area of useful optics, the bowl, where all power measurements should be made. This area is surrounded by a carrier, an area of the lens that has no optical function. A plus lenticular lens has the appearance of a fried egg, with the yolk corresponding to the bowl and the egg white to the carrier (Figure 6-45A). This lens type is sometimes worn by aphakes. Aphakic lenses are also made in a full-field or nonlenticular form (Figure 6-45B).

The minus lenticular lens (Figure 6-46A) appears to have had its very thick outer edge removed. If the front surface is flat (plano power when read with the lens clock) and the lenticular area on the lens back surface is also flat, the lens is termed a myodisc (Figure 6-46B).

Verification of Invisible Bifocals

Invisible bifocals may be divided into two categories: blended bifocals and progressive addition lenses. Both types are invisible in the sense that a segment line cannot be seen on the surfaces of the lenses. The principles of design of

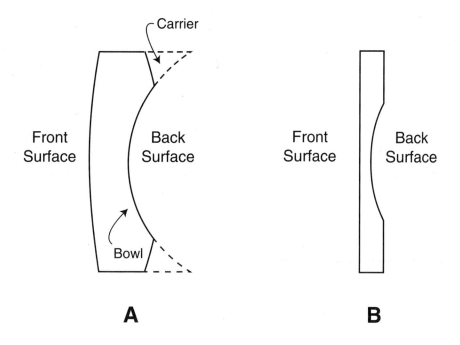

FIGURE 6-46—High minus power spectacle lenses. A. Minus lenticular. B. Myodisc.

the two types of lenses differ considerably, however, and their verification is discussed separately below.

Verification of Blended Bifocals

Blended bifocals are one-piece glass or plastic bifocals. The junction between the distance and near portions has been smoothed and polished (blended) to make the segment difficult to see. These lenses are easily identified because the blended zone is visible as a ring of distortion or poor optics surrounding the segment when the lens is held in front of a patterned surface (Figure 6-47).

Powers of blended bifocals are verified in the same manner as for other bifocal types. The only precaution to be observed is that power measurements should not be made through the blended zone.

Segment height and the near PD are difficult to verify for a blended bifocal. Segment height is measured to the top of the blended zone surrounding the segment. This point can be found by viewing a patterned surface through the lens. The point at which the distortion of the pattern ends at the top of the bifocal should be marked with a felt-tipped pen, and segment height is measured to this mark. The near PD is verified in a similar manner by marking the nasal and temporal edges of the blended zones, then measuring from the temporal edge of one segment to the nasal edge of the other.

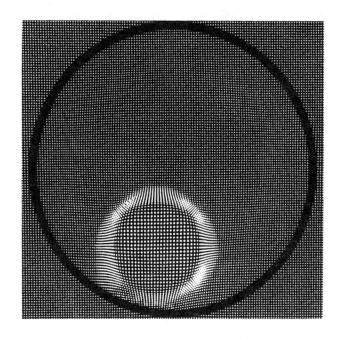

FIGURE 6-47—A blended bifocal as viewed against a patterned background. The blurred or distorted area is the blended zone surrounding the segment. (Courtesy of Varilux Corp., Oldsmar, FL.)

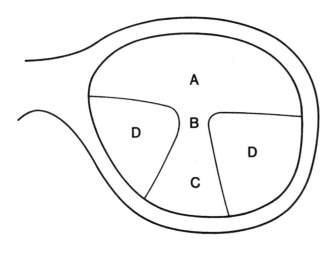

FIGURE 6-48—Design of a progressive addition lens. A. Distance portion. B. Progressive corridor, where the change from the distance power to the near power occurs. C. Near portion. D. Areas of poor optics.

Verification of Progressive Addition Lenses

The PAL is a unique concept in lens design. The front surface of a progressive addition lens is aspheric, with the curvature of the surface increasing from the top to the bottom of the lens. This change in curvature results in a gradual increase in lens power from the distance power in the upper portion of the lens to intermediate powers in the middle of the lens to the add power in the lower portion. A patient wearing a PAL can have clear vision at all distances just by looking through the proper part of the lens. The transition from the distance to the near power occurs along a narrow corridor in the middle of the lens. On either side of this progressive corridor and on either side of the add (near) portion of the lens are areas of poor optics. Figure 6-48 illustrates the design of a PAL.

Because of the variations in power across the surface of a PAL, lens power and prism must be verified at specific places. In addition, each lens must be properly positioned in the frame if a patient is to be able to use the lenses correctly. Most, but not all, new PALs received from the optical laboratory will be marked with temporary verification marks that show where measurements are to be made. Most PALs are also etched with permanent semivisible markings that identify a lens by name and manufacturer and allow an unmarked lens to be remarked for measurement of powers. Each lens manufacturer uses its own marking system. Representative PALs are listed in Table 6-1.

Figure 6-49 illustrates the markings commonly found on a new PAL received from the optical laboratory. The semicircle in the upper portion of the lens, the cross, the small dot, and the circle in the bottom portion of the lens are all removable ink markings. There are also two sets of permanent markings, not visible under normal lighting conditions, etched onto the lens front surface. These are the small circles, numbers, and letters labeled "d" in the figure. The "s" under the nasal circle is the manufacturer's trademark. This marking, which varies from manufacturer to manufacturer, assists in identifying a lens by trade name. Some manufacturers will use small squares, triangles, diamonds, or other shapes instead of the small circles. These markings can also be used to identify a lens. The "1.50" under the temporal circle is the add power. Some manufacturers will use two digits rather than three to specify add power. For example, the number "22" indicates an add power of +2.25.

TABLE 6-1. Representative progressive addition lenses

Trade name	Manufacturer
Truvision	American Optical
Truvision Omni	American Optical
AO Pro	American Optical
Line Free	Orcolite[a]
Zoom	Pentax[b]
Life	Rodenstock
Progressiv S	Rodenstock
P-6	Seiko[c]
Elegance	Signet Armorlite[d]
Kodak	Signet Armorlite
Adaptar	Silor
Super No-Line	Silor
VIP	Sola
XL	Sola
Comfort	Varilux
Gradal	Zeiss[e]

[a]Orcolite, Division of Optical Radiation Corp., Azusa, CA.
[b]Pentax Vision, Inc., Hopkins, MN.
[c]Seiko Optical Products, Inc., Mahwah, NJ.
[d]Signet Armorlite, Inc., San Marcos, CA.
[e]Carl Zeiss Optical, Petersburg, VA.

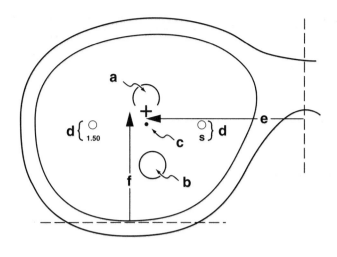

FIGURE 6-49—Temporary and permanent verification marks of a generic progressive addition lens. The arrows and letters a–f are not part of the markings, but have been added for purposes of illustrations.

Permanent markings are best found by holding the lens back surface a few inches away from a bright light source such as a frosted incandescent light bulb. (The lens must be clean.) View the light reflected from the lens surfaces as the lens is tilted back and forth. The markings will be visible on the lens front surface, one set on the temporal side, the other on the nasal side.

PAL powers are verified using the temporary markings. Distance power is measured with the semicircle (labeled "a" in Figure 6-49) centered on the lensometer lens stop and the lens back surface against the stop (as distance power is normally measured). Add power is measured through the small circle "b" in the bottom portion of the lens. The lens front surface must be against the lens stop, and the add power will be the difference between the power measured through the small circle and the power remeasured through the semicircle, with the lens front surface also against the stop. The add power measured should match that engraved on the lens under the permanent circles. Prism power is measured for each lens individually by centering the small dot "c" on the lens stop with the lens back surface against the stop. The lensometer target may be distorted because the prism dot is within the progressive corridor, but this distortion should not affect the accuracy of the measurement. The amount of horizontal or vertical target deflection from the reticle center will be the prism in the lens. ANSI standards for lens power and prism errors should be used (see the section on ANSI standards in this chapter).

Lens positioning in the frame is verified using the cross on the PAL surface (the *fitting cross*). Unlike other multifocal types, segment heights and the near PD are not used when ordering a PAL. Instead, the fitting cross of each lens is usually positioned so it is directly in front of the patient's pupil in straight-ahead (distance) gaze. On the order form, the cross positioning for each lens is given by the split distance PD and a measurement commonly termed the *fitting height*, the distance from the bottom of the frame box to the center of the pupil. The distance from the center of the frame bridge to the center of the cross (see the arrow labeled "e" in Figure 6-49) should match the split PD ordered for each lens. The vertical distance from the lowest part of the lens bevel to the center of the cross (see the arrow labeled "f" in Figure 6-49) should match the fitting height ordered. It is generally recommended that both measurements be accurate to within ±0.5 mm of the values ordered, although the ANSI Z80.1-1995 standards allow a ±1.0 mm error.

Once a PAL spectacle prescription has been verified, the temporary verification marks should not be removed because these marks will be used to align the lenses on the patient during dispensing. After dispensing procedures are completed, the temporary marks can be removed with rubbing (isopropyl) alcohol.

It is often necessary to verify a PAL from which the temporary marks have been removed. To do this, it is necessary to remark the lens using a verification card (Figure 6-50). First, find the two etched permanent circles on the lens and mark them with a felt-tipped pen. Next, hold the lens convex side down over one of the large circles on the card, and align the marked circles with the small circles. Trace over the verification marks on the card, remarking the lens. (The circles labeled "L" and "R" indicate where add power is to be measured for the left and right lenses, respectively.) Once the lens is remarked, distance power, add power, prism, the split PD, and the fitting height may all be measured as previously described.

It may be difficult to find the permanent markings on an older PAL. The markings wear

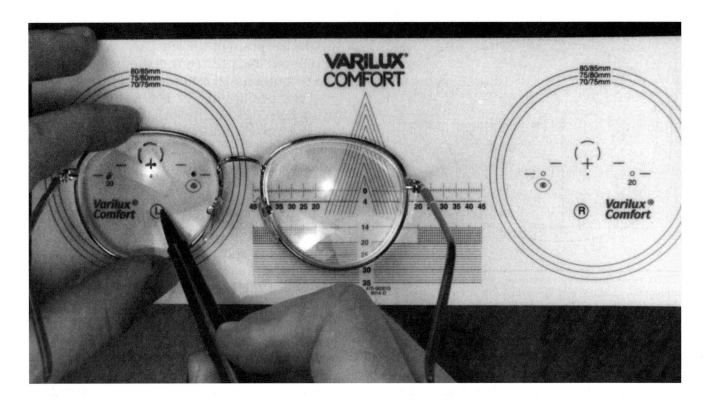

FIGURE 6-50—Verification card being used to remark an unmarked progressive addition lens. The permanent markings on the lens have been aligned with the small circles on the card.

off with time, and scratches can make the markings difficult to see. A few manufacturers use a marking system that glows when exposed to a UV source (a "black" light) but which is not otherwise visible. The markings are traced while the lens is held under the source. If markings cannot be found using other methods, check the lens under a UV source.

Although it is generally a simple task to identify a PAL by trade name or manufacturer using the permanent markings on the lens, it is difficult to keep track of the markings used by the many different manufacturers. One solution to this problem is the Progressive Lens Identifier Chart prepared by the Optical Laboratories Association (Merrifield, VA). This chart presents drawings of the temporary and permanent markings of most available PALs (Figure 6-51), allowing a lens to be identified easily.

American National Standards Institute Standards

Because there are recognized limitations to spectacle lens manufacturing accuracy, the optical laboratory must be allowed some margin of error when making spectacle lenses. The standards used are those developed by ANSI and are referred to as ANSI Z80.1-1995—American National Standard for Ophthalmics—Prescription Ophthalmic Lenses—Recommendations. ANSI is not a governmental organization, and the standards it proposes are not legally binding, but most optical laboratories and optometrists comply with ANSI standards. (Exceptions are the drop-ball test for dress lenses and the industrial eyewear standard, both of which are governmental requirements.) The Appendix at the end of the chapter summarizes the ANSI Z80.1 standards. A copy should always be kept near the lensometer. When spectacles are received from the laboratory, the lenses must be verified for accuracy. Each component should be correct within the error tolerance determined from the ANSI standards, as discussed in the sections that follow.

Example 4

The use of ANSI standards is best demonstrated by an example. Suppose that spectacles with the

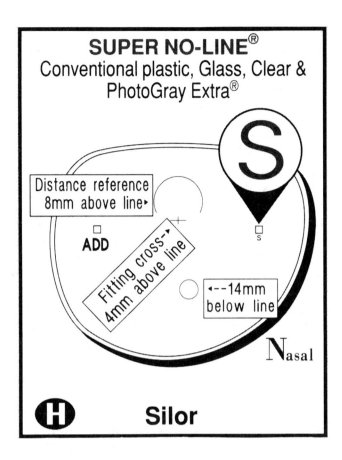

FIGURE 6-51—A diagram from the Progressive Lens Identifier Chart, illustrating the markings, both temporary and permanent, of a Silor Super No-Line progressive addition lens. (Courtesy of the Optical Laboratories Association, Merrifield, VA.)

following parameters are ordered from the optical laboratory:

O.D. + 2.00 –1.75 x 110

O.S. + 2.00 –0.75 x 095

+ 2.50 Add O.U.

Glass D-25 Bifocal, 16 mm high O.U.

PD 65/61

Sphere and Cylinder Power

Sphere and cylinder power accuracy tolerances are given in Appendix 6-1, section 5.1.2. The two lists of tolerances—one for single-vision and multifocal lenses, the other for progressive addition and aspheric lenses—are complex in appearance but are somewhat simpler to apply in practice. For the most commonly used lens powers (less than 9.00 D for the meridian of highest absolute power and less than 4.00 D of cylinder), the tolerances are ±0.12 D, with the tolerance increasing to ±0.18 D for a few cases. The error tolerance for commonly used lens powers therefore becomes ±0.12 D. An error of ±0.25 D or more would be cause for rejection of a pair of spectacles. The power accuracy tables need be consulted only when dealing with lenses of unusual (very high) power.

Two specific error tolerances must be met when verifying the sphere and cylinder power of a lens. First, each principal meridian must be correct within ±0.12 D. Acceptable sphere powers (the first, or more plus, focus when measuring power with the lensometer) for both the right and left lenses in Example 4 would be +1.87, +2.00, or +2.12 D. If a sphere power of +1.75 D or +2.25 D was measured for either lens, this would be cause for rejection, and the spectacles would be returned to the laboratory to be remade. The second or more minus focus of the lensometer, which is used for determining cylinder power, must also be accurate within ±0.12 D. The right lens in Example 4 has a power of +2.00 –1.75. Its second focus should be at +0.25 (1.75 D more minus than the first focus). Acceptable readings for this meridian would therefore be +0.37, +0.25, or +0.12 D. The left lens should have a power of +1.25 in its second principal meridian (+2.00 minus 0.75). Acceptable readings would be +1.37, +1.25, or +1.12 D.

Second, the difference between the two principal meridian powers (which is the amount of cylinder power in the lens) must be accurate to within ±0.12 D. Acceptable cylinder powers in Example 4 would be –1.62 to –1.87 D for the right lens and –0.62 to –0.87 D for the left lens.

Cylinder Axis

Using section 5.1.3 of Appendix 6-1, acceptable cylinder axes in Example 4 for the right lens would be from 108 to 112 degrees (±2 degrees for a 1.75 D cylinder) and from 90 to 100 degrees for the left lens (±5 degrees for a 0.75 D cylinder). Note that the higher the lens cylinder power, the more accurate the required axis positioning. Fairly large errors are allowed for small cylinders.

Add Power

Multifocal add power error tolerances are given in section 5.1.4 of Appendix 6-1. For add powers between 0 and +4.00 D, the tolerance is ±0.12 D. Acceptable measured add powers in Example 4 would be +2.37, +2.50, and +2.62 D.

Segment Positioning

The two parameters to be verified are segment height and segment inset (or near PD). According to section 5.2.3 of Appendix 6-1, each segment height should be within 1 mm of what was ordered, but the two segments should not differ in height by more than 1 mm (assuming that equal segment heights were ordered). Segment heights of 15 mm for both lenses, 16 mm for both lenses, or 17 mm for both lenses would be acceptable in Example 4, as would a segment height of 15 mm for the right lens and 16 mm for the left lens. A segment height of 17 mm for the right lens and 15 mm for the left lens would not be acceptable, however, although each would be within the single-lens tolerance.

As noted in section 5.2.4 of Appendix 6-1, near PDs should be within ±2.5 mm of the ordered values. Measured near PDs between 58.5 and 63.5 mm would be acceptable in Example 4. The segments should be positioned symmetrically in the frame.

ANSI standards also exist for tilt of the segments, a cosmetic concern. According to section 5.2.5 of Appendix 6-1, the segment top should not be tilted by more than 2 degrees. This parameter is difficult to measure in practice. The best advice is to reject the spectacles if the tilt results in a poor cosmetic appearance.

Lens Positioning (Prism)

The best tolerances to use when checking for lens positioning or prism errors are the mounted pair tolerances. As noted in section 5.1.5 of Appendix 6-1, the tolerance for vertical prism error for lenses mounted in a frame is $\frac{1}{3}\Delta$. The total amount of vertical prism present in a pair of spectacles is best measured (as previously described) by centering the lensometer target on the reticle first for the lens with more power in its vertical meridian, then moving to the other lens without changing the lens vertical position on the lens table. For Example 4, since no vertical prism was ordered, up to $\frac{1}{3}\Delta$ of measured vertical prism would be acceptable, either BU or BD, right lens or left lens. A tolerance for vertical PRP positioning (±1.0 mm) is also available but is not used as often.

Horizontal lens positioning errors are described in the ANSI Z80.1 standard both as PD error tolerances and as horizontal prism error tolerances. Probably the best method of verifying horizontal positioning is to first verify that the PD is correct. If an error is found, it is necessary to determine how much prism is created by the error. To verify that the PD is correct, each lens is dotted at its PRP (the point with the prescribed prism) using the lensometer inkmarking system. The separation of the two dots should match the patient's PD. According to section 5.1.5 of Appendix 6-1, the dot separation should be within ±2.5 mm of the PD that was ordered. For Example 4, PDs between 62.5 and 67.5 mm would be acceptable.

When lenses are received with a PD that is incorrect, it is necessary to determine how much horizontal prism is created by the error. If the lenses are of low power, large errors in the PD can be present without much of a horizontal prism error. Small PD errors can create large amounts of prism error if the lenses are of high power. To measure the amount of prism created by a PD error, mark each lens with a felt-tipped pen at the desired PD (see Figure 6-31). Center each mark on the lens stop and measure the amount of horizontal prism created, as previously described. The amounts of horizontal prism at the two marks must then be properly added to determine the total prism in the spectacles. Horizontal prisms in the same directions add, and prisms in opposite directions subtract. As an example, suppose that $\frac{1}{2}\Delta$ BO was measured at the mark on the right lens, and $\frac{1}{4}\Delta$ BI was measured at the mark on the left lens. The total horizontal prism in the spectacles would be $\frac{1}{4}\Delta$ BO. If $\frac{1}{2}\Delta$ BO was measured at the right lens mark and $\frac{1}{4}\Delta$ BO was measured at the left lens mark, then the total prism would be $\frac{3}{4}\Delta$ BO.

According to section 5.1.5 of Appendix 6-1, the total horizontal prism measured should not differ from the total prescribed by more than $\frac{2}{3}\Delta$. For Example 4, since no prism was prescribed, a total measured horizontal prism of up to $\frac{2}{3}\Delta$ BI or $\frac{2}{3}\Delta$ BO would be acceptable.

A note of caution: Even if the amount of horizontal prism in a pair of spectacles is found to be outside tolerances, it is not wise to send the spectacles back to the laboratory to be remade automatically. Many patients can tolerate some horizontal prism, and in some cases, the extra prism will actually be of benefit to the patient. It is always best to check with the optometrist before returning the spectacles.

VERIFICATION OF SPECTACLE FRAMES

Frame Size

The size of the spectacle frame must be verified as being correct as part of the normal verification procedures for spectacles received from the optical laboratory. The three dimensions to verify are the eyesize, the bridge size, and the temple length.

Frame eyesize is usually the A dimension of the frame as specified using the boxing system. Frame bridge size is usually the boxing system DBL dimension. Both are commonly stamped on the temple of the frame. If numbers are not stamped on the frame, then the A and DBL dimensions must be measured with a PD rule (Figure 6-52). To measure the A dimension, place a PD rule horizontally across the eyewire opening with its zero mark aligned with the temporal-most extent of the lens bevel. The distance across the lens to the nasal-most extent of the lens bevel will be the A dimension in millimeters. (It may usually be assumed that the lens bevel will extend about 0.5 mm into the frame eyewire on each side of the lens, as shown by the dotted lines in Figure 6-52.) The frame DBL dimension is similarly measured as the minimum horizontal separation of the two lens bevels.

When the A and DBL dimensions of a frame are measured, it will sometimes be found that the dimensions do not match the ordered eye size and bridge size. This does not necessarily mean that the wrong frame was supplied. Instead, it may mean that the frame manufacturer did not use the boxing system to specify frame dimensions. A "frame book" can be used to determine if a manufacturer is using the boxing system. Frame books are compilations of manufacturers' literature on spectacle

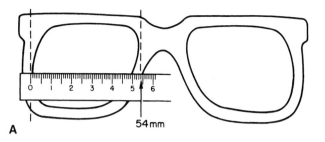
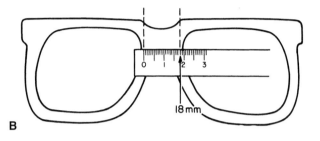

FIGURE 6-52—A. Measurement of the A dimension of a frame. The A dimension is the widest horizontal dimension of the lens opening as measured from the tips of the eyewire grooves. These grooves extend approximately 0.5 mm into the frame material, as shown by the dotted lines. B. Measurement of the distance between lenses (DBL) dimension of a frame. The distance between lenses is the smallest distance between the eyewire grooves.

frames that contain information on available sizes and colors of almost all frames made. Using Figure 6-53 as an example, the A dimensions of the Polo Classic V frame do not match the eyesizes listed. Therefore, the manufacturer was not using the boxing system to specify frame sizes.

The temple length of a frame is usually, although not always, specified as the distance from the center of the temple hinge barrels to the end of the temple (Figure 6-54). It may be specified in either millimeters or inches, usually in multiples of 5 mm or in multiples of ¼ inch, and is commonly stamped on the temple.

Figure 6-55 illustrates a procedure that can be used to measure temple length if temple length is not stamped on the temple. Place a PD rule along the top of the temple and position it so that the zero mark is aligned with the center of the hinge barrels. Slowly roll the ruler around the temple bend until it again lies flat against the temple. Temple length will be the PD rule reading opposite the temple end.

144 Chapter 6

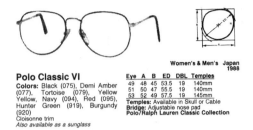

FIGURE 6-53—Availability information for the Polo Classic VI frame from Optique du Monde. (Courtesy of Frames, Data, Inc.)

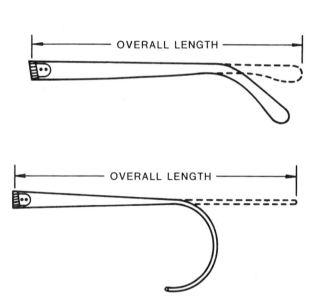

FIGURE 6-54—The most commonly used method for specifying temple length. Temple length is the distance from the center of the barrel hinges to the end of the temple. The upper illustration is of a "skull"-type temple. The lower illustration is of a "riding bow," "comfort cable," or "relaxo" temple designed to wrap around the ear.

Frame Color

Until familiarity is achieved with frame colors, the color of a plastic spectacle frame received from the optical laboratory is best verified by comparison to a sample. Color should be matched to a sample frame that is an exact duplicate of the frame received (same frame name and manufacturer), since frame colors are not standardized among manufacturers.

Metal frame colors are more easily verified. A frame ordered in the color yellow, yellow

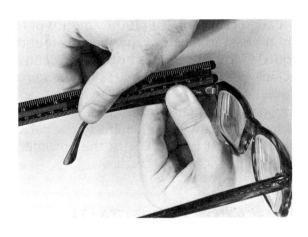

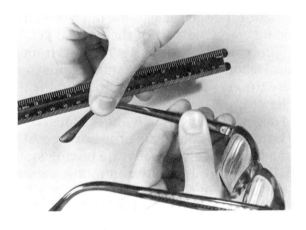

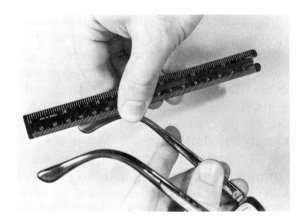

FIGURE 6-55—Measurement of temple length with an interpupillary rule. In the top photograph, the zero mark of the rule has been aligned with the center of the hinge barrels. In the middle photograph, the rule is being rolled around the temple bend. At bottom, the rule is again flat against the temple. The temple length is 145 mm, or 5¾ inches.

gold, pink, pink gold, or gold should appear gold in color. A frame ordered in the color white, white gold, or silver should appear silver in color. Other metal frame colors are best verified against a sample frame because the frame color cannot always be predicted from the manufacturer's color name.

Frame Shape

The shape of a frame (or lens) does not usually need to be verified, since most plastic and metal frames are available in only one lens shape. Several lens shapes may be available for some rimless and semirimless frames, however. Verify the lens shape against information presented in the frame book.

Temple Type

The style of temple received should be verified, since some frames are available with more than one temple type. Two common temple types are shown in Figure 6-54.

Bridge Type

The frame bridge type received should be verified against the order form. Although most plastic frames are available in only one bridge style, some metal frames are available with the choice of either adjustable pads or a formfit bridge.

Frame Quality

New spectacle frames received from the optical laboratory, frame manufacturer, or importer should not be damaged or defective. Scratches, dents, or unpolished areas are cause for rejection. One commonly found plastic frame defect is a pitting of the surface caused by overheating during insertion of the lenses. Hinges should be tightly attached to the frame front and temples, and lenses should fit tightly into the frame eyewires. Any frame that is found to be damaged should be returned for replacement.

New spectacles received from the optical laboratory should also have been adjusted by laboratory personnel to the "standard alignment" position. This position is a beginning point for frame adjustments, and a frame that is in standard alignment is usually easier to adjust to a patient's face than a frame that is out of alignment. A frame in standard alignment has the following three characteristics: (1) Both lenses will be in the same plane (i.e., the eyewires will not be twisted around the bridge), (2) the frame will have a small amount of pantoscopic tilt, and (3) the temples will be parallel to each other and will extend back from the frame front at a 90-degree angle to the front. If a new pair of spectacles received from the optical laboratory is grossly out of adjustment, it should be realigned to the standard alignment position at the time of verification. This will save time later when the glasses are dispensed to the patient.

CONCLUSION

Using the procedures described in this chapter, the paraoptometric can increase the efficiency of the optical dispensary and provide quality control for the eyewear received from the optical laboratory.

SUGGESTED READING

Brooks CW, Borish IM. System for Ophthalmic Dispensing (2nd ed). Boston: Butterworth-Heinemann, 1996.

Optical Laboratories Association. Perspectives on Lenses. Merrifield, VA: Optical Laboratories Association, 1996.

Appendix: Summary of ANSI Z80.1-1995 American National Standard for Ophthalmics– Prescription Ophthalmic Lenses–Recommendations*†

5.1 OPTICAL TOLERANCES

5.1.2 Minimum Requirements on Distance Refractive Power (Back Vertex Power)

Lenses shall comply both with the tolerances on each principal meridian, A, and with the tolerances of the cylinder, B, as specified below.

Single-vision and multifocal lenses

Meridian of highest absolute power	Tolerance on each meridian (A)	Tolerance on nominal value of the cylinder (B)			
		0.00 up to 0.75	>0.75 up to 4.00	>4.00 up to 6.00	>6.00
0.00 up to 3.00	±0.12	±0.09	±0.12	±0.18	±0.25
>3.00 up to 6.00	±0.12	±0.12	±0.12	±0.18	±0.25
>6.00 up to 9.00	±0.12	±0.12	±0.18	±0.18	±0.25
>9.00 up to 12.00	±0.18	±0.12	±0.18	±0.25	±0.25
>12.00 up to 20.00	±0.25	±0.18	±0.25	±0.25	±0.25
>20.00	±0.37	±0.25	±0.25	±0.37	±0.37

NOTE: The distance refractive power imbalance between a pair of lenses in each meridian shall not exceed two-thirds the sum of the tolerances for each lens for that meridian.

Progressive and aspheric lenses

Meridian of highest absolute power	Tolerance on each meridian (A)	Tolerance on nominal value of the cylinder (B)			
		0.00 up to 0.75	>0.75 up to 4.00	>4.00 up to 6.00	>6.00
0.00 up to 3.00	±0.12	±0.12	±0.18	±0.18	±0.25
>3.00 up to 6.00	±0.12	±0.12	±0.18	±0.18	±0.25
>6.00 up to 9.00	±0.18	±0.18	±0.25	±0.25	±0.25
>9.00 up to 12.00	±0.18	±0.18	±0.25	±0.25	±0.25
>12.00 up to 20.00	±0.25	±0.18	±0.25	±0.25	±0.25
>20.00	±0.37	±0.25	±0.25	±0.37	±0.37

NOTE: The distance refractive power imbalance between a pair of lenses in each meridian shall not exceed two-thirds the sum of the tolerances for each lens for that meridian.

---

*Reproduced with permission from American National Standard for Ophthalmics–Prescription Ophthalmic Lenses Recommendations, ANSI Z80.1-1995. Merrifield, VA: Optical Laboratories Association, 1995.
†Section numbers throughout the appendix refer to the section in ANSI Z80.1-1995 in which the standard appears.

5.1.3 Tolerances on the Direction of Cylinder Axis

Nominal value of the cylinder power (D)	Up to 0.37	>0.37 up to 0.75	>0.75 up to 1.50	>1.50
Tolerance of the axis (degrees)	±7	±5	±3	±2

5.1.4 Tolerance on Addition Power for Multifocal and Progressive Addition Lenses

Nominal value of addition power (D)	Up to 4.00	>4.00
Nominal value of the tolerance on the addition power (D)	±0.12	±0.18

NOTE: If the manufacturer applies corrections to compensate for the as-worn position, then the tolerances apply to the corrected value and this corrected value must also be stated in the documentation.

5.1.5 Tolerances on Prism Reference Point Location and Prismatic Power

For Single Lenses

The prismatic power tolerances specified below shall be met at the prism reference point (PRP). In all cases, the tolerances shown apply to lenses with and without prescribed power. A PRP placement error of ±1.0 mm in any direction is permissible.

Prismatic power (Δ)	Tolerance (Δ)
0.00 up to 2.00	±0.25
More than 2.00 up to 10.00	±0.37
More than 10.00	±0.50

For Mounted Pairs

Prismatic imbalance from processing between mounted lenses in the vertical direction shall not exceed 0.33Δ. A variation of 1.0 mm in vertical level is permissible.

Prismatic imbalance from processing between mounted lenses in the horizontal direction shall not exceed 0.67Δ. A variation of ±2.5 mm from the specified distance interpupillary distance is permissible.

5.1.6 Base Curve

When specified, the base curve shall be supplied within ±0.75 D. The base curve shall be given using an assumed index of refraction of 1.530.

5.1.7 Warpage

The cylindrical surface power induced in the base curve of a lens as a result of finish processing in the laboratory should not exceed 1 D. This recommendation need not apply within 6 mm of the mounting eyewire.

5.1.8 Localized Errors

Localized power errors or aberrations caused by waves, warpage, or internal defects, which are detected by visual inspection, are permissible if no measurable or gross focimeter target element distortion or blur is found when the localized area is examined with a focimeter. Areas outside a 30-mm diameter from the distance reference point, or within 6 mm from the edge, or beyond the optical area of a lenticular, need not be tested for local power errors or aberrations. Progressive power lenses are exempt from this requirement.

5.2 GEOMETRIC TOLERANCES

5.2.1 Tolerance on Center Thickness

The center thickness shall be measured at the prism reference point of the convex surface and normal to this surface. It shall not deviate from the nominal value by more than ±0.3 mm.

NOTE: The nominal thickness of the lens may be specified by the prescriber or be the subject of agreement between prescriber and supplier.

5.2.2 Segment Size Tolerances for Multifocals

The segment dimensions (width, depth, and intermediate depth) shall not deviate from the nominal values by more than ±0.5 mm.

The difference between the segment dimensions in the mounted pair shall not exceed 0.7 mm.

5.2.3 Segment Vertical Location

The segment height shall match within ±1.0 mm of specification. In the case of progressive addition lenses, the fitting cross height shall be within ±1.0 mm of specification.

The difference between the segment heights or fitting cross heights in the mounted pair shall not exceed 1.0 mm.

5.2.4 Segment Horizontal Location

The distance between the geometric centers of the segments in a mounted pair shall be within ±2.5 mm of the specified near interpupillary distance. The inset of both lenses shall appear symmetrical and balanced unless monocular insets are specified. The geometric center of an E-line (fullwidth) multifocal segment is defined as the thinnest point on its ledge.

NOTE: In the case of progressive addition lenses, the near reference point is set by the lens design. Progressive lenses are fit with reference to the distance interpupillary distance and the fitting point and are therefore exempt from this requirement.

5.2.5 Segment Tilt

For the case of a segment with a straight-edged top, the tilt of its horizontal axis shall be less than 2 degrees.

5.3 MECHANICAL TOLERANCES

5.3.1 Eyewire Closure

The eyewire closure of the lens mounted in the frame shall be sufficient to prevent the lens from rotating.

5.3.2 Impact Resistance

5.3.2.1 Prescription Impact-Resistant Dress Eyewear Lenses

All lenses shall be capable of withstanding the impact test described in Section 6.6. Laminated, plastic, and raised-ledge multifocal lenses that may be damaged by impact test procedures may be certified by the manufacturer as conforming to the initial design testing or statistically significant sampling as specified by Title 21, Code of Federal Regulations, 801-410.

All monolithic (not laminated) glass lenses shall be treated to be resistant to impact.

5.3.2.2 Special Corrective Lenses

Certain lenses prescribed for specific visual needs are not suitable for the drop-ball technique of testing. Wherever possible, such lenses should be treated to be resistant to impact; however, impact testing requirements are waived. These lens types include

- Prism segment multifocals
- Slab-off prisms
- Lenticular cataracts
- Iseikonics
- Depressed segment one-piece multifocals
- Biconcaves, myodiscs, and minus lenticulars
- Custom laminates and cemented assemblies

5.4 TRANSMISSION AND ATTENUATION TOLERANCES

5.4.1 Spectrally Attenuating Materials

Manufacturers of materials which directly transmit optical radiation shall make spectral transmittance characteristics available to processors, fabricators, and to the professions. How the data was obtained by the manufacturer shall be described.

5.4.2 Ultraviolet Attenuating Lenses

Manufacturers of lenses who claim specific ultraviolet (UV) attenuating properties shall state the average percent transmittance between 290 and 315 nm (UV_B) and between 315 and 380 nm (UV_A).

5.5 PHYSICAL QUALITY AND APPEARANCE (SURFACE IMPERFECTIONS AND INTERNAL DEFECTS)

In a zone of 30 mm diameter centered around the distance reference point and over the whole area of the segment, if the segment is equal to or less than 30 mm (for segments over 30 mm, the inspection area shall be a 30-mm diameter zone centered around the near reference point), the lens shall not exhibit any pits, scratches, grayness, bubbles, cracks, striae, or watermarks that are visible and that would impair function of the lens. Outside this zone, small isolated material, surface defects, or both are acceptable.

6.6 IMPACT-RESISTANCE TEST METHOD

The impact resistance of lenses subject to individual test shall be measured with a 15.9 mm (5/8 in. ± 0.0001 in.) diameter steel ball weighing not less than 16 g (0.56 oz) dropped from a height of not less than 127 cm (50 in.), or an equivalent impact.

6.9 LOCALIZED ERROR TEST METHOD

View a high-contrast grid pattern of dark and light lines through the lens, scanning the lens area by area. The lens should be held approximately 305 mm (12 in.) from the eye for weak plus or minus lenses. For strong plus lenses, the eye should be placed near the focus. The target should be placed at least 305 mm (12 in.) from the lens.

Virtually any straight-edged object is suitable for viewing waves through minus lenses. A grid pattern, as viewed through the lens, should appear smoothly curved and gradually distorted from the center of the field outward.

Localized ripples or distortions that are visible to the unaided eye are an indication of a possible significant aberration, however. The area should be marked for evaluation in a focimeter. Localized ripples or distortions that are invisible to the unaided eye may be disregarded.

7 / Ophthalmic Dispensing

Marian C. Welling

Dispensing is the art of manipulating a frame so that it holds ophthalmic lenses in such a manner that the visual needs of the patient are optimally met. The frame must not only be cosmetically pleasing, it must also be comfortable to wear and keep the lenses in their proper position for a variety of physical activities.

A series of basic frame adjustment techniques is used to meet these objectives. Essentially, these are manual skills that require practice, along with an understanding of the concepts of frame fit and frame construction.

HOW TO FIT A FRAME

The first and most important step in good dispensing is a good frame fit. If a frame does not fit well, there is no adjustment that will make it comfortable and keep it in place on a patient's face. A good frame fit is critical to patient comfort and also to the proper functioning of the lenses in the frame. These basic rules of proper frame fit are designed to be incorporated with frame styling guidelines. These rules do not change even though frame styles change.

Rules for Proper Fit

1. *The width of the frame, from endpiece to endpiece, should be approximately equal to the width of the facial bone structure just above the cheek bones* (Figures 7-1 and 7-2). This keeps undue stress from being placed on the endpieces and hinges of the frame. The endpieces and hinges receive more wear and tear than any other frame parts because tension is placed on them whenever the frame is put on or removed. This should also help keep the sides of the temples from pressing into the sides of the head, a condition that causes the frame to be pushed down to the end of the nose. When placing the frame on the patient, it should be an open square. Do not spread the temple to accommodate a broad face.
2. *The longer the face, the greater the vertical depth of the frame should be* (Figure 7-3); *the shorter the face, the smaller the vertical depth should be* (Figure 7-4). This elemental rule of proportion keeps a frame eyewire from touching the eyebrows or the cheeks. A frame that touches cheeks or eyebrows not only discolors and wears out from contact with the oils and acid in the skin, but also moves on the face every time the wearer changes his or her facial expression.
3. *The bridge of the frame should rest flat on the sides of the nose, evenly distributing the weight of the frame.* Only the flat smooth surfaces of the bridge of the frame should touch the face, so there is no facial contact with edges that can leave red marks and break the skin.
4. *The temple should extend 40 mm behind the top of the ear and follow the contour of the face.* The temples act as frame stabilizers. The wide flat side of the temple holds the frame in place by touch, not pressure, against the skull behind the ear, following the contour of the ear. As a general rule, comfort cable temples are fit 15 mm longer than the traditional skull temple.

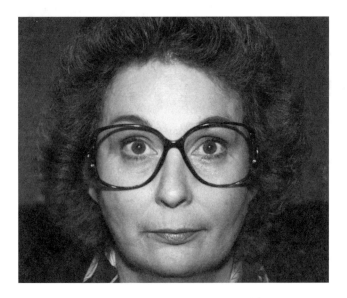

FIGURE 7-1—This frame is too wide for the facial bone structure.

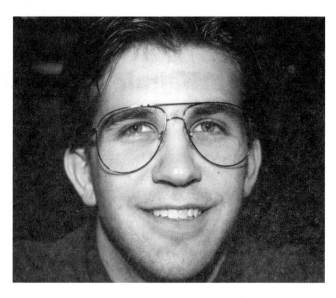

FIGURE 7-3—The longer the face, the greater the vertical depth of the frame.

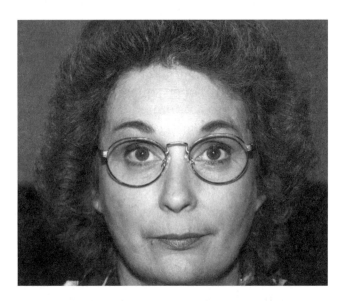

FIGURE 7-2—The width of this frame is too narrow for the facial bone structure.

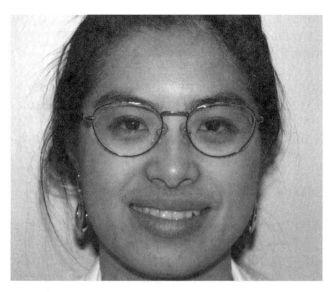

FIGURE 7-4—The shorter the face, the smaller the vertical depth of the frame.

HOW TO ALIGN A FRAME

The next step in dispensing a frame is to put the frame in standard alignment. Standard alignment of a frame is the process of making a frame symmetric. Standard alignment allows frames to "feel good" when the patient tries them on. Patients not only want a frame that looks good, but they also want it to feel good. They tend not to purchase a frame that is out of adjustment even if you assure them that it can be adjusted. The frames on your frame boards should always be kept in standard alignment. Maintaining alignment is an ongoing process as frames tend to lose alignment the more they are tried on.

Standard alignment is also the perfect starting point for frame fittings and adjustments because its main feature is symmetry. An aligned frame is very close to the perfect adjustment for

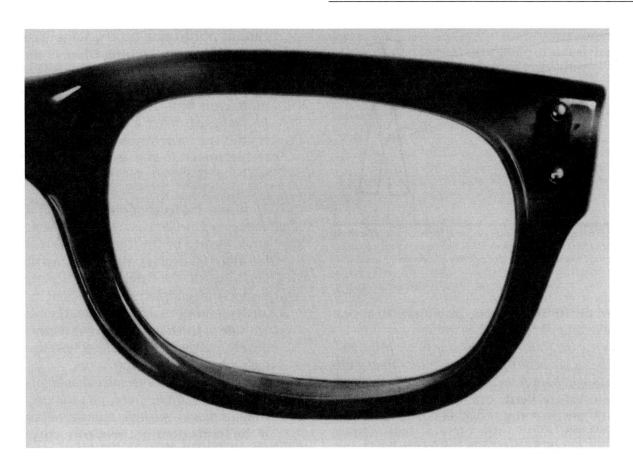

FIGURE 7-5—A rolled lower eyewire in a plastic frame. (Reprinted with permission from CW Brooks, IM Borish. System for Ophthalmic Dispensing [2nd ed]. Boston: Butterworth-Heinemann, 1996;125.)

most patients. Most adjustments are to temple tension and bends to customize the fit.

Steps for Standard Alignment

The steps to achieve standard alignment of a frame are easy to follow, and the time it takes is well worth it, both in terms of frame sales and time spent adjusting frames.

1. *Start with the frame front. Check for rolling of the eyewire* (Figure 7-5). If it is rolled, remove the lens or demo lens and straighten the eyewire. Use heat if it is a plastic frame. Make sure the bevel is straight and will hold the lens securely when it is reinserted. When checking a nylon suspension rimless frame, make sure the nylon cord is tight enough to hold the lens firmly in place.
2. *Next, look for X-ing of the bridge* (Figure 7-6). This is done by viewing the frame from both the sides and the top. The eyewires will not be aligned if the bridge is X-ed. If it is, you must carefully rotate the bridge area only until the eyewires are aligned. When working with a plastic frame make sure that the heat is confined to the bridge area.
3. *If the eyewires are out of alignment but the bridge is not X-ed, you must bend the bridge area evenly without rotating it until the eyewires are equal.* A frame should have face form so that it will follow the curve of the face.
4. *To make sure the frame front is even, you should lay your interpupillary distance (PD) rule across the ocular side of the frame front just below the temples at the endpiece.* When the PD rule is touching both endpieces, it should be equidistant from the frame at its two nasal points just above the nosepads (Figure 7-7).
5. *Temple alignment follows front alignment.* The front is aligned first because a misalignment

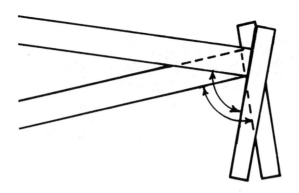

FIGURE 7-6—X-ing of the bridge as viewed from the side. (Reprinted with permission from CW Brooks, IM Borish. System for Ophthalmic Dispensing [2nd ed]. Boston: Butterworth-Heinemann, 1996;147.)

of the front can cause the temples to appear asymmetric when they are not.

6. *View the frame from the side to see if the endpieces are bent up or down, rather than going straight back from the frame front.* If the endpieces are bent, one temple will appear higher than the other. The bent endpiece must be repositioned. Once again, with a plastic frame heat must be used, but be careful not to pull on the temple itself as that will loosen the hinge.
7. *If the temples are not even when viewed from the side but the endpieces are straight, the temple hinge is bent. The hinges themselves must be realigned.* This a cold bend (i.e., the frames are not heated) regardless of the frame material and is easiest to achieve with wide-jawed temple angling pliers (Figure 7-8).
8. *Make sure the temples meet the front at a 90-degree angle when viewed from the top.* If the angle formed by the front and the temples is less than 90 degrees, the endpieces must be bent out. If the angle is greater than 90 degrees, the endpieces must be bent in. These angles must be exactly equal on the right and left side of the frame. Any asymmetry here is greatly exaggerated in terms of how the frame feels when someone tries it on.
9. *Fold the frame. The temples should fold evenly across the frame front, and the tips of the temples should touch the eyewire, not the lens.* If the frame does not fold correctly, or the temple rubs the lens, the temple hinge

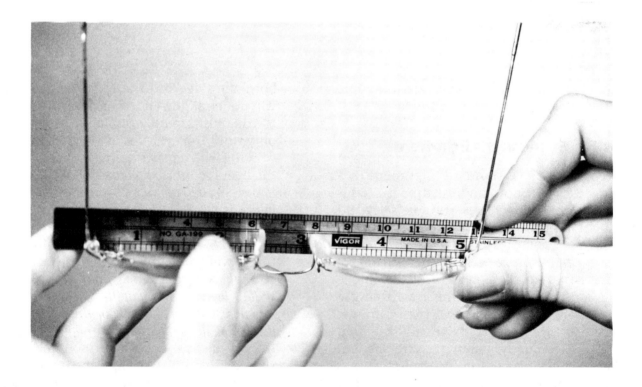

FIGURE 7-7—Using an interpupillary distance rule to make sure that the frame front is even. This is also known as vertical alignment or four-point touch. (Reprinted with permission from CW Brooks, IM Borish. System for Ophthalmic Dispensing [2nd ed]. Boston: Butterworth-Heinemann, 1996;180.)

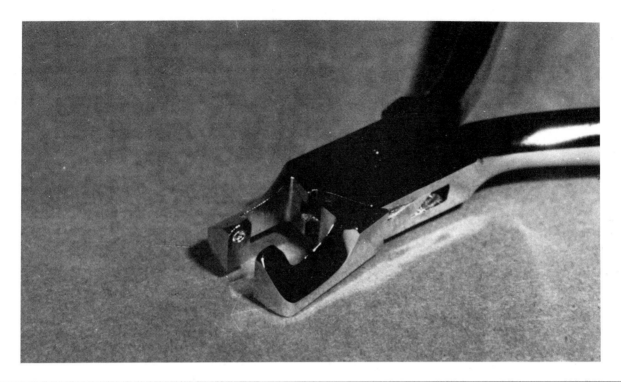

FIGURE 7-8—Temple-angling pliers. (Reprinted with permission from CW Brooks, IM Borish. System for Ophthalmic Dispensing [2nd ed]. Boston: Butterworth-Heinemann, 1996;157.)

must be rotated in or out until both sides are equal. This, like all hinge bends, is done cold, with hinge-angling pliers.

Following these steps will lead to a frame that "feels good" when it is tried on and will also make your frame adjustments when dispensing the frame minor and simple. Standard alignment is the starting point for all frame adjustments.

HOW TO ADJUST A FRAME

After the frame is aligned, the frame fit is customized through a series of adjustments that adapt the frame to the particular wearer (Table 7-1). When discussing frame adjustments it is necessary to standardize terminology. "In" means toward the center or midpoint of the bridge area of the frame; "out" means towards the temples of the frame. "Up" means toward the top of the eyewire; "down" means toward the bottom of the eyewire when you are looking at the frame as though it was on the wearer's face.

Using the recommended pliers rather than fingers for making frame adjustments protects the frame. Pliers allow you to use more leverage when making a bend, and they control where the bend will be made without putting unwanted stress on solder joints and hinges or weaker frame points (Table 7-2).

There are several parts of a frame that are bent to accommodate a wearer's facial structure. The order in which these adjustments are made

TABLE 7-1. Frame adjustment tips

1. If one eyewire is closer to the face than the other, the endpiece bends must be equalized.
2. If one eyewire is higher on the face than the other, the temple hinge angles must be equalized.
3. To keep frames from sliding down the nose, the temple bend should be a 45-degree angle at the top of the ear.
4. To properly stabilize the frame, the temple should lay flat against the skull behind the ear without touching the ear itself.
5. If the temples press into the sides of the head in front of the ear, the glasses are being pushed off the nose. Widen the endpiece angles to avoid this problem.

TABLE 7-2. Pliers worth their weight in gold

Pliers	Description
Pad-angling pliers	Used to angle nosepads without putting pressure on the solder joints of the guard arms. Correct pad angles allow the weight of the frame to be distributed equally with no cutting edges
Nylon-jawed pliers	Allows endpiece bends in both plastic and metal frames to be made without marring the finish
Wide-jawed hinge angling pliers	Allows for angling of hinges without stress being placed on solder joints or hidden hinges becoming loose
Round-flat jawed pliers	Ideal for both guard arm bends and endpiece bends
Needle-nose pliers or long handled tweezers	Essential to facilitate the placement of tiny screws in hard-to-reach places

Note: A good set of optical screwdrivers, wrenches, and files should round out your tool kit.

is important to a successful outcome. At this point, the frame is put on the wearer, and the actual amount the frame that is bent at each of its adjustment points is determined in relation to the wearer's facial structure.

1. *The endpieces are bent in or out to leave approximately 2 mm of space between the flat side of the temple and the side of the wearer's head.* This bend is made using fiber-jawed pliers in order to protect the frame finish. If the frame is plastic, the endpiece is heated first. After the endpiece is heated, be careful not to pull on the temple, as this will loosen the hinge. Metal frame bends are made cold.

   The endpiece bend is the most common adjustment made in frames. This is because the endpiece bends stretch out when the frames are put on and taken off. When frames loosen with wear, it is this bend that must be tightened. The endpieces must be bent in to tighten a loose frame.

2. *The frame hinge must be angled down to add approximately 15 degrees of pantoscopic tilt to the frame.* Pantoscopic tilt is the angle that the frame front makes with the temple when viewed from the side (Figure 7-9). When the frame is on the wearer, the bottom of the eyewire should be closer to the cheeks than the top of the eyewire is to the eyebrows. Pantoscopic tilt is added to both plastic and metal frames by bending the hinge down with hinge-angling pliers. This is a cold adjustment, since you are actually bending the metal hinge itself regardless of frame material.

   Pantoscopic tilt is needed in a frame in order for the wearer to achieve the proper optics through their lenses by placing the lenses as close to the patient's eyes as comfortably possible and to obtain the widest possible field of view through a multifocal lens.

3. *If the frame has adjustable nosepads, they are angled to follow the slope of the wearer's nose.* If there are no adjustable pads, proceed directly to step 4. Adjustable pads are angled with pad-angling pliers. There are three nosepad angles that correspond to the slopes of a nose.
   a. *Frontal angle.* The tops of the pads should be angled inward approximately 15 degrees.
   b. *Splay angle.* The edge of the pads closest to the frame front should be angled inward approximately 15 degrees.
   c. *Vertical angle.* The bottoms of the pads should be angled toward the frame front when viewed from the side.

   These angles are added while you are viewing the frame just as if it was on the wearer's face. Once these angles are in place, the nosepads should rock into position on the wearer's nose. The wide, flat pad surface should evenly touch the nose. None of the pad edges should be digging into the nose.

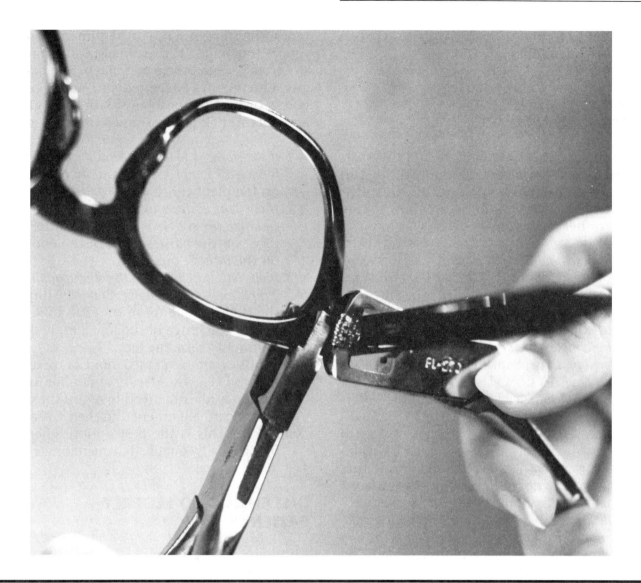

FIGURE 7-9—Using angling pliers to change the pantoscopic angle. (Reprinted with permission from CW Brooks, IM Borish. System for Ophthalmic Dispensing [2nd ed]. Boston: Butterworth-Heinemann, 1996;158.)

There should be 1 mm of space between the nosepad and the eyewire when you view the frame on the wearer. The guard arm that attaches the nosepad to the eyewire of the frame is bent in or out with needle nose pliers to achieve this.

4. *Bow the temples slightly inward so that they begin to touch the skull just in front of the ears.* This is done by shaping the temple between the thumb and index finger. Plastic temples are heated first. The flat side of the temple should touch the skull just in front of the ear and extend to the end of the temple.
5. *Place a 45-degree angle bend at the point on the temple that coincides with the top of the ear.* This is done after heating the point on the temple that must be bent. Metal frames have a plastic cover at this point; they are carefully heated prior to bending also. This bend is made with the fingers rather than with pliers. It should be a true 45-degree angle rather than a curve in the temple. This bend in the temple keeps the frame from sliding forward.
6. *The temple should be angled in so that its flat side touches the skull behind the ear.* The temple should be close to the cartilage of the ear but never touch it. To achieve uniform touch behind the ear, it is often necessary to add a mastoid bend to the temple to coincide with the depression in the wearer's mastoid bone. This is done by heating the temple behind the bend and making a

depression in it with your thumb, between the bend and temple end.

CARE AND HANDLING INSTRUCTIONS

The dispensing is now complete, and the wearer is ready to leave with comfortably fitting and correctly positioned frames. At this time, it is important to explain to the wearer how to care for his or her new eyewear.

1. *Frames should be put on and taken off using two hands, one on each temple just behind the hinge.* The frame should first be tilted up over the ears and then pulled straight off or put straight on.
2. *The temples should be folded and the frame stored in a case.* Explain how to place glasses in a case. To store glasses in hard cases, the temples are placed outside, and the flap is snapped over the temples. To store glasses in slip cases, the wide side of the glasses goes to the wide side of the case. If no case is available, wearers should at least make sure that the frame is not resting on the lens surfaces; the lens side should always be facing up.
3. *The frame should be cleaned daily with a mild, nonabrasive soap such as dish detergent and warm water.* Special attention should be given to the bridge and nosepad areas.
4. *Lenses should be cleaned as often as necessary, but at least once a day.* Lenses should always be wet with warm water before they are wiped off with a soft cloth. It is acceptable to use facial tissues to wipe the lenses as long as they have been wet first. Special lens cleaners are not necessary. Warm water and a mild soap work well even on coated lenses. Coated lenses need warmer water (even hot water) and soap to cut the grease that collects on their surfaces. Commercial lens cleaners are fine as long as they do not contain alcohol or other chemicals that can damage frame finishes or lens coatings.

FOLLOW-UP ADJUSTMENTS

Even normal wear can cause a frame to lose its adjustment over time. When this happens, repeat the steps in standard alignment and customize the frame fit again. Inspect all frames for stress cracks and brittle material before making any adjustments. Make patients aware of any cracks or possible problems with their glasses and obtain their permission to adjust them.

1. *If the frame is too loose, bend the endpieces in to increase temple tension* and increase curve on temples behind ears.
2. *If one lens is closer to the face than the other, equalize the endpiece bends.* Bend the endpiece on the close side in or the endpiece on the far side out.
3. *If one lens is higher than the other, equalize the temple angles at the hinge.* Bend the hinge of the high temple up in order to lower the lens or the hinge of the low temple down, in order to raise the lens.

If the frame is aligned, none of these conditions will exist. An easy option for follow-up frame adjustments is to return the frame to standard alignment and then customize the fit. This is the best option when the frame is badly out of adjustment or very old.

DISPENSING TO ELDERLY PATIENTS

Although the basic principles of fitting and adjusting frames are the same for all age groups, there are problems unique to adjusting the frames of older patients. These differences are due to the physical differences brought about by the aging process, which alters the necessary frame manipulations slightly.

The frame adjustment process changes because of the aging of the skin on the face. As it ages, the skin thins and loses subcutaneous fat, causing folds and wrinkles. There is a loss of connective tissue that leaves the skin less elastic. These changes are pronounced in the region of the nose, the area that supports the entire weight of the frame. The frame weight is more likely to irritate or abrade the skin on the nose of the aged patient, and the healing process is slowed in the elderly. Consequently, there are special steps to take to adjust elderly patients frames to make them more comfortable.

Use adjustable nosepads. If the frame does not have them, guard arms and pads can be

TABLE 7-3. Tips for lens minimizing
Using high-index lens materials alone will not result in thin, cosmetically pleasing lenses. The high-index lens materials must be combined with the following steps for maximum lens thinness and the best cosmetic value.
1. Center the eye in the frame, both vertically and horizontally. 2. Choose a lens shape as close to round as possible. 3. Use antireflection coatings. 4. Use a hide-a-bevel edge finishing. 5. Do not roll the lens edges. 6. Do not polish the lens bevel. 7. Use a pale edge tint in a shade complimentary to the frame. 8. Use a frame with a turn-back endpiece. 9. Fit the bridge carefully. 10. Do not forget to use aspheric designs to minimize high plus lenses.

added to the frame. Adjustable pads have the advantage of flexibility. You can change their position on the patient's nose at regular intervals so no one point abrades from constantly bearing the weight of the frame.

The nosepads should be made of silicone for several reasons. It is very soft and flexible for comfort. It is also "breathable." The skin below it gets oxygen and becomes less likely to abrade. It will also allow an already abraded nose to heal more quickly.

Extra-large nosepads will distribute the frame weight over a greater area, putting less weight on any given point. There are also adjustable nosepads with a saddle-type connecting top that spreads the frame weight across the crest of the nose as well as on the sides of the nose.

If the patient does not want adjustable nosepads, you can add press-on silicone pads to the bridge area of a plastic frame. This redistributes the frame weight, provides a cushioning effect, and adds the "breathability" factor necessary for healthy skin to a rigid bridge.

The elderly patient's temples should be bent so that they do not touch the cartilage of the ear itself, but have their flat edge evenly against the skull, following the contour of the ear but never touching it.

If the patient wears a behind-the-ear hearing aid, the temple should be angled around it. Select a narrow temple that is perhaps a bit longer on the hearing aid side, being careful to avoid contact that would cause unpleasant pressure on or even dislodge the hearing aid.

Remember that temples are stabilizers that hold the frame securely in position by touch along the skull behind the ear. They are not meant to be wrapped tightly around the ear itself. That will bring about irritation and abrasions.

Also, lenses should be as thin as possible to reduce the weight of the frame on the nose. There are several steps that may be taken to maximize lens thinness (Table 7-3).

DISPENSING TO CHILDREN

The bone structure of children is different from that of adults; these differences require the use of different frame adjustment techniques when fitting them with frames.

As a general rule, children's heads are more round. To accommodate this, the angle the endpiece makes with the temple may need to be bent so that it is greater than 90 degrees. It is usually preferable to angle the endpieces out to reduce endpiece stress than to fit a larger eyesize. Children's eyes are close-set, and a large eyesize gives a child a disproportionate look. Remember, the temples should not dig into the side of the head, which would cause the frame to slide down the nose. This adjustment will also put less pressure on the endpiece of the frame itself. (The endpiece is the major stress point of the frame.) Spring hinges are also a good choice because they relieve much of the stress placed on the endpieces when the glasses are being put on or taken off.

Children often have very long eyelashes. To keep the eyelashes from touching the lenses, 15–20 degrees of pantoscopic tilt should be added to the frame. This is approximately 5 degrees more than an adult's frame would have.

Children are usually extremely active and tend toward rough playing. This necessitates a frame that is held securely in place. To achieve this, the sides of the temples behind the ears are bent snugly into the skull. This is done by adding a slight bowing to the temple shaft. The bend in the temple can also be angled down closer to the ear itself than normal. These adjustments will hold the frame more securely in place. The use of an elastic sport band may also be suggested.

Riding bow temples can be used on toddlers and small children so that they cannot remove the glasses themselves. They also provide extra stability.

The bridge of a child's nose does not fully develop until puberty, so adjustable guard arms with nosepads help support the frame on the face and keep it from sliding down the nose. Do not use the super soft, flexible nosepads on children's frames because they have the same texture as soft candy and children may chew them off the guard arm attachment.

Finally, a good manufacturer's warranty is an essential part of selecting a child's frame, since no matter how perfect the frame adjustment or how durable the frame material, a child will probably break it. There is no such thing as a childproof frame.

SUGGESTED READING

Brooks CW, Borish IM. System for Ophthalmic Dispensing (2nd ed). Boston: Butterworth-Heinemann, 1996.

8 / Basic Pretesting Procedures

Mary Jameson

The comprehensive primary care optometric examination involves taking a thorough patient history and collecting an extensive battery of preliminary test results. The contemporary optometrist will typically employ two or more paraoptometrics (assistants or technicians) to ensure maximum efficiency, accuracy, and thoroughness in the collection of these data. By "delegating" preliminary procedures to a competent paraoptometric, optometrists may effectively and safely extend their practice capabilities to a larger patient population. For delegation of such patient care responsibilities to work best, it is important to establish a few concepts that serve to enhance the practitioner/paraoptometric relationship. Four are suggested here.

1. *The role of the paraoptometric.* Optometric assistants and technicians are integral members of the optometric care team. By reason of either or both their training and experience, they are knowledgeable and skilled in gathering data, performing tests, making preliminary assessments, and working in many areas of patient care. Teamwork and mutual respect between the doctor and the paraoptometric are crucial to an integrated approach to patient care. Continuous communication throughout the day is vital in order to clearly understand which areas of patient care are appropriately delegated.
2. *Sequence and method of testing.* A minimum data base should be established for all initial and established comprehensive exams and for various levels of follow-up visits. A consistent sequence of testing will minimize the likelihood that important data will be overlooked. Initially and periodically, the doctor and the paraoptometric should carefully compare their testing technique to ensure consistency.
3. *The location of testing.* If the office has two examination lanes, the paraoptometric may use one while the doctor uses the other, and the patient may not have to be moved. If there is only one lane, a specific, appropriately equipped room must be designated in which the paraoptometric may function in privacy.
4. *Method of recording.* The patient medical record is a legal document, and entries in it must be accurate, thorough, and legible. A "fill-in-the-blanks" type of record form may be useful because it provides headings, thus helping prevent data being overlooked. This format is especially useful in ensuring consistency of records in a practice setting where several practitioners and paraoptometrics are working together. In addition, commonly used abbreviations should be agreed on and published in the office glossary of abbreviations.

PATIENT HISTORY

One of the most important procedures in any eye examination is the patient history. This point is often missed because of the seemingly "nontechnical" nature of history. The history, however, is the point in the data gathering in which we determine the chief complaint and ask many key questions, which may often provide a fairly accurate preliminary diagnosis. The patient history may be instrumental in planning a useful testing regimen. Because the patient history and interview is a time-consuming process, the paraoptometric's role also serves to free the doctor to spend more time on other, more complex areas of patient management. After the initial history, it is often useful for the paraoptometric to consult with the doctor prior to further testing and data collection in order to focus this activity. The doctor may also then make better use of his or her time as the remainder of the patient care sequence unfolds.

Technique

The performance of a patient history can be compared to performing an interview. First, the patient should be made to feel comfortable. You should display a cordial and caring attitude toward the patient. The goal, which should be explained to the patient, is to elicit information necessary for the doctor to investigate, diagnose, and manage the patient's condition.

Your interview should begin with an introduction. Greet the patient in a friendly and professional manner. It is preferable to go into the reception area to greet the patient rather than to call the patient to come forward to a desk or through a doorway. Generally, unless the patient is well known to you, it is best to address the patient formally and not by his or her first name. If you have a question about how a patient would like to be addressed, ask the patient. Then note it in the chart for future reference for the doctor and staff. You may desire to greet the patient with a handshake in order to establish a professional, formal bond.

Move with the patient to an examination lane or other area of the office designated for history taking. It should be a quiet area, away from office traffic, where there will be no interruptions. The patient will be more likely to respond to your questions truthfully in a private setting, knowing that he or she has your full attention and that others in the office are not listening to your conversation. This approach is more than good data collection technique; it helps to establish patient rapport (Figure 8-1).

Explain to the patient that you are going to be asking some questions about her or his general health and ocular history and that this information is an important part of the examination. Since your approach to the patient sets the tone of the interview, be sure to maintain eye contact with the patient, and be alert and attentive. It is usually best to refrain from writing down the responses until the patient has finished responding, and often more than one history point can be "remembered" and written down in groups. To save time, write down only the positive responses to any questions. Negative responses are easier to remember and may be added to the history form at the end of the interview. The goal is to interview the patient in a relaxed and easy manner, retrieving all the necessary information to assist the doctor in the diagnosis, while communicating a caring and professional attitude.

The case history will almost always open with a form of the question, such as, "Why are you here?" "What brings you in today?" or "What is the main purpose of your visit today?" The doctor must know the patient's reason for the visit, or chief complaint, in order to address the patient's needs appropriately. The response should be recorded in the patient's own words, with quotation marks around the response. The response should not be rephrased or interpreted by the paraoptometric before recording. It may need to be investigated further for clarification, but the patient record must reflect precisely what the patient said.

After eliciting the chief complaint, the questions asked during a patient history are fairly standard. Doctors often have a specific list of key history questions. The three generally accepted methods of history taking are *open-ended*, *outline*, and *checklist*.

In the open-ended approach, the interviewing is the least structured. General questions are asked, and the unrestricted patient response is simply recorded. This form of interview is time-consuming and may lead to a dead end in the pursuit of data if not carefully controlled. For these reasons, the open-ended question is usually used only for the chief complaint.

In contrast, the outline method uses an examination form with topical headings in

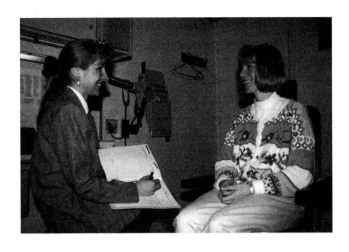

FIGURE 8-1—A private setting is conducive to effective communication.

order to stimulate questions concerning a standard set of categories. For example, the headings might include the following:

Chief complaint

Last eye exam—when? by whom?

Prescription history

Patient perception of vision (subjective)—distance and near

Ocular health—self, family

Ocular symptoms

General health—self, family

Last physical exam—when? physician name

Medications—what? when taken? what for?

Allergies—drugs? environment? seasonal? other?

Occupation/hobbies—visual tasks involved

A small amount of space is usually provided next to each categorized history area for writing notes about patient responses.

The third case history type is the checklist format. The checklist may include the same headings as above, but under each heading is a comprehensive list of more detailed items to which the responses required are usually "yes" or "no." This is perhaps the safest method, as a well prepared list can cover all necessary information. This type of case history is the easiest to delegate. The patient may be given this form on a clipboard to be completed in the waiting area before the examination.

Although thorough, the checklist method of history taking usually gives little detail about the patient's problems or complaints, and it should be supplemented by probing pertinent positive responses. The procedure of orally taking a checklist history allows patients to give yes or no responses and then describe or amplify a complaint in terms most familiar to them.

It is important for the interviewer to allow the patient to tell his or her story while maintaining control of the interview. Keep the patient on track by asking specific clarifying or probing questions about vague terms, such as spots, flashes of light, and fatigue. Ask the patient to describe the symptom in more detail so you can have a better idea of what the patient is experiencing. This may require prompting the patient without actually suggesting answers to the patient. This approach enables the paraoptometric to encourage the patient to elaborate regarding his or her problems.

The following is a list of characteristics that will enable the patient to clarify her or his condition:

Frequency—how often the patient has had this problem

Onset—when the problem typically first occurs

Progression—how the problem begins, unfolds, resolves

Duration—how long the problem typically lasts

Location—specifically where in the body the problem occurs

Aggravating or alleviating factors—what makes it worse or better

Any associated symptoms or attributions—what causes it

Family history is also important, since heredity may be a factor in many diseases, such as diabetes and high blood pressure. The paraoptometric should record the relationship of the patient for any positive family history responses. For example, MGM + HBP means that the patient's maternal grandmother has high blood pressure.

Systemic diseases and any medications taken for their treatment are important to note because of ocular effects that may be related to either the disease or the medication. It is often useful to be able to look up these medications to find such side effects. The *Physician's Desk Reference, Facts and Comparisons*, or another similar reference are excellent resources for this information.

It is usually a good idea to avoid using medical terminology when explaining results to the patient. Terms such as "myopia" and "astigmatism" may sound threatening to a patient and may be misunderstood. Tell the patient that it is fine to ask questions about any unfamiliar terms or phrases. Usually defer answering questions about patient concerns until all data are collected and assessments have been made by the doctor. Explaining results too early in the examination may lead to incorrect information and patient confusion. You should answer a patient's questions only when you understand clearly why he or she is asking. Be sure that your reply is accurate and appropriate. It is up to both the paraoptometric and the doctor to determine and assume roles in patient education.

Appropriate recording of patient history data is extremely important. The patient medical record is a legal document, and it can be reviewed by anyone to whom the patient gives permission. All pertinent data must be recorded accurately and legibly. In addition to recording positive responses to questions, it is always necessary to record significant negatives as well, such as (–)DM (no diabetes mellitus) or (–)HBP (no high blood pressure).

By learning as much as possible about the patient during the case history, the doctor and the paraoptometric will be better able to meet the needs of the patient for eyewear, contact lenses, or treatment of an ocular condition. The case history is the time to establish a rapport with the patient and to put the patient at ease so that she or he will feel comfortable with the rest of the examination. Good interviewing skills and techniques, combined with the caring, professional manner of the paraoptometric, will help the practitioner address the patient's concerns and provide a high level of care and service to the patient.

VISUAL ACUITY

Typically, the first data collected after the history are visual acuity. The *Dictionary of Visual*

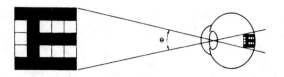

FIGURE 8-2—The Snellen system. (Reprinted with permission from SS Bates. Fundamentals for Assisting in Primary Care Optometry. New York: Professional Press/Fairchild, 1983.)

Science defines *visual acuity* as "acuteness or clearness of vision which is dependent on the sharpness of retinal focus, the conductivity of the nerves, and the interpretive faculty of the brain." Both aided and unaided visual acuity (VA) are measured and recorded: (1) to provide data on the quality of a patient's unaided (uncorrected) vision, (2) to quantify the patient's habitual visual status (with current prescription), and (3) to provide criteria by which to strive to achieve best quality vision.

VA charts are designed with several lines of letters, with the largest letters at the top and a decreasing letter size with each descending line. The standard VA chart was designed by Snellen, and it bears his name. The letters of each line subtend an angle of 5 minutes of arc when viewed at a specific distance. Each letter may be broken down into five parts, each part forming a one-minute angle with the eye (Figure 8-2).

The smallest line read by the patient is the line that is recorded as the VA. Distance VAs are recorded using Snellen notation, which is a fraction with two numbers (i.e., 20/40). The first number, or numerator (in this case, the "20"), represents the testing distance in feet or meters. The second number, or denominator (in this case, the "40"), is the distance at which the letter subtends a 5-minute angle in feet or meters. This may also be referred to as the letter size.

Since 20 feet is the customary testing distance, the numerator is usually 20, that is, 20/something. An acuity of 20/20 means that the letter designed to be read at 20 feet is being read at 20 feet. The fraction 20/30 means that the patient is reading a letter designed to be read at 30 feet at 20 feet, indicating decreased VA. In metric notation, 6/6 is the same as 20/20; 6/9 is the same as 20/30; 6/12 is the same as 20/40; and so forth.

TABLE 8-1. Height of 6/60 (20/200) E for various testing distances	
Distance	Height
6 m (~20 ft)	87 mm
5 m (~16 ft)	73 mm
4 m (~13 ft)	58 mm
3 m (~10 ft)	44 mm
Source: Reprinted with permission from T Grosvenor. Primary Care Optometry (2nd ed). New York: Professional Press/Fairchild, 1989;139.	

The numerator 20 should be used only when the testing distance is 20 feet. In cases when the patient has to walk toward the chart to read a letter, the distance at which the patient was first able to read the big E is recorded. If the big E is a 20/400 letter, and if the patient is able to read it at 15 feet, the VA is recorded as 15/400 (15-foot test distance, 400-size letter).

For calibration purposes, the 20/200 letter on a standard Snellen chart should always be 87 mm high for a test distance of 20 feet (Table 8-1). Near VAs measured with the Reduced Snellen near point card will be recorded with the Snellen notation, followed by the testing distance (i.e., 40 cm, since the numerator is supposed to be the testing distance). Other near point cards, such as the Lighthouse Continuous text card, the "J" card, and the Jaeger "M" card, use metric or letter notations for recording (i.e., J1 at 40 cm; 0.40/1 m).

While taking VAs, you might find that the patient is able to read all of the 20/25 line and only two letters on the 20/20 line. This may be recorded as 20/25+ or 20/25+2. If the patient consistently misread one letter on the 20/20 line, this may be recorded as 20/20– or 20/20–1. Again, consistency in recording in the office is very important, and the doctor and paraoptometric should make sure they are both recording in the same manner.

There are many new research-oriented acuity charts now being used in practice. Charts such as LogMAR, Bailey-Lovie, and Pelli Robson are based on differential spacing, vanishing contrast, or logarithmic variations in size. These charts almost always contain Snellen equivalents for consistency of recording.

Most of the different visual acuity charts available use rows of letters that the patient is asked to read. Other charts are designed for patients who do not know the alphabet. A Tumbling E chart consists of the letter E facing different directions. The Landolt C, Landolt Ring, and Broken Ring charts consist of incomplete rings or Cs in different positions. Like the letters on the Snellen chart, the figures decrease in size farther down the chart. The patient is asked to tell you the direction the E is facing or the position of the break in the ring. These types of charts may also be used with children. Lighthouse Cards make use of pictures of objects such as birds, houses, and birthday cakes. For examples of different acuity charts, see Figures 8-3 through 8-6.

Technique

The chart itself should be well illuminated for proper testing conditions. The recommended illuminance level for the distance and near test charts is 12–20 foot-candles.[1] Room illumination may vary from a darkened room to a well lighted room based on practitioner philosophy, testing method, or the patient's habitual visual environment. Whatever the room illumination, it is very important that all personnel in the office use the same conditions for measuring VAs.

Distance VAs are measured at 20 feet (or 6 m). Near visual acuities are measured at 16 inches (or 40 cm). Both are measured with and without the patient's current spectacle prescription, monocularly (each eye separately) and binocularly (both eyes together). In an examination room shorter than 20 feet, a mirror system may be used to create an optical 20-foot distance.

There is no one correct sequence of testing, but it is generally agreed that unaided testing should be done first at a given distance so the patient does not memorize the chart. One sequence is the following:

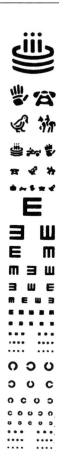

FIGURE 8-3—The American Optical children's acuity slide or optotype. (Reprinted with permission from T Grosvenor. Primary Care Optometry [3rd ed]. Boston: Butterworth-Heinemann, 1996;160.)

Distance, without Rx

Distance, with Rx

Near, without Rx

Near, with Rx

In this sequence, the room/chart illumination (i.e., dim room with bright chart illumination for distance testing; bright room with bright chart illumination for near) and handling of the near point card changes just once, but the patient's eyewear is off, on, off, and on again. Another sequence is the following:

Distance, without Rx

Near, without Rx

Near, with Rx

Distance, with Rx

In this sequence, the patient is handling eyewear less, but you must adjust the lights and charts more often.

Once you have established a sequence that is comfortable for you, adjustments to lights, charts, and patient instructions will become routine.

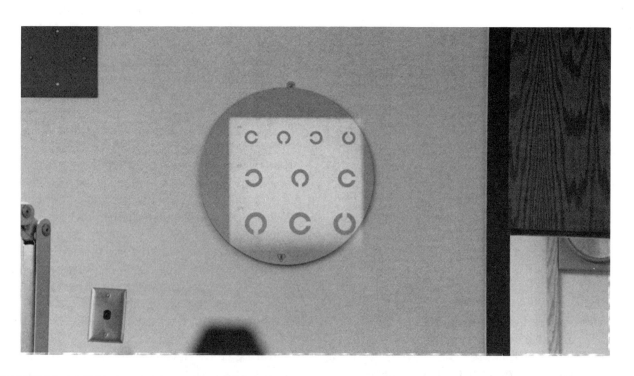

FIGURE 8-4—Landolt Cs.

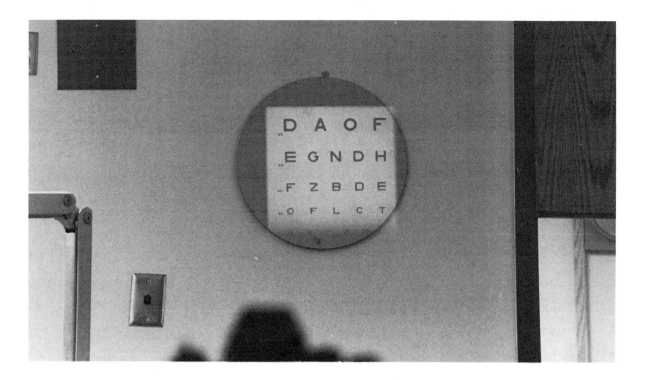
FIGURE 8-5—Snellen chart.

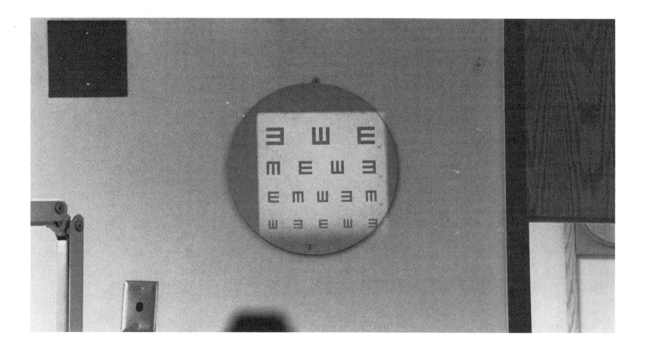
FIGURE 8-6—Tumbling Es.

You will also determine if it is more comfortable for you to hold the occluder (or paddle) or for the patient to hold it. It is generally convenient for the patient to hold the occluder for distance VAs while the examiner adjusts the chart, and for the examiner to hold it for near VAs while the patient holds and adjusts the near point card (Figure 8-7). In either case,

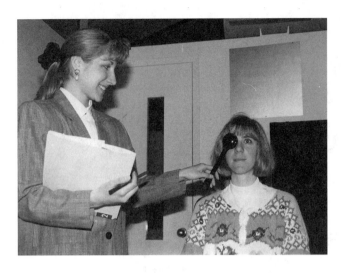

FIGURE 8-7—Testing distance visual acuities. Note the paraoptometric is occluding the patient's eye while observing the patient through the procedure.

make sure you clean the occluder between patients.

Keep your attention on the patient, not the chart. Do not allow the patient to squint or look around the occluder. This may alter test results. Also remind the patient that there are no right or wrong answers. He or she should just report what he or she sees. While you may "push" a bit to get best acuity, the patient should not try to guess, and you should never reveal how the patient is performing.

If you are using a wall chart, one in which the patient is able to view the entire chart at once, the patient will pick a row of letters he or she is comfortable reading. If your chart is projected, you will be able to isolate groups of lines or a single line of letters. Start with large letters. If you start with letters the patient cannot see, he or she may think that something is wrong with his or her vision. Patient responses will enable you to move quickly to the appropriate line.

One technique, assuming that the patient is binocular, is to test the right eye first. Cover the left eye by holding or having the patient hold the occluder. Ask the patient to read the smallest line of letters she or he can. Once she or he has done so, have the patient move the occluder to cover the right eye, and repeat to measure the VA of the left eye. Then ask the patient to remove the occluder and to read the smallest line she or he can with both eyes.

Another technique is to have the patient look out at the big "E" with both eyes, with no correction. Ask if he or she can see it. If yes, ask if it is clearer, brighter, or sharper with the right eye or left eye as you move the occluder from one eye to the other. If the patient reports that it is better with one eye, measure the monocular VA of the blurrier eye first. Proceed to the other eye, and then to both eyes.

If the patient is unable to read the largest letter on the chart, have the patient walk toward the chart until she or he can read it. Measure the distance from the chart to the patient. This distance will be recorded as the numerator of the VA measurement.

To measure near VAs, start without correction. Have the patient hold the near point acuity card where it is comfortable to hold it, and where he or she likes to hold his or her work. It may be appropriate to ask the patient to close his or her eyes and physically position the near point card where it is comfortable. Having the patient hold the card also ensures that glare from the overhead light is not a factor.

The examiner should hold the occluder in front of the nontested eye and have the patient read the smallest print possible. Continue to the other eye and for both eyes in the same manner as for distance acuities. Measure the distance that the patient is holding the card with a tape measure. This is recorded with the acuity measurement.

If the patient wears a prescription for near, VAs are then repeated with the correction. If the patient wears multifocals, make sure the card is being viewed through the near segment. If the patient moves the card closer or farther away when viewing through the near correction, measure the distance again, and record it with the VA measurement (Figures 8-8 and 8-9).

COLOR VISION

Color vision evaluation is an important part of an optometric examination. It may be used to detect both genetic and acquired color vision anomalies. Acquired color vision changes may result from cataracts, retinal disease, or optic nerve problems, and may also be caused by drugs or the side effects of medical therapy. To be effective, testing is performed monocularly,

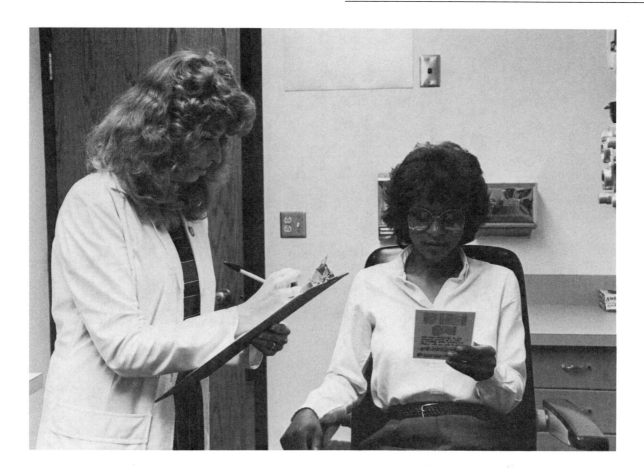

FIGURE 8-8—Testing near visual acuities.

because acquired color vision defects are often monocular.

Most color vision evaluation in optometric practice is done simply to determine whether or not a color vision defect exists. Further testing may be done to classify the specific type of defect.

Color vision evaluation is most commonly done using pseudoisochromatic plates (PIPs). These booklets have specially designed plates with numbers, symbols, or designs on the pages. The colors of the background and foreground figure vary in hue and brightness. An individual with normal color vision will be able to identify the figure on each plate as it differs from the background. For someone with a color vision defect, the figure is indistinguishable from the background or only partially seen. The PIPs that are commonly used are the American Optical Pseudoisochromatic Plates, Ishihara, Dvorine, and Standard Pseudoisochromatic Plates (Figure 8-10).

Using PIPs, color vision is evaluated under specific illumination. Daylight from the northern sky is the ideal illumination, but since that is not always practical, the Macbeth Illuminant C lamp should be used instead.

Color vision is usually evaluated at the reading distance of 30 inches (75 cm). If a patient needs to wear a correction to see the color plates, watch for dark tints in the lenses, which may alter color perception and, therefore, the results of testing. Patients should be tested with clear lenses.

The patient should be given a limited amount of time to complete the color test, viewing the plates for only a few seconds before responding. If a longer time is allowed, a patient with a color vision defect may be able to use other clues, such as brightness, to name the figure.

The other types of color vision testing most commonly done in practice are the Farnsworth D-15 Dichotomous Test and the Farnsworth-Munsell 100 Hue test. The D-15 is available in the

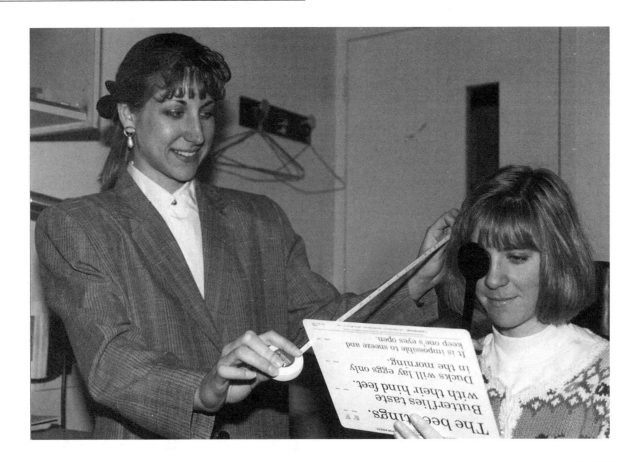

FIGURE 8-9—Measuring the patient's working distance. Note that the patient is holding the occluder for ease of measuring.

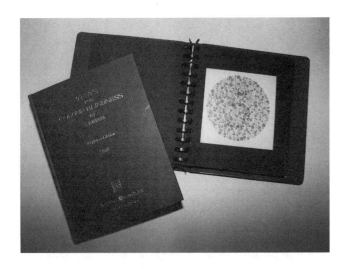

FIGURE 8-10—Ishihara Color Vision Plates.

highly sensitive desaturated format or in the much less sensitive saturated format. It is a set of 15 colored discs. The patient is asked to arrange the discs in color sequence to follow the stationary disc at one end of the tray. The 100 hue test is of the same basic design using a total of 85 discs in four separate trays. The patient is asked to arrange the colored discs in the proper sequence in each tray. The order in which the patient places the discs in the trays is recorded on a special form. These tests detect and classify red-green and blue-yellow defects, and both are done using standard daylight illumination. It is critical that the patient be instructed not to touch the face of the discs (Figures 8-11 and 8-12).

Three other color vision tests are available but are not commonly used in practice. First is the Farnsworth lantern test, which has been used for military and transportation qualification. It requires the patient to identify colors of light.

The Nagel Anomaloscope is an effective, but expensive, color vision test. It may be used to diagnose and classify red-green color defects. In this test, the patient looks into the instrument, which looks similar to a lensometer, and turns dials to match a standard of yellow light with a mixture of red and green. The readings on the dials indicate the specific color vision problem.

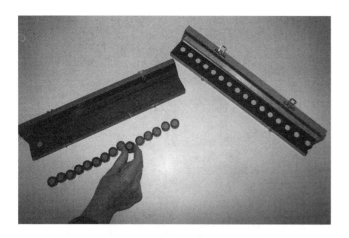

FIGURE 8-11—The Farnsworth D-17 Dichotomous Test for color vision.

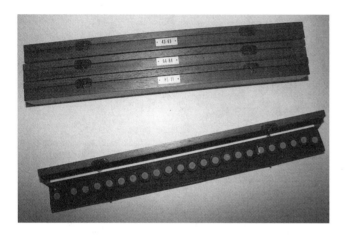

FIGURE 8-12—The Farnsworth-Munsell 100 Hue test.

The Holmgren Wool Test is a color matching test using strands of colored yarn. The patient selects strands of yarn and matches them to the same color in a book. Although, it is readily apparent to the examiner when the patient is unable to match the colors, this test remains highly unreliable. The dyes are not always standardized and, with age and handling, the yarns become faded and dirty (Figure 8-13).

Although not widely used in practice now, computer software packages that produce color vision tests on a monitor should be available in regular clinical settings soon.

The recording of color vision tests will vary depending on the procedure being performed. An example of a recording method for PIPs is to write the number of correctly identified plates, a slash mark, and then the number of plates tested for each eye, including the name of the test used: for example, OD 11/12; OS 12/12; Ishihara.

The paraoptometric should be familiar with several terms associated with color vision. There are two types of retinal receptors: rods and cones. The rods are primarily responsible for night vision and peripheral vision, and the cones are primarily responsible for day vision, central visual acuity, and color vision. Cones receive light at certain wavelengths and perceive it as color. If some of the cones are not working properly, color vision defects result. Color vision anomalies are often incorrectly called color blindness. Because true color blindness, or the inability to distinguish color at all, is extremely rare, "color deficiency" or "anomalous color perception" are more appropriate terms.

There are three main classifications of color vision: *trichromatism, dichromatism,* and *monochromatism.* Trichromatic color vision is considered normal color vision. A person with trichromatic vision uses the three primary colors of red, green, and blue to match a color sample. An *anomalous trichromat* still uses the three primary colors but in different proportions to match a color sample. The types of anomalous trichromatism are: *protanomalous,* a red weakness; *deuteranomalous,* a green weakness; and *tritanomalous,* a blue-yellow weakness. Deuteranolmalous trichromatism is the most common of all color vision defects.

A dichromat uses two primary colors to match color samples. The types of dichromats are the *protanope,* who has a red deficiency; the *deuteranope,* who has a green deficiency; and the *tritanope,* who has a blue-yellow deficiency.

A monochromat is an individual who sees everything in the same color. Monochromatism is also called *achromatism.* It is an extremely rare congenital color vision defect.

STEREOPSIS

Stereopsis, or stereoacuity, is the ability to see or appreciate depth using both eyes. Because the eyes are laterally displaced with respect to each other (i.e., interpupillary distance [PD]), a slightly different perception is appreciated by each eye. When the two pictures are fused perceptually in the brain, a three-dimensional perception results. This ability to appreciate depth

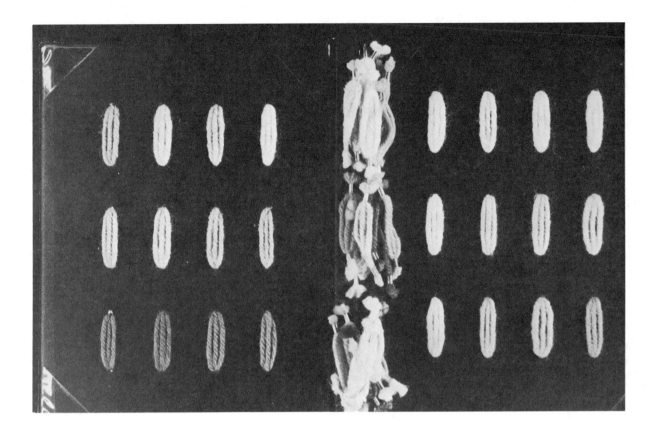
FIGURE 8-13—The Holmgren Wool Test.

is something we are born with; it is not a learned process. It may be reduced by either or both decreased VA and binocular problems.

Stereopsis is the highest degree of depth perception. It is recorded in seconds of arc. The lower the number, the better the stereopsis.

A number of tests are available to measure stereopsis. Several are booklets with specially designed plates that are polarized. The right and left eye will see the same picture, but the picture will be in slightly different positions. When the patient wears cross-polarized filters, which separate the pictures, the patient should see a three-dimensional image.

Several booklets are designed to measure *stereopsis at near*. One of the most commonly used tests is the Titmus Stereotest. It is also called the Stereo Fly because the test for gross stereopsis is a picture of a fly. The patient is asked to touch the fly's wings. Another test is the Bernell Stereo Reindeer, in which the test for gross stereopsis is a picture of a reindeer (Figures 8-14 and 8-15). The patient is asked to touch the antlers on the reindeer. By moving the booklet, the reindeer's nose can be made to wiggle. Other stereotests available include the Randot Stereotest and the Random Dot E Stereotest. Each book comes with a set of instructions that should be followed (Figure 8-16).

Stereopsis testing should always be done with the patient's best correction because stereopsis requires good visual acuity. The test should be done under good illumination in a well lighted room. The patient should hold the book at approximately 16 inches, or 40 cm away, and position it in such a way as to avoid glare from the overhead light on the plates. The test booklet should be kept free of fingerprints or smudges by wiping with a soft cloth. A pointer may be used by the patient to indicate the raised object instead of his or her finger (Figure 8-17).

Each booklet has a series of plates that check suppression and measure from gross to fine stereopsis. The suppression check on the Stereo Fly consists of the letters R and L appearing in the lower right and left corners of one plate. The R can be seen by only the right eye,

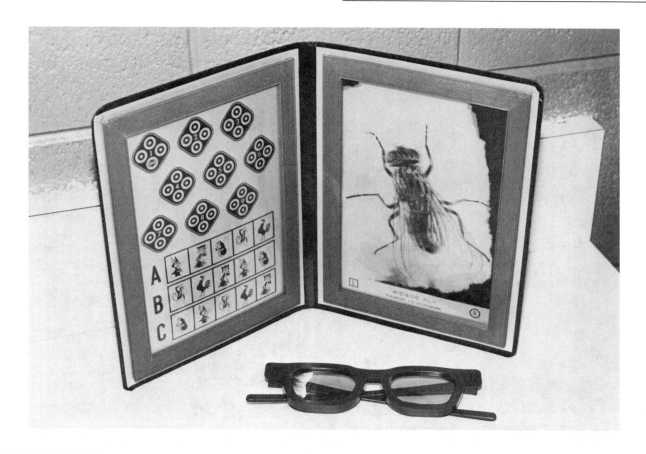

FIGURE 8-14—Stereo Fly and Polaroid glasses.

and the L can be seen by only the left eye. If the patient sees both letters, he or she is using both eyes. A patient who reports seeing only one letter is using that eye only to see and is not binocular. Further testing with the booklet cannot be done on a patient who reports seeing only one of the letters.

Also in each booklet is a test for *gross stereopsis*. The Titmus Stereo Fly, for example, evaluates stereopsis to approximately 3,000 seconds of arc. The patient is asked to touch or "pinch" the fly's wing. The patient's finger should not touch the booklet; it should be slightly above the page. If the patient touches the page, she or he is not seeing the image as three-dimensional, and thus demonstrates that she or he does not have gross stereopsis.

Another part of the stereotest is designed to test *intermediate stereopsis*. It may also be used for demonstration purposes and to test children. In the Titmus test, for example, there are three rows of animals, and the patient is to report or point to the animal that appears to be closer or seems to be "popping off the page." In descending rows, the figures are closer to the page, and a higher degree of stereopsis is necessary to identify the raised figure. The cat in the first row, the rabbit in the second, and the monkey in the third row subtend 400, 200, and 100 seconds of arc, respectively.

Fine stereopsis is measured in the same way. A series of figures are presented that sequentially get closer and closer to the page. Remember to reassure the patient that there are no right or wrong answers, that you are simply taking a measurement, and that it is okay if the figures seem flat on the page toward the end of the test. The last figure on the Titmus test, for example, subtends 40 seconds of arc.

In some cases, the patient may not be able to give a correct response when holding the booklet properly, though it has been determined that stereopsis is present. Have the patient move the book around a bit or hold the booklet upside down. With the booklet upside down, the patient should report the circles

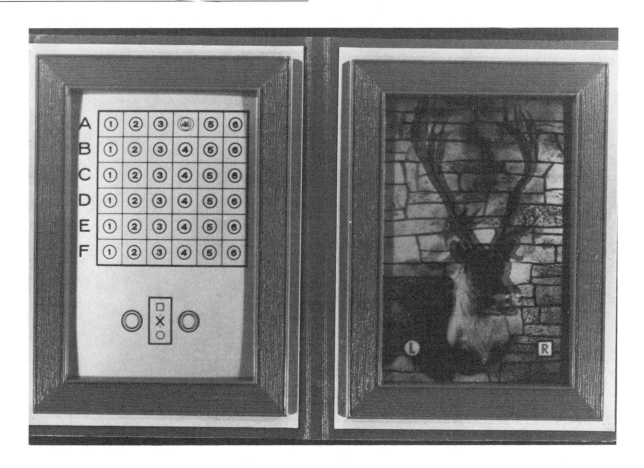

FIGURE 8-15—Bernell Stereo Reindeer.

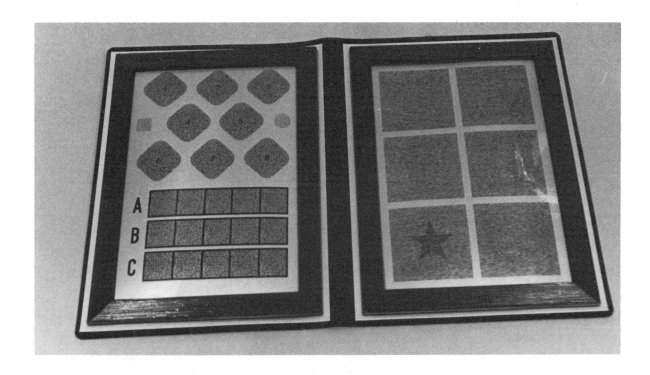

FIGURE 8-16—Randot Stereotest.

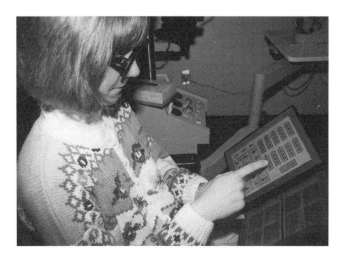

FIGURE 8-17—Patient performing the Titmus stereotest.

receding into the page, not standing off of it. This procedure may be used to validate patient responses as well.

For *distance stereopsis*, the American Optical Vectographic Project-o-Chart slide is used to measure stereopsis at 20 feet (6 m). The slide fits into the projector and contains tests for acuity, astigmatism, fusional vergence, and other conditions, as well as for stereoacuity. The stereopsis test consists of four rows of circles with five circles in each row. The patient wears polarized filters over his or her best distance correction. He or she reports the one circle in each row that appears to be closer when compared to the other circles in the row. The top row measures stereopsis of 240 seconds, and the bottom row measures stereopsis of 30 seconds.

Recording stereopsis includes the measurement in seconds of arc and the name of the test used.

NEAR POINTS OF ACCOMMODATION AND CONVERGENCE

Accommodation is simply defined as the focusing ability of the eyes. *Convergence* is the act of the eyes turning inward toward the nose. Accommodation and convergence, along with *pupil constriction,* are a linked triad of near-point actions of the eyes. As an object of regard is brought toward the eyes, the eyes will converge (turn in), the lens will accommodate (increase power), and the pupils will constrict.

The purpose of evaluating the *near point of accommodation* (NPA) of a patient is to check the ability of the eyes to focus at near. The purpose of evaluating the *near point of convergence* (NPC) of a patient is to measure the ability of the two eyes to work together.

As a target is brought toward a patient's nose, the eyes will turn in, or converge, trying to maintain a single image. As the target gets closer to the nose, it will first become blurry. As the target is moved closer, the eyes will no longer be able to maintain a single image. The eyes, or one eye, will turn out, and the target will then appear to be doubled. This is called *breaking fusion*, and the distance from the target to the nose may be measured. This is the near point of convergence. If the target were then placed on the nose and brought back out along the midline, the patient would be able to reconverge his or her eyes and see a single, fused target. This is called the *recovery point*.

Determining the binocular NPA and NPC may be done as one continuous test. The distance from the nose to the blur, break, and recovery points are simply measured and recorded.

The patient should be wearing his or her near spectacle correction. The room and the target should be well illuminated. Face the patient. A small fixation target is used. The patient should be asked to look at the fixation target, which is held at the midline and slightly below the horizontal meridian. Instruct the patient to look at the target and tell how many targets he or she sees. If the patient says "two targets," move the target further back until he or she sees one.

Slowly move the target toward the patient, asking the patient to try to keep it clear and single and to report when it becomes blurry. Stop when the patient says it is blurry and ask if he or she can clear it. If so, slowly continue moving the target. When he or she can no longer clear it, measure the distance from the target to the bridge of the nose. This is the *blur point*, or NPA.

Continue moving the target slowly in toward the nose, asking the patient to try to maintain a single image. You should be carefully observing the patient's eyes, watching for an eye to turn out. When the patient reports that the target appears double, or when you see one

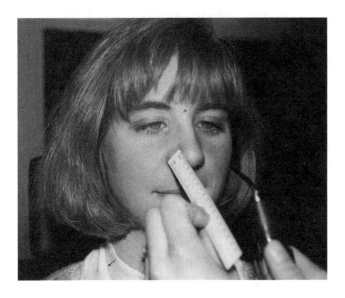

FIGURE 8-18—Measuring the near point of accommodation and convergence.

eye lose fixation on the target, measure the distance from the target to the bridge of the nose. This is the *break point*, or NPC. If the patient does not report *diplopia* at the time of the eye turn, he or she is suppressing that eye, and that should be noted on the patient record. You should also record which eye you observed turn outward. If the patient can keep the target single all the way to the nose, record "to nose" for the NPC.

Place the target on the nose and slowly move it away along the midline. Ask the patient to report when it becomes single again. As you observe the patient's eyes, you may notice when he or she fuses on the target. That point at which the patient reports the target as single again is the *recovery point*, and is measured from the bridge of the nose in centimeters.

The data recorded are blur, break, and recovery points and which eye turned outward (Figure 8-18).

AMPLITUDE OF ACCOMMODATION

Amplitude of accommodation (AA) is a calculation of the measured focusing ability of the eye, converted into diopters (D). This is done monocularly and binocularly. Accommodative amplitude is most often done as part of a series of near point tests in the examination room using the phoropter with the best correction and a target suspended from the near-point rod in front of the phoropter.

As a pre-examination procedure, a common technique for determining AA is through the push-up method, the same as for measuring NPA. As described above, a fine detail target is brought along the midline toward the patient's habitual near correction. The point from which the target blurs to the bridge of the nose is measured in centimeters. The binocular measurement may simply be the NPA as measured above. In monocular testing, one eye is occluded. To test for fatigue of accommodation, the procedure may be repeated three times on each eye and three times using both eyes.

Once the NPA is determined, the centimeter value is converted to diopters. The following formula is used to convert the NPA to AA:

$$\text{Diopters} = \frac{100 \text{ cm}}{\text{measured distance in centimeters}}$$

For example, if the near point of accommodation is 12 cm, the amplitude of accommodation is 8.33 D ($^{100 \text{ cm}}/_{12 \text{ cm}}$ = 8.33 D).

The measurements and conversions should be recorded for each eye and for both eyes together.

The expected amplitude of accommodation decreases with age. Hofstetter's formula for average expected AA is the following:

$$18.5 - 0.30(\text{age}).$$

For example, a 15-year-old would be expected to have a 14 D AA (15 years multiplied by 0.30 equals 4.5, subtracted from 18.5 equals 14 D). A 45-year-old, on the other hand, would be expected to have a 5 D AA (45 multiplied by 0.30 equals 13.5, subtracted from 18.5 equals 5 D).

This formula is for the average expected AA and assumes a range for minimum and maximum expected AA. Another system that is used to obtain the expected amplitude of accommodation is Donder's table.

COVER TEST

Cover tests are used to evaluate the alignment of the eyes. There is much terminology relating to the alignment of the eyes, which is reviewed first. *Ortho* refers to the eyes being in perfect or straight-ahead alignment. *Phoria* refers to a tendency of an eye or the eyes to deviate from ortho. *Tropia* refers to an actual deviation of an eye (see Chapter 13).

Although the eyes may be able to point to a target and perceive it as single, their position at rest (or when they are not being stimulated to fusion) is important in determining the quality of binocularity. A person's eyes may be constantly working to maintain fixation, causing fatigue and headaches. A person may be suppressing, or not using the vision in one eye, although the person appears to be fixating. Discovering binocular problems such as these is very important.

There are two parts to the cover test: the *unilateral cover test*, also called the *cover-uncover test*; and the *alternating cover test*. The unilateral cover test is used to detect the presence of a tropia (strabismus). The alternating cover test determines the direction of the phoria or tropia, but it cannot differentiate between them. The procedure, although technically simple to perform, requires a trained eye to detect very slight movements of the eyes.

In the unilateral cover test, the patient, wearing his or her habitual distance correction, is asked to look at a single letter on the distance visual acuity chart. This letter is usually one line larger than the patient's corrected visual acuity. The position of the examiner is important during the cover test procedure. Both the covered and uncovered eye should be observable without blocking the patient's view of the acuity chart.

Place the occluder in front of the patient's right eye for 2–3 seconds. Look for movement of the left (uncovered) eye. Remove the occluder and observe the left eye for any consequent movement. This should be repeated several times, covering and uncovering the right eye while observing the left eye. Repeat this procedure for the right eye, covering the left eye while observing the right eye. You should also note if the covered eye moves when it is being covered (behind the occluder) or when it is uncovered.

If there is no movement of the uncovered eye, there is no tropia present, and the position is noted as ortho. If movement is noted, the patient has a tropia. If the right eye moves when the left eye is covered, it is a *right tropia*. If the left eye moves when the right eye is covered, it is a *left tropia*. If the both eyes move when the other eye is covered, it is an *alternating tropia*.

If the uncovered eye moves in to fixate, it was turned out when both eyes are uncovered. The eye's habitual posture is therefore out (exo). Outward or temporal movement of the uncovered eye indicates that its habitual posture is in (eso). Upward movement indicates habitual down (or inferior) posture (hypo), and downward movement indicates habitual up (or superior) posture (hyper).

The alternating cover test determines the direction of the phoria or tropia. The patient is instructed to look at a letter on the distance acuity chart. The examiner covers the patient's right eye with the occluder and holds it in place for approximately 1 second. It is then moved to cover the left eye. The examiner observes the right eye for movement. The occluder is held over the left eye for approximately 1 second and then moved back to cover the right eye. The examiner observes the left eye for any movement. The procedure is repeated several times before stopping.

If there is no movement, the eyes are said to be *orthophoric*, or in the straight-ahead position. If the eye moves in to pick up fixation as it is uncovered, the habitual position is out, and the patient is *exophoric*. If the eye moves out to pick up fixation after it is uncovered, it is *esophoric*. If no movement is noted on the unilateral cover test, but movement is detected on the alternating cover test, then a phoria is present.

Both the cover-uncover test and alternating cover test should be repeated at near (40 cm) using a letter in a row one line above the patient's corrected acuity on the reduced Snellen acuity chart.

PURSUITS (THE BROAD H TEST) AND SACCADES

Pursuits are movements of the eyes as they follow a moving target. Saccades are jumping movements from one target to another. Both of these skills are necessary for visual tasks involved in reading, driving, and sports.

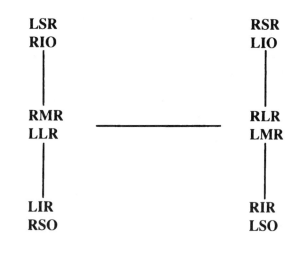

FIGURE 8-19—Eye muscles evaluated for different positions of gaze.

The two procedures described below evaluate whether the extraocular muscles in each eye are functioning properly. The chart in Figure 8-19 shows the extraocular muscles involved when moved to each position of gaze. If the results of these tests show a problem, the doctor will further investigate to determine which muscles are not functioning properly and why, and, if possible, prescribe a management plan to ensure functional binocularity.

To evaluate pursuits, the Broad H Test is commonly used. You face the patient, with the room and the target well-illuminated. The patient removes her or his eyewear, as a frame may interfere with full range of motion. Hold a target, such as the target used for NPA/NPC, approximately 40 cm directly in front of the patient. Instruct the patient to follow the target with his or her eyes without moving his or her head. The target is moved in an H pattern. Starting at the midline, move the target horizontally to the right side of the patient approximately 12 inches, then up, then down, then back up to the midline. Move the target across the midline to the patient's left side approximately 12 inches left of center, then up, and then down, then back up to the midline (Figure 8-20).

You should observe the smoothness of movement, the accuracy of following the target, and the extent of movement of the eyes. The eyes should move approximately 30–40 degrees in each direction. Note if one or both eyes lag behind or if the patient reports doubling, pain, or discomfort.

When recording the results, note whether the eye movements were "smooth and full," "jerky," or "incomplete." If the eyes did not turn in a particular direction, indicate that direction when recording. The practitioner will determine the muscle that is affected. Check with the practitioner for her or his preferred method of recording.

To evaluate saccadic eye movements, two targets are required, but they do not have to be fine detail targets. One may be the same as used for pursuits, and each should be easily identified. For example, if you use a reduced Snellen chart on the end of a paddle for one target, the other target may be the tip of your pen.

Testing conditions are the same as for pursuits. You present two targets to the patient, approximately 40 cm in front of the patient and approximately 30 cm apart horizontally. Ask the patient to look from one to the other, saying, for example, "Look at the chart, now the pen, now the chart, now the pen," and so on. You will repeat this sequence in the vertical meridian and in both directions of an "X" pattern.

You should observe and record the accuracy of the eye movements, whether the eyes are able to locate and fixate on the targets accurately, or if the eyes tend to overshoot (go past and come back to) or undershoot (not go far enough and must continue to move to reach) the target.

INTERPUPILLARY DISTANCE

The interpupillary distance is the distance between the centers of the pupil of each eye. It is commonly abbreviated PD and is measured in millimeters. This measurement is needed to center the phoropter lenses in front of the patient's eyes during the examination. It is also necessary for the proper alignment of the optical centers of ophthalmic lenses in a patient's eyewear to match her or his line of sight.

There are different methods to measure a patient's binocular PD. A simple, commonly used procedure involves taking two measurements for the PD. One measurement is for *dis-*

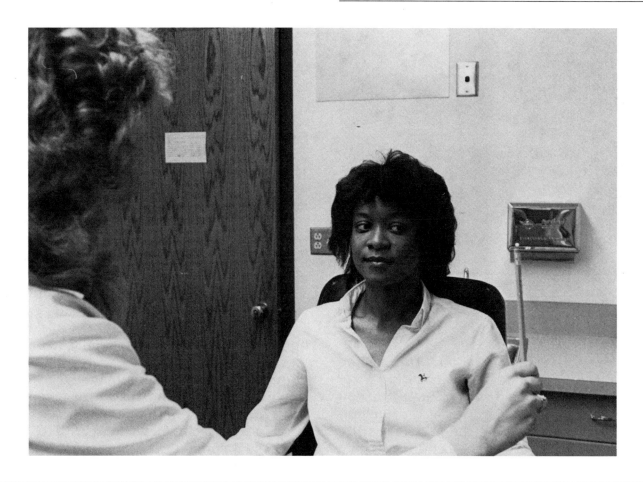

FIGURE 8-20—Observing version movements.

tance PD. This is taken with the patient's two eyes directed in the straight ahead position, as if looking at a object in the distance. The other is a *near PD* measurement. This is taken with the patient's eyes slightly turned in, as when reading or doing near tasks.

The examiner is positioned facing the patient, approximately 40 cm away. The examiner holds a millimeter rule in the right hand between the thumb and index finger. The other three fingers may be used to steady the hand against the patient's face. Place the rule at the spectacle plane of the patient, resting it gently on the bridge of the nose. Close your right eye and instruct the patient to look into the open left eye. Line up the zero point of the millimeter rule with the temporal edge of the patient's right pupil. Next, open your right eye and close your left eye. Instruct the patient to look into your open (right) eye. Take the reading from the millimeter rule that is directly in line with the nasal edge of the patient's left pupil. Finally, close your right eye and open your left eye. Have the patient look into your open left eye while you check to make sure that the zero point is still lined up correctly (Figure 8-21).

Having the patient look from one eye to the other simulates distance viewing, because the patient is looking straight ahead with each eye, just one at a time.

Near PD measurement is done at the same time in the same position. The patient is instructed to look at your open left eye. The zero point on the ruler is aligned with the temporal edge of the patient's right pupil. Next, look to the patient's left eye. Because the patient is looking at your open eye at 40 cm, her or his eyes are converging for near. The measurement is read from the ruler scale where it intersects the nasal edge of the patient's left pupil. This is the near PD. It is usually 3–5 mm less than the distance PD.

Instead of using the edge of the pupil, the center of the pupil (as determined by the reflection of a penlight), or the limbus of each eye

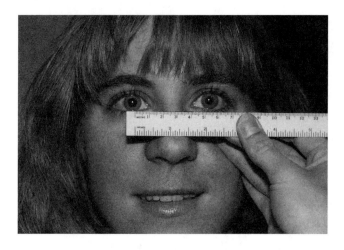

FIGURE 8-21—Measuring interpupillary distance.

may be used as reference points. This may be useful if the patient has a very dark iris.

The PD is recorded as a fraction, with the distance measurement written as the numerator, or top number, and the near PD as the denominator, or bottom number (for example, 68/64.) Errors in the PD measurement may occur if the examiner's PD varies greatly from the patient's PD, if the examiner is too close to the patient, if the patient or examiner moves his or her head, or if the patient is not looking into the examiner's pupil.

The *monocular PD* is the measurement from the center of the pupil to the center of the bridge of the nose. Because most people do not have perfectly symmetric faces, there is often a difference between the monocular PDs. When prescribing progressive addition lenses, monocular PDs are often required.

Monocular PD measurement may be done after measuring the binocular PD. To determine the center of the pupil, the reflection of a penlight is useful. Using the center of the pupil of the right eye as a reference point, note the reading on the millimeter rule at the center of the nose. This is the right monocular PD. Subtract this reading from the binocular PD to calculate the monocular PD for the left eye. For example:

Distance binocular PD = 68

Right monocular PD = 36

Left monocular PD = 32

Several companies manufacture gauges to measure the PD. These usually measure monocular or split PD. Pupillometers and rulers are also acceptable means of measuring PDs.

EYE DOMINANCY

The dominant eye is the eye that is usually used for monocular viewing or for sighting. Eye dominance may also be called *eye preference*. Information on the dominant eye is useful to the optometrist when prescribing a correction. In a monovision fit of contact lenses, for example, the dominant eye is corrected for distance vision, and the nondominant eye is corrected for near vision.

Eye dominance is also pertinent in a developmental evaluation. The patient's hand and foot dominance may also be ascertained. Cross-dominancy, when the dominant eye is opposite the dominant hand, may affect a patient's coordination.

Numerous techniques may be used to determine the dominant eye. These procedures are easy to perform, take very little time, and are done in a well lit room. Many people are not aware that they have a dominant eye and are often fascinated by these simple exercises described below.

With most procedures, instructions are give to the patient before the test begins about the purpose of the test. With eye dominance, it is best not to tell the patient until you are finished. Thinking about the purpose of the test may influence the result.

One method is to have the patient point to an object in the distance. Sometimes, when asked to point at an object, the patient will close one eye and sight through only one eye, the dominant eye. If the patient keeps both eyes open, the examiner occludes one of the patient's eyes. If the patient does not move his or her finger, the viewing eye is the dominant eye. If the patient moves his or her finger, the covered eye is the dominant eye.

Another procedure uses an index card with a 2- to 3-cm hole in the middle. The patient is asked to hold the card with both hands on her or his lap. Go to the opposite side of the room facing the patient, and ask the patient to raise the card straight up in front of her or his face and look at you through the hole in the card. You will be looking at the patient's dominant eye.

A slightly modified version of the above method uses the patient's hands instead of the card. Stand next to the patient, and show the patient how make a triangle using his or her hands, with overlapping thumbs forming the bottom of the triangle and fingers overlapping. (You want the hole to be small enough so he or she will be using only one eye.) Ask the patient to lay his or her hands on his or her lap. Go to the opposite side of the room facing the patient, and ask the patient to raise his or her hands straight up in front of his or her face and to look at you through the triangle. You will be looking at the patient's dominant eye. This is the most common way to test eye dominance (Figure 8-22).

If the patient falters, such as brings the card (or hands) up at the midline and moves to one side or the other, have the patient replace the card on her or his lap, and repeat the test.

Eye dominance is recorded by simply writing which eye is used for observation of the target. If either or both hand and foot dominance was asked, record that information also.

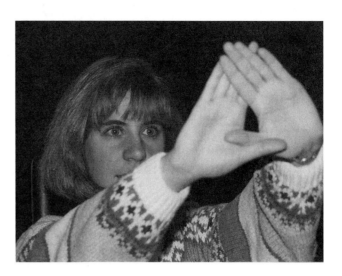

FIGURE 8-22—Determining eye dominancy.

BLOOD PRESSURE MEASUREMENT

Uncontrolled high blood pressure can have serious untoward effects on a person's vision. Measuring a patient's blood pressure at the optometrist's office not only may be the patient's entry point into the health care system, it may also alert the doctor and patient to a potential health problem that can affect the patient's entire well-being as well as his or her vision.

Blood pressure is defined as the force exerted against the arterial walls during the left ventricular contraction (heart beat) and relaxation (heart at rest). The *systolic pressure* is the first and largest number of a blood pressure measurement. It reflects the amount of force on the artery walls when the heart beats. The *diastolic pressure* is the second, smaller number. It reflects the amount of force when the heart is at rest. High blood pressure in adults is a consistently elevated blood pressure of at least either or both 140 mm Hg systolic and 90 mm Hg diastolic.

Blood pressure assessment is performed with a *sphygmomanometer* and a *stethoscope*. The sphygmomanometer has a cuff that consists of an airtight, flat rubber bladder covered with cloth that extends beyond the bladder to various lengths. Two tubes are attached to the bladder. One is attached to the manometer, which registers the pressure, and the other is attached to a bulb that is used to inflate the bladder with air. Cuffs are available in different sizes to assure a proper fit. If a cuff is not the right size for the patient, the blood pressure measurement will be inaccurate.

There are two types of sphygmomanometers: *aneroid* and *mercury*. The aneroid manometer uses a pressure gauge with an indicator on a dial to measure the blood pressure. A mercury manometer uses mercury to measure the blood pressure. Both the mercury and aneroid manometers give accurate results when they are working properly and are used correctly.

The stethoscope is an instrument that carries sounds from the body to the examiner's ear. There are electronic blood pressure meters on the market that translate blood pressure into "beeps," making a stethoscope unnecessary. These are helpful for patients who wish to take their own blood pressure.

To take a blood pressure measurement, begin by determining the proper cuff size for the patient. Make sure that the patient is relaxed for this procedure. Explain the purpose of the procedure. The patient should be sitting comfortably, with his or her arm slightly flexed and supported at heart level with palm of hand facing up. Expose the upper arm and place the cuff

1 inch above the brachial artery pulse or the inner crease of the arm. Wrap the cuff around the arm snugly, centering the arrows marked on the cuff over the brachial artery. Fasten the cuff securely. Locate the pulse of the brachial artery and place the stethoscope disc firmly over it. Do not apply heavy pressure, as this will distort the sounds. Close the valve of the pressure bulb. Inflate the cuff to 30 mm Hg above the patient's normal systolic level. (If you do not know the patient's systolic pressure, palpate the radial artery, and inflate the cuff to a pressure 30 mm Hg above the point at which radial pulsation disappears. Deflate the cuff and wait 30 seconds.)

Slowly release the valve, releasing the air at a rate of 2–3 mm Hg/second. Note the point on the manometer at which the first clear sound of two consecutive beats are heard. This is the first phase of the Korotkoff sounds. The point at which this occurs is the systolic pressure measurement. Continue deflating the cuff gradually, noting the point on the manometer at which the sounds become muffled. This is the diastolic pressure. Note the point on the manometer at which the sounds disappear. Allow the cuff to deflate quickly, remove the cuff, and record the findings according to the practitioner's policy. If you are going to repeat the procedure, wait 30 seconds before attempting again (Figure 8-23).

Hypertension has minimal symptoms. Early detection and treatment may save a person's life. Blood pressure measurement can be performed quickly and easily on each patient and provides for full-scope health care by the eye care provider.

VISUAL SKILLS

Visual skills testing is designed to measure a patient's visual performance on a battery of tests. There are several different visual skills testing instruments. The four instruments that have the most widespread use are the Keystone Telebinocular, Stereo Optical's Biopter, the Titmus Vision Tester, and the Bausch & Lomb Orthorater. The instruments and their individual tests look slightly different, but all the instruments test basically the same visual skills.

Most visual skills test batteries include visual acuity, fusion, lateral and vertical phorias, stereopsis, and color vision. Some tests are designed for distance vision, some for near vision, some for monocular vision, and some for binocular vision. These tests are also usually designed to be easily administered and understood by patients.

Visual skills are usually intended to be used with the patient wearing her or his current prescription. For distance tests, the instrument should be set for distance, and the patient should be viewing through his or her distance prescription. For near tests, the instrument should be set for near, and the patient should be viewing through her or his near prescription.

Visual skills tests may provide valuable information to the doctor on how well the patient's eyes are working together before the complete eye examination. They may also function as a screening tool.

In this chapter, there cannot be a complete description of the tests available for each of the visual skills instruments, but each instrument provides an instruction manual that fully explains each test and various techniques particular to that instrument.

CONCLUSION

To become proficient in any or all of the above tests, the paraoptometric must first become knowledgeable in the purposes and techniques of these procedures and then must practice administering them. In this chapter, suggested methods are provided, but variations may be made to allow the testing to be smoother, more efficient, and more comfortable for the examiner. Working with the doctor to learn and refine testing techniques will add to the consistency and teamwork in the office.

The order in which the procedures are presented in this chapter is a suggested sequence of performance. The less you handle equipment, change lights, and move around the room, the more efficient the examination will be. For example, we may assume that you will always begin with history and VAs. While the patient is wearing his or her near correction, the room and overhead lights are on, and the patient has the occluder in hand, it is logical to follow near VAs with color vision testing. Then take the occluder, hand the patient the Polaroid filters, switch books, and do stereopsis. Then position

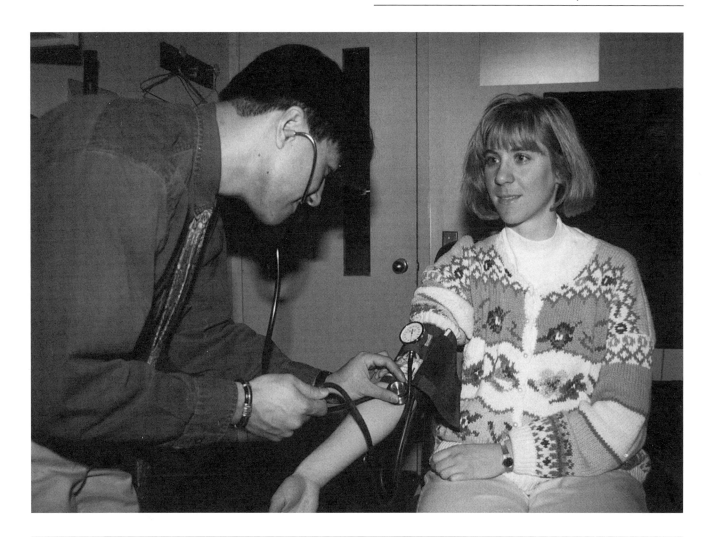

FIGURE 8-23—Measuring blood pressure.

yourself in front of the patient. If your near point targets are on the ends of your PD rule and occluder, you need only these two instruments for NPA/NPC, cover tests, pursuits/saccades, and PD measurement. Lastly, determine eye dominancy. Then put the instruments away, and you're done.

With practice, patience, and persistence, you can develop these skills to become an expert pre-examiner and an integral part of the optometric care team.

REFERENCE

1. Woo GCS, Long WF. Recommended light levels for clinical procedures. Optom Monthly 1979;70:722.

9 / Specialty Testing

Lynn E. Konkel and Sharon Overgaard

The purpose of this chapter is to discuss the most commonly delegated special testing procedures used in the optometric examination, as well as some of the less commonly delegated procedures. It is meant as a study guide for the paraoptometric, who, along with the optometrist, may practice these skills. The role of the paraoptometric is that of a gatherer of information to assist the optometrist in the diagnosis and treatment plan for the patient. The paraoptometric is not to interpret or diagnose a patient's condition from these tests, only to gather the data for the optometrist.

KERATOMETRY

Keratometry is the measurement of the corneal curvature. The cornea supplies approximately two-thirds of the refracting power of the eye (43.00 D). The more curved the cornea, the more power it will have. When measuring the cornea, the minimum and maximum meridians of curvature or power are measured. Usually, these meridians refer to the meridians at the vertical and horizontal. The keratometer measures approximately a 3-mm area of the central cornea. The instruments used to measure this curvature are called *keratometers* or *ophthalmometers*. The readings or measurements from these instruments are commonly referred to as *K readings*.

The procedure for measuring corneal curvature will vary slightly with different instruments and may vary significantly when using automated keratometers. This discussion centers around the Bausch & Lomb (now Reichert) Keratometer (Figure 9-1). The paraoptometric should first adjust the eyepiece for his or her eye to ensure accurate readings. The instrument should be turned on, the white occluder turned down in front of the instrument barrel, and the eyepiece turned counterclockwise as far as it will turn. The paraoptometric looks into the instrument and observes the black cross (Figure 9-2). While looking at the now blurry black focusing cross, slowly turn the eyepiece clockwise until the cross is in sharp, clear focus. As soon as the black cross is in focus, stop turning the eyepiece. The eyepiece should not be turned back and forth to get the cross in focus, since this will stimulate the accommodative system and result in an incorrect eyepiece setting. If you miss the focus point of the black cross, you should simply start at the beginning of the procedure with the eyepiece turned all of the way in the counterclockwise direction. When the cross is in focus, note the reading on the outside of the eyepiece. The steps to focus the eyepiece are repeated several times and the readings noted. If the results are about the same each time, the eyepiece is properly adjusted. Once this has been done, each time the same instrument is used, simply set the eyepiece focus by turning the eyepiece to the proper setting.

Before seating the patient, clean the chin and forehead rests with isopropyl alcohol. Seat the patient comfortably—the patient's head should be firmly against the headrest, and the patient's chin should be in the chin rest. The

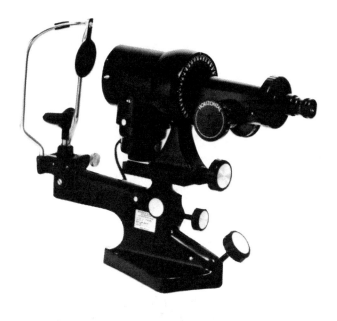

FIGURE 9-1—The Bausch & Lomb (Reichert) Keratometer. (Reprinted with permission from SS Bates. Fundamentals for Assisting in Primary Care Optometry. New York: Professional Press/Fairchild, 1983).

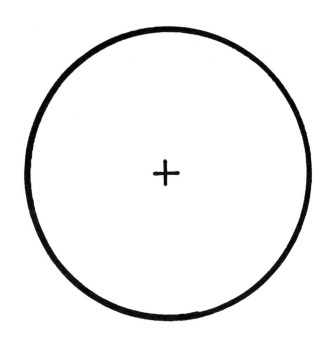

FIGURE 9-2—Cross used for focusing the keratometer.

eye not being tested should be occluded. Explain to the patient that you are going to measure the curvature of his or her eye and that he or she needs to look straight down the barrel of the instrument. Once you align the instrument, the patient will see an image of his or her own eye directly down the center of the barrel. Release the locking knob of the instrument located on the left side and swing the instrument in front of the eye being tested. The instrument should be raised or lowered until the pin at the side of the lamp house is aligned with the patient's outer canthus when looking outside the instrument (Figure 9-3). Also, while looking at the patient's eye, adjust the instrument until the white circle is reflected off the cornea and the glow of the instrument lamp is centered around the patient's eye. Instruct the patient to look down the instrument at the reflection of his or her eye. At this time, the paraoptometric looks into the instrument for the first time since focusing the eyepiece and locates the mires, which are three white circles with plus and minus signs surrounding the circles (Figure 9-4). Using the instrument-focusing knob directly below the eyepiece, the paraoptometric should focus the circles until they are sharp and clear (see Figure 9-4). The circles should then be aligned so that the black focusing cross is in the center of the lower right circle (called the *focusing circle*). This alignment is done by moving the instrument right or left and using the instrument elevation knob to move the circles up and down. The focusing circle should be kept single at all times by turning the focusing knob. Once the mires are focused and centered, tighten the instrument-locking knob so that the barrel of the instrument will stay in the set position. If during the balance of the test procedure the mire pattern should shift, simply release the locking knob, reposition the mires, and set the lock.

Locating the Cylinder Axis

Once the mires are centered, you must locate the major meridians of power. To do this, turn the horizontal measuring drum (large knob on the left side of the instrument housing) until the plus signs between the two lower circles are barely separated (Figure 9-5). If the horizontal bars of the plus signs are not aligned tip to tip as in Figure 9-5, you must rotate the axis grip until the horizontal bars of the plus signs are aligned tip to

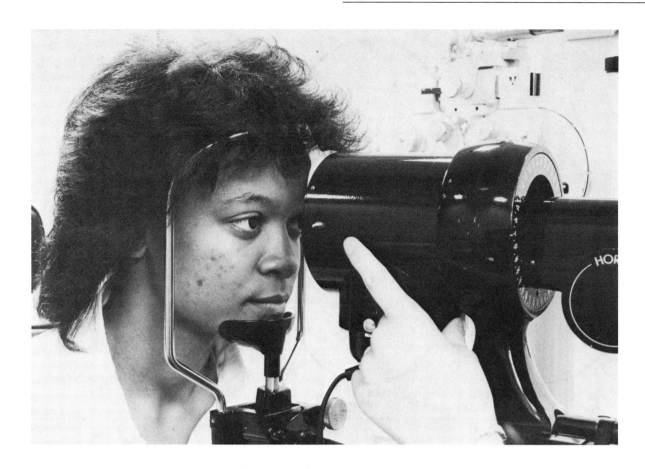

FIGURE 9-3—Aligning the lamphouse pin with the patient's canthus.

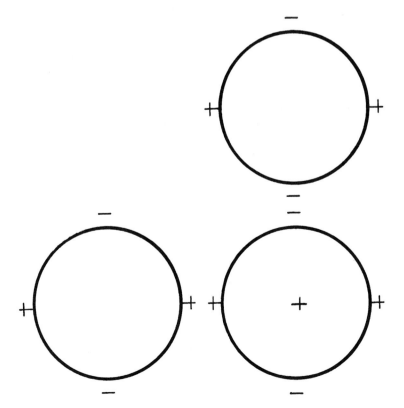

FIGURE 9-4—The keratometer mires.

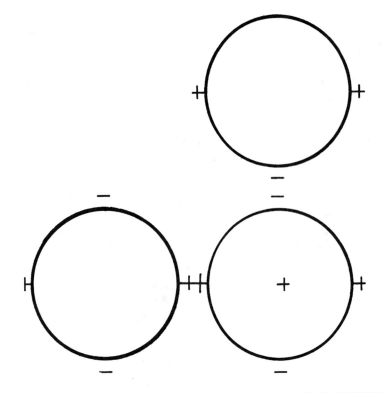

FIGURE 9-5—Axis grip has been rotated for correct alignment.

tip. Once again, you must keep the focusing circle clear and single at all times.

Measuring the Power of the Major Meridians

Once the plus signs between the two lower circles are aligned, turn the horizontal measuring drum until the two plus signs overlap, keeping the focusing circle sharp and clear by turning the focusing knob simultaneously. When determining the horizontal measurement, it is important to keep the area of the plus signs of the focusing circle sharp and clear. The entire focusing circle may not become sharp and clear at the same time if the patient has a significant amount of astigmatism. Now switch hands, placing your left hand on the focusing knob and your right hand on the vertical measuring drum found on the right side of the instrument. Shift your gaze to the minus signs between the two vertical circles, and, with your left hand, focus the minus signs. With your right hand, turn the vertical measuring drum until the minus signs are overlapped (Figure 9-6). Remember that the plus signs and minus signs will **not** focus simultaneously if the patient has corneal astigmatism. The paraoptometric should maintain a sharp image of the plus signs when superimposing them and a sharp image of the minus signs when superimposing them.

Recording Keratometry Findings

Many times, multiple readings are performed for each eye and averaged together. When the paraoptometric has taken the last reading for a given eye, the patient may sit back while the paraoptometric records the findings. The results are recorded directly from the instrument, using the horizontal measuring drum and axis indicator and the vertical measuring drum and axis indicator. The horizontal power reading is taken first, from the drum on the left side of the instrument, and the meridian of that power is obtained from the horizontal hash mark found on the axis indicator. The vertical power reading is then recorded from the right-hand vertical measuring drum. The axis is also recorded for the vertical meridian. An example of the results would be:

O.D. 42.50 @ 175; 43.50 @ 085

O.S. 43.00 @ 005; 43.75 @ 095

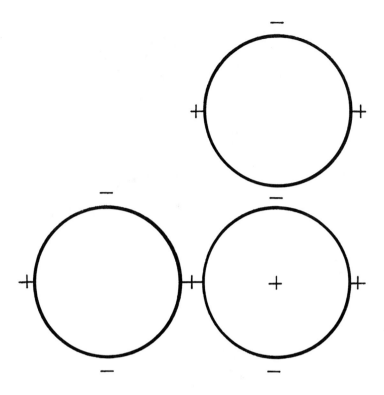

FIGURE 9-6—Mires in proper focus, with horizontal and vertical power measured.

The amount of corneal astigmatism may be determined by taking the difference between the horizontal and vertical powers. In the above example, the corneal astigmatism would be –1.00 x 175 or +1.00 x 085 in the right eye and –0.75 x 005 or +0.75 x 095 for the left eye.

Most keratometers and ophthalmometers function in similar ways, but the mire patterns on the instruments vary somewhat. When using an instrument that you are not familiar with, determine what parts of the mire pattern are used to measure the horizontal and vertical meridians. Results may be recorded as in the example above or as the optometrist prefers.

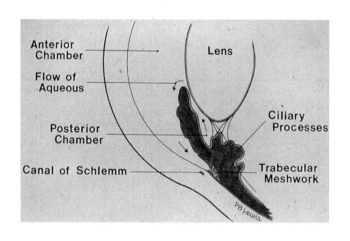

FIGURE 9-7—Aqueous humor flowchart.

TONOMETRY

Tonometry is the measurement of intraocular pressure (IOP). IOP measurements are taken with an instrument called a *tonometer*. Some of the more common types of tonometers include Schiötz, Goldmann, and the noncontact tonometer.

Pressure inside the eye is caused by aqueous humor, which is fluid in the anterior portion of the eye. Aqueous humor is constantly being produced in the ciliary body and flows between the lens and posterior iris, through the pupil, past the front of the iris, and out the eye via the canal of Schlemm (Figure 9-7). If the aqueous humor is produced and not allowed to exit the eye at a normal rate, this increase in fluid within the anterior chamber causes the pressure inside the eye to increase. The retinal nerve layer and the optic disc may be affected by this increase in intraocular pressure, causing visual

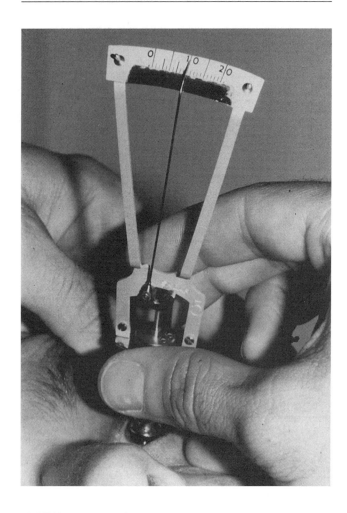

FIGURE 9-8—The Schiotz tonometer. (Courtesy of Liberty Optical P.A.C.E. Program, Newark, NJ.)

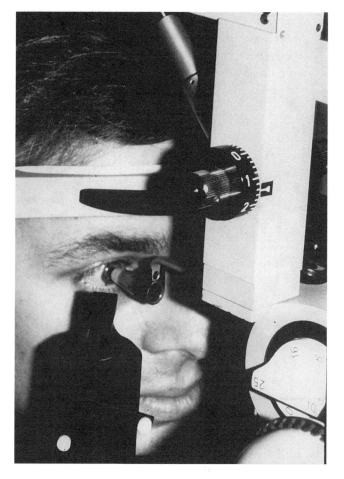

FIGURE 9-9—Goldmann tonometer. (Courtesy of Liberty Optical P.A.C.E. Program, Newark, NJ.)

field loss. The increase in intraocular pressure and damage of the visual field is known as *glaucoma*. The measurement of IOP, therefore, plays a role in the detection and treatment of glaucoma. A word of caution: A person with low or normal IOP may have a type of glaucoma known as *low-tension glaucoma*. The measurement of IOP is just one of many tests to determine whether a person has glaucoma. The optometrist will also evaluate the patient's anterior chamber angle, appearance of the optic disc to include the cup/disc ratio, and visual fields.

There are two main types of tonometers: *indentation* and *applanation*. Indentation tonometry is performed with the Schiötz tonometer. The Schiötz has a foot plate that rests directly on the anesthetized cornea, with a plunger in the center. The plunger holds a series of weights used to create the force to indent the cornea (Figure 9-8). The amount of indentation is read from a scale, and this measurement is converted into millimeters of mercury (mm Hg), the unit for measuring IOP. The more the cornea indents, the lower the IOP, and the more rigid the cornea, the higher the IOP.

Applanation tonometry is performed most commonly with a Goldmann or noncontact tonometer. In applanation tonometry, usually a predetermined area of the cornea is applanated or flattened. IOP is determined by how much pressure is required to flatten this specific area.

The Goldmann tonometer is attached to a slit lamp and is considered the standard in tonometry (Figure 9-9). It requires the use of a corneal anesthetic and fluorescein (this may be given in combination using a diagnostic drug called Fluress). The anesthetic and fluorescein are instilled in the eye, and the tonometer probe is positioned so that it is centered on the cornea. The examiner looks into the slit lamp and sees two green semicircles of fluorescein. A knob on

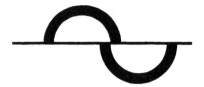

FIGURE 9-10—Appearance of Goldmann tonometer mires when tonometer is correctly centered and cornea is applanated. (Reprinted with permission from T Grosvenor. Primary Care Optometry [3rd ed]. Boston: Butterworth-Heinemann, 1996;182.)

the side of the tonometer is turned, increasing the pressure on the eye until the inner edges of the two semicircles touch (Figure 9-10). The IOP measurement is obtained when the scale reading on the instrument is multiplied by ten.

The noncontact tonometer (NCT) (Figure 9-11), uses a puff of air to flatten the cornea. A corneal anesthetic is not required for this procedure. The instrument is designed so that its lights and mirrors electronically translate the amount of time it takes the puff of air to flatten the corneas into millimeters of mercury of pressure. A digital readout displays the amount of pressure. The patient's chin must be in the chin rest and the forehead against the forehead rest. The patient is instructed to look at the red dot in the instrument without moving her or his eyes. The paraoptometric focuses and centers the red dot within the black ring with the use of the joy stick and elevation control knob. When the red dot is properly aligned within the black ring and focused, the air puff may be released by depressing the trigger button. The NCT may be startling to some patients; therefore, the puff of air should be demonstrated on their hand before taking the measurement. The newer noncontact tonometers emit a lower volume of air, which is less startling to patients, as with Reichert's Expert Noncontact Tonometer (Figure 9-12).

Each tonometer has specific calibration procedures, and these should be followed when using the instruments.

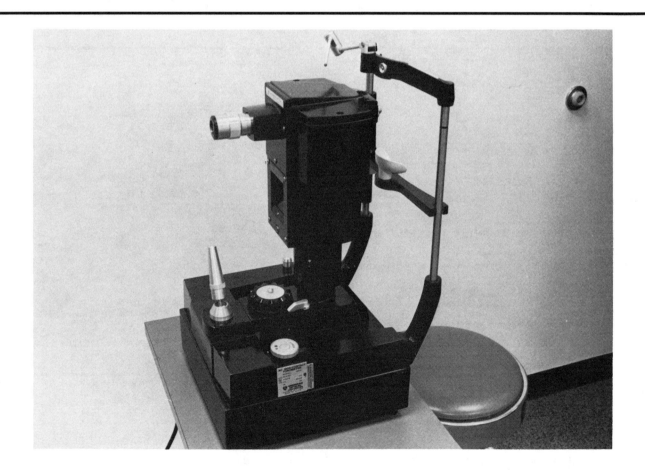

FIGURE 9-11—The American Optical Noncontact Tonometer.

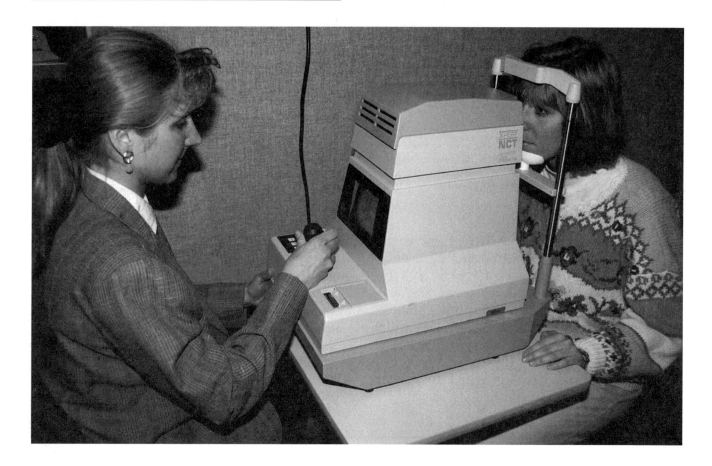

FIGURE 9-12—The Reichert's Expert Noncontact Tonometer.

Tono-Pen

The Mentor Tono-Pen X-L is an electronic, handheld tonometer (Figure 9-13). It has the advantages of being portable, fast, and comfortable to hold. It is as accurate as Goldmann tonometry and is battery operated and lightweight.

The tip of the Tono-Pen is made of stainless steel, and this probe houses a solid-state strain gauge. The gauge acts to convert the intraocular pressure to an electronic signal that is read out on the liquid crystal display (LCD).

Another advantage of the Tono-Pen is that it contains a microprocessor that analyzes, stores, and compares four valid readings. The Tono-Pen's electronics then calculate the mean IOP and indicate the reliability on the LCD.

To use the Tono-Pen, first prepare the instrument. Clean the tip with compressed gas each morning of use. Then cover the probe tip with an unused Ocu-Film tip cover. Calibrate the instrument each morning by following the directions included with the instrument.

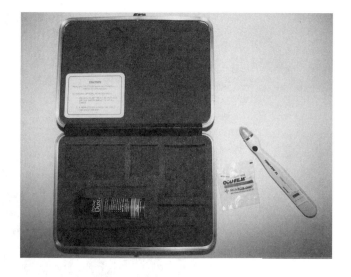

FIGURE 9-13—The Mentor Tono-Pen X-L.

Prepare the patient by instilling one drop of topical anesthetic into the eye to be examined. Typically, both eyes are measured for IOP. The patient may be seated or lying down to take a mea-

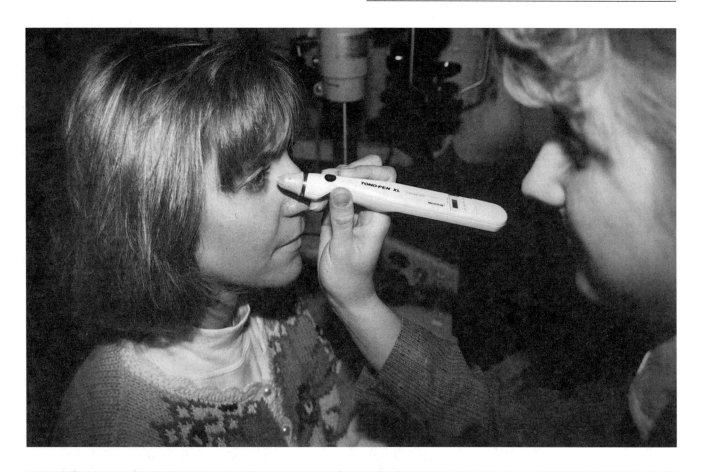

FIGURE 9-14—Proper position for holding the Tono-Pen.

surement. Have the patient look straight ahead. Hold the Tono-Pen as you would hold a pencil, depress the activation switch for a moment, and then release it. The probe will indicate when it is ready to take a reading (Figure 9-14).

Touch the central cornea lightly and briefly several times (Figure 9-15). Make sure not to indent the cornea. When a valid reading is made, you will hear a "click" sound. After four valid readings, you will hear a "beep" sound or tone. The averaged measurement will appear on the LCD.

If you are using the Tono-Pen in your office, make sure to familiarize yourself with the instruction manual supplied with the device. Its in-depth descriptions include unpacking instructions, battery installation, instructions for use, LCD interpretation, and maintenance.

GLARE TESTING

A bright source of light such as sunlight may produce glare that can reduce the quality of

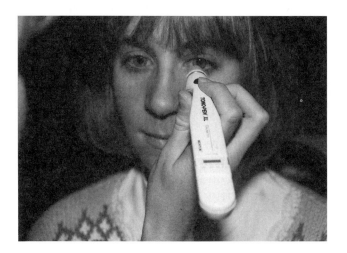

FIGURE 9-15—Touching the central cornea lightly several times.

sight. Glare may distort the patient's vision and produce *photophobia*. A patient may read the Snellen acuity chart without difficulty, yet when exposed to normal daylight conditions be unable to see clearly due to glare. This may indi-

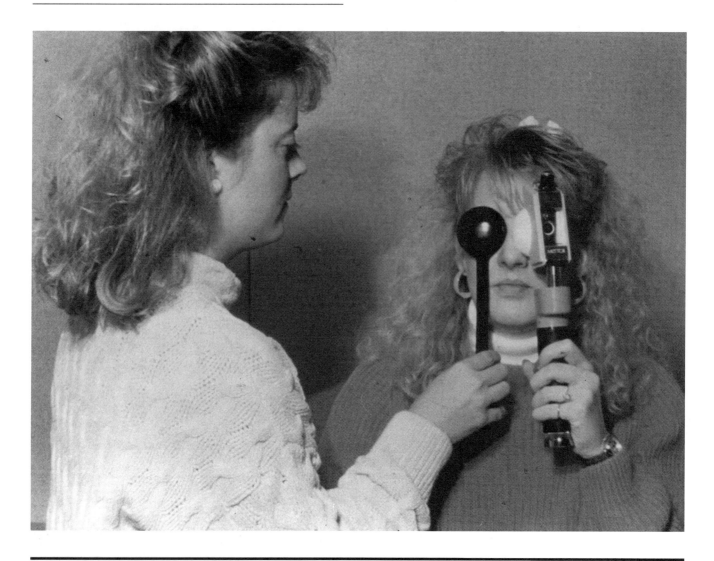

FIGURE 9-16—Brightness Acuity Tester. (Courtesy of Davis Duehr Dean, Madison, WI.)

cate the patient has a cataract or other ocular opacities. Glare testing is used to determine if sensitivity to glare is contributing to a patient's visual symptoms. The Brightness Acuity Tester (Figure 9-16) is one of the ways to test or evaluate a patient's true visual acuity in three different degrees of lighting.

CONTRAST SENSITIVITY

The contrast of dark and light between an object and its surroundings is necessary for a person to perceive objects visually. No one can see an object in absolute darkness. This concept is referred to as *contrast sensitivity*. The patient may have sharp visual acuity when in fact a cataract, corneal opacity, or other eye disease is reducing his or her contrast sensitivity. For patients with these medical conditions, "normal" vision is like looking through fog. Contrast sensitivity testing helps determine a need for surgery for those patients who have sharp visual acuity yet are unable to view objects clearly. A method for testing contrast sensitivity is to present the patient with a chart showing letters or symbols in varying amounts of faint gray print rather than the sharp black or white found on most standard vision charts.

POTENTIAL ACUITY METER

The potential acuity meter (Figure 9-17) is a small light source with a visual acuity chart and a lens. When a patient has reduced visual acuity caused by a cataract, this test will assist the

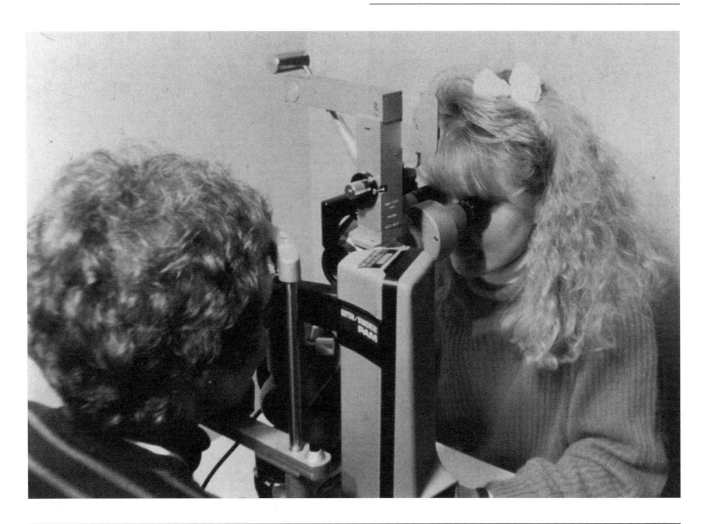

FIGURE 9-17—Potential Acuity Meter is attached to the slit lamp. (Courtesy of Davis Duehr Dean, Madison, WI.)

doctor in determining the patient's potential visual acuity without the cataract. The light in the instrument will project through the patient's pupil around any opacity in the lens to the retina. The patient is asked to identify the smallest line he or she can see. The patient's response is then recorded. This office test will help the doctor and patient decide if cataract surgery will be beneficial or if there is a possible macular problem that may limit the patient's visual acuity even if the lens is removed.

FUNDUS PHOTOGRAPHY

Fundus photography refers to color photos taken of the posterior portion of the patient's eye. The fundus contains the retina, optic disc, and retinal vessels. Figure 9-18 shows the fundus with the camera centered on the optic disc,

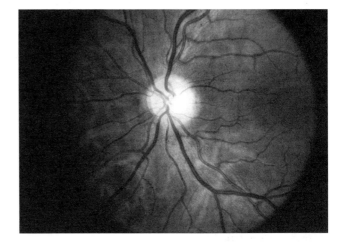

FIGURE 9-18—A normal fundus. The photo is centered around the optic nerve. (Courtesy of Davis Duehr Dean, Madison, WI.)

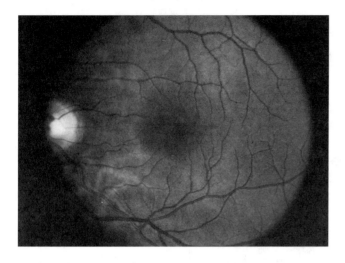

FIGURE 9-19—A normal fundus. The photo is centered around the macula. (Courtesy of Davis Duehr Dean, Madison, WI.)

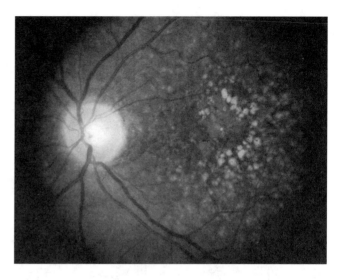

FIGURE 9-20—Macular degeneration (dry form) with drusen. (Courtesy of Davis Duehr Dean, Madison, WI.)

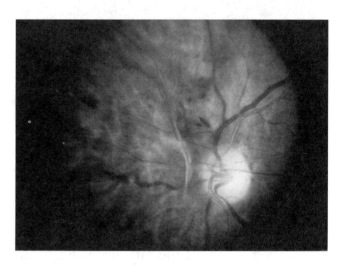

FIGURE 9-21—Diabetic retinopathy with neovascularization and a retinal fold. (Courtesy of Davis Duehr Dean, Madison, WI.)

the bright spot in the center of the picture. Also shown in Figure 9-18 are the retinal arteries and veins and the macula, the darker area to the right of the disc. In Figure 9-19, the camera is centered around the macula, illustrating how the retinal vessels lead up to the macula but end in the center of the macula (called the *fovea*). A fundus camera projects regular light and uses 35-mm film. There are two types of fundus cameras that may be used: *normal* (30-degree round photographs) or *wide-angle* (60-degree oval photographs). The type used depends on the extent of the retinal area involved. In addition to the normal fundus, photographs may be taken of pathology. These may include macular degeneration (Figure 9-20), a condition in which a patient's central vision is lost; diabetic retinopathy (Figure 9-21), which involves leakage of the retinal vessels; and retinal detachments, with holes, tears, or both in the retina. These photographs are extremely beneficial in revealing subtleties that may be difficult to identify during an eye examination.

OPHTHALMIC ULTRASONOGRAPHY

The process of using the reflection or echo of high-frequency sound waves to determine the outlines of ocular and orbital structures is called ophthalmic ultrasonography. With ultrasound, we are able to detect the presence of abnormalities within the eye, such as tumors, and to determine their size and position within the eye. Two types of ultrasound are used in optometry: *A-scan* (A-mode) and *B-scan* (B-mode).

A-scan uses sound waves traveling in a straight line to determine the position and the distance between structures within the eye. The main use of the A-scan is to determine the length of the eyeball, which is used to determine the proper power of the intraocular lens to be implanted in the eye once a cataract has been removed. Before an A-scan is performed,

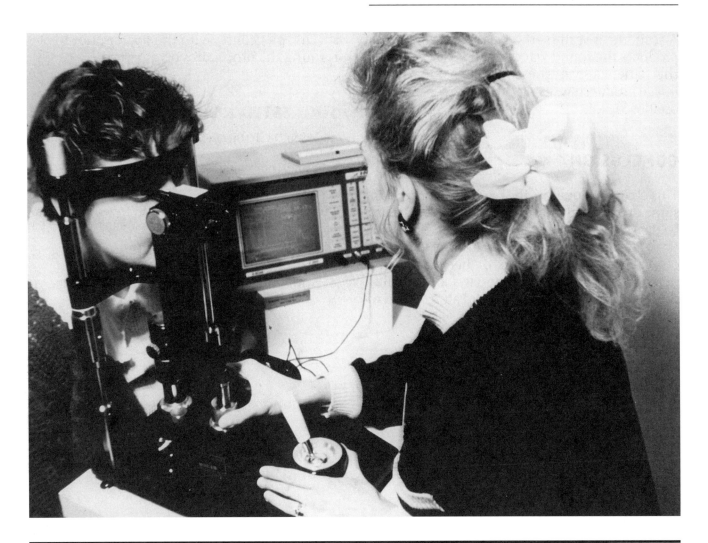

FIGURE 9-22—A-scan. (Courtesy of Davis Duehr Dean, Madison, WI.)

the patient's eye must be anesthetized with a topical anesthetic drop. Once the patient's name, birthdate, and other data have been entered, you may proceed with the A-scan. The probe is attached to a device that delivers adjustable sound waves to the eye. The probe is placed on the center of the cornea to obtain a reading (Figure 9-22). The measurement will be displayed on the screen, and the appearance of spikes and distance between them may be correlated to locations within the eye such as the cornea, anterior chamber, iris, lens, vitreous, and retina (Figure 9-23).

B-scan emits radiating sound waves. This technique provides a two-dimensional reconstruction of ocular and orbital tissues. B-scan is beneficial in detecting and measuring the size and position of tumors within the eye. As with

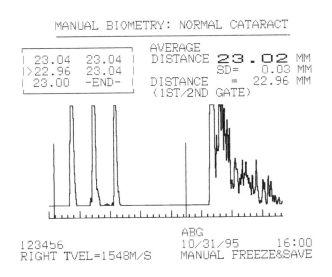

FIGURE 9-23—A-scan results.

A-scan, the B-scan method uses a probe tip that produces the sound waves when it is touched to the patient's eye. The two-dimensional echo image produced is displayed on the screen of an oscilloscope.

CONCLUSION

This chapter acquaints the paraoptometric with some of the special testing procedures that may be delegated as part of a complete eye examination. The doctor will decide which procedures to delegate depending on his or her manner of practice and applicable state laws and regulations. The paraoptometric should always review specific procedures with the doctor prior to performing the procedures on a patient.

SUGGESTED READING

Anderson DR. Testing the Field of Vision. St. Louis: Mosby, 1982.

Bates SS. Fundamentals for Assisting in Primary Care Optometry. New York: Professional Press/Fairchild 1983.

Carlson NB, Kurtz D, Heath DA, Hines C. Clinical Procedures for Ocular Examination. Norwalk, CT: Appleton & Lange, 1990.

Stein HA, Slatt BJ. The Ophthalmic Assistant (5th ed). St. Louis: Mosby, 1988.

Trobe JD, Glasser JS. Visual Fields Manual. Gainesville, FL: Triad Scientific Publishers, 1983.

10 / Visual Fields

Kathryn J. Wood and Van B. Nakagawara

The *Dictionary of Visual Science* defines the *visual field* as "the area or extent of physical space visible to an eye in a given position." The measurement of this field is performed with the eye in a fixed (visual axis directed toward a fixation point) position. The extent of the monocular visual field usually measures 60 degrees superiorly, 75 degrees inferiorly, 105 degrees temporally, and 60 degrees nasally.[1] The visual field of both eyes forms an oval that extends approximately 200–210 degrees laterally and 130–135 degrees vertically[2] (Figure 10-1).

The visual field may be represented as a map that is divided by *horizontal meridians* (0 and 180 degrees) and *vertical meridians* (90 and 270 degrees). These meridians intersect perpendicularly at the central point of fixation, separating the field into four quadrants. *Radial meridian lines*, defined by a distance in degrees from the horizontal meridian, are normally added at 15-degree intervals (Figure 10-2). *Circles of eccentricity*, concentric circles defined by their distance in degrees from the point of fixation, may also be included (Figure 10-3).

Every point on the visual field corresponds to a point on the retina, and its sensitivity to light may be measured. The fovea has the highest sensitivity/lowest threshold (requiring a small/weak target to evoke a response), whereas the peripheral retina has the lowest sensitivity/ highest threshold (requiring a large/bright target to evoke a response).[3] Approximately 15 degrees temporal to fixation is the *physiologic blind spot*, which represents the area in the retina occupied by the optic nerve head. Since there are no retinal receptors (cones and rods) in this area, the physiologic blind spot forms an absolute *scotoma* (vision entirely absent) in the visual field.

There are two ways to present the target while evaluating the visual field: *kinetic* and *static*. The target is in motion in kinetic presentation. For example, a target of fixed value (size/brightness) is moved from selected radial meridians, from nonseeing to seeing or seeing to nonseeing, until it is first detected or no longer perceived by the patient. The target is stationary in static presentation. The static targets may be presented by either a *threshold* or *suprathreshold* method. In static threshold perimetry, every test point is evaluated by a "bracketing" or "staircase" process. A target adjusted to a level slightly greater than the expected sensitivity is presented at a test point. If seen, it is then dimmed in increments until it is no longer seen, and then brightened in increments until it is first seen by the patient. If the target is not seen, it is brightened in increments until seen, then dimmed in increments until no longer seen.[4] (Note: In either case, the intensity of the last detected target is designated as the threshold value.) In static suprathreshold perimetry, targets are presented at predetermined locations in the visual field by two methods: suprathreshold (target value is adjusted to a level assumed to be above threshold for all points tested) and threshold related (target value is adjusted to a level slightly greater than the expected sensitivity for any given point tested). That area of the visual field in which a

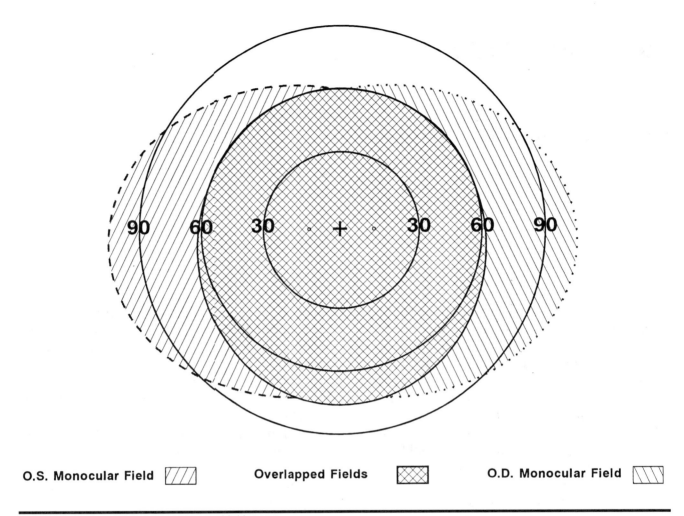

FIGURE 10-1—Overlapping monocular visual field.

target of a given value is visible, using either kinetic or static presentation, is an *isopter* (iso = equal, opter = sight).

Visual field testing performed on an instrument that has a hollow hemisphere, a rotatable semicircular, or arc-shaped, band with the eye located at the instrument's center of curvature, is called *perimetry*.[5, 6] Testing conducted on a flat surface, with the eye located at a known distance from the screen along a line that is perpendicular to the center of the surface (the fixation point) is called *campimetry*. Clinical visual field testing using either perimetry or campimetry will generate a topographic representation of sensitivity to given target values and will also search for any scotomas (areas of absent vision or depressed sensitivity). Scotomas may be identified by their depth, diameter, and location.[2]

Instruments for testing the visual field may be classified as *manual* (involving the skill of the paraoptometric) or *automated* (having the capability of operating independently). Manual examination of the visual field permits interaction between the patient and the paraoptometric. This interaction, based on the replies and behavior of the patient, allows the paraoptometric to introduce adaptations and refinements as the test proceeds. This interaction, however, will lessen the degree of standardization. Automated visual field testing, which ranges from simpler techniques to complex computerized programs, will follow a similar procedure regardless of the responses or behavior of the subject. As a result, the automated examination is standardized, and one test may be meaningfully compared to another.[7] Unfortunately, the subjective refine-

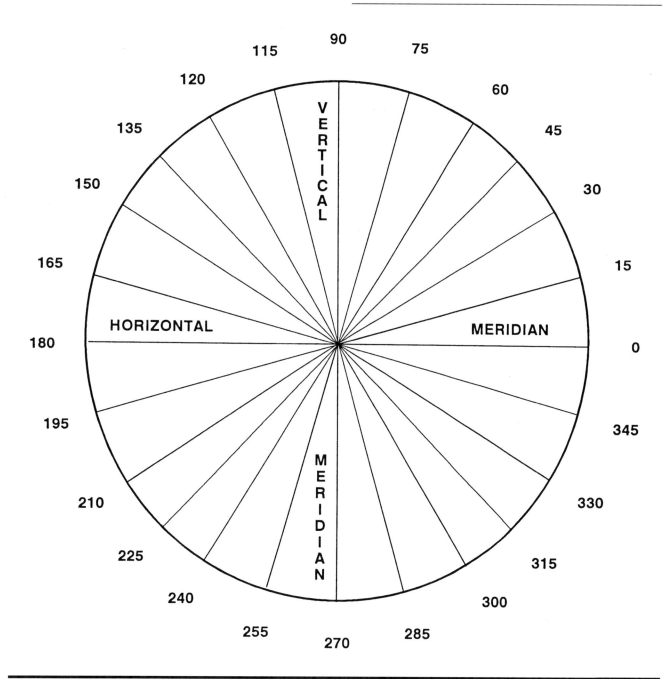

FIGURE 10-2—Mapping the visual field: radial meridians.

ments of the testing procedure by the paraoptometric are lost.

CONFRONTATION TESTING

Confrontation testing is used as a rapid, quantitative screening of the visual field, suitable only for eliciting gross defects in the visual field.[2] No equipment is required other than an occluder and hand-held targets. Normalcy of the paraoptometric's visual field is required to evaluate the adequacy of the patient's responses, however. The paraoptometric monitors the patient's fixation by direct observation and compares her or his visual field with that of the patient's. At a distance of 2 feet, the paraoptometric faces the patient while both are either standing or sitting. The patient and paraoptometric have opposite eyes occluded and fixate on each other's open eye (Figure 10-4). The paraoptometric moves the test object

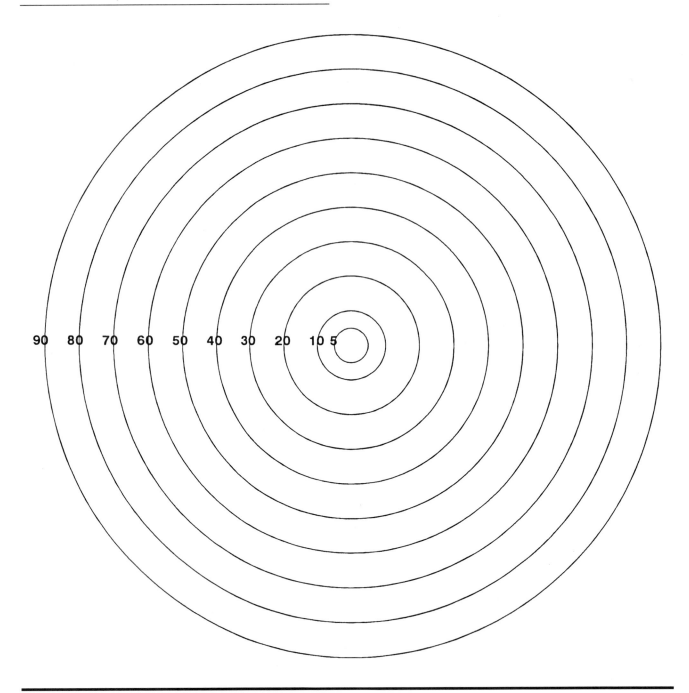

FIGURE 10-3—Mapping the visual field: circles of eccentricity.

(e.g., finger, mounted test target) from the periphery of the patient's visual field in one of the meridians and moves across to the other end of the meridian. The patient is instructed to respond at the point where the test object is first seen and also at any subsequent points of either or both disappearance and reappearance. The target should be brought in at least eight times, two times in each quadrant. The entire procedure is repeated for the other eye. If the paraoptometric notes a loss in the visual field by the confrontation method, additional testing with more sophisticated test methods should be performed to determine the extent of the field loss. If there are no field losses, standard recording terminology is WNL (within normal limits) or negative (indicating no abnormalities).

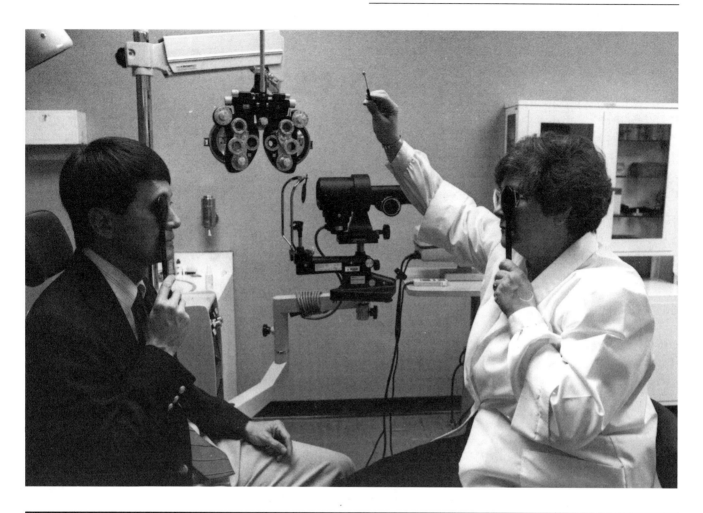
FIGURE 10-4—Performing confrontation field testing.

TESTING INSTRUMENTS

Harrington Flocks Visual Field Screener (Burton Screener)

The Harrington Flocks Visual Field Screener (also known as the Burton screener) requires 3–5 minutes to test both eyes (Figure 10-5). Because of its simple design and application, a paraoptometric may administer the test with a minimum of training. Since the procedure is standardized, the examination should remain unchanged regardless of where or by whom it is administered. The test uses the principle of tachistoscopic, or flash, presentation of simple, abstract patterns of dots and crosses, which act as visual stimuli to various parts of the visual field. The instrument will plug into any convenient electrical outlet. It consists of a bound book of 20 pattern cards with an Amsler grid (discussed later in the section on the Amsler grid) on the back cover, a box

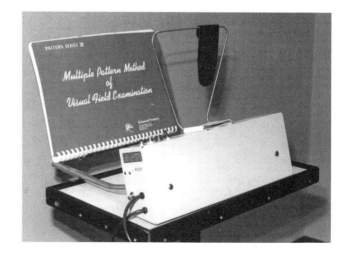
FIGURE 10-5—Harrington Flocks Visual Field Screener.

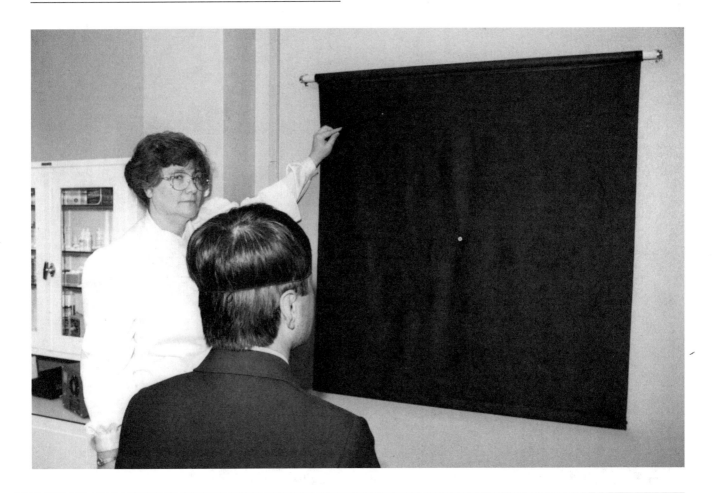

FIGURE 10-6—Visual field testing with a tangent screen.

containing a black-light tube, and a chin rest to fixate the patient's eye at a distance of 333 mm from the cards. The pattern cards are printed with white fluorescent sulfide ink so that under ordinary room lighting only the black central fixation dot is visible. When illuminated by a flash from an ultraviolet light source of 0.25-second duration, the test pattern is visible. There are 33 areas of the visual field within the central 25 degrees that are evaluated. These combined patterns will encompass most of the visual field defects (e.g., nasal step, arcuate scotomas). The patient is instructed to respond by describing the exposed pattern (e.g., "three" or "three dots"). The first 10 cards are shown to the right eye, and the second 10 cards are shown to the left eye. If one part of a pattern is missed, that test pattern is repeated. (A pattern missed twice by a patient is noted on the recording chart.) If a defect is identified during the test, its location and character simplify any follow-up visual field testing.

Automated Screeners

Most automated perimeters used in clinical practice today have the capability to do a screening strategy. *Suprathreshold screening*, one of the simplest strategies used, presents all test targets at one predetermined intensity. This provides information about whether a given test target was or was not seen at that level of intensity. No information about the extent or depth of any defect is provided.

Tangent Screen

A tangent screen is a black or gray nonreflective, matte-finished cloth, such as felt or velvet (Figure 10-6). Testing may be performed at 0.5, 1, or 2 m (measuring about 50, 30, and 20 degrees, respectively, of the visual field), although the most common test distance is 1 m.[8] The screen may be entirely unmarked or it may be stitched in semivisible black or gray thread for ease in testing and transcribing results. These markings include the vertical and horizontal meridians, radial meridians (marked at 30-degree intervals); concentric circles (which may be marked at 5, 10, 20, and 30 degrees, depending on screen size); and two blind spots, one on each side of fixation. The white central fixation target may vary in size from 1 mm to 100 mm (the size used depends on the patient's visual acuity). Three wand-mounted test targets are available: spherical beads; circular flat discs; and self-luminous targets, such as the Jenkel-Davidson Lumiwand. These targets vary in size from 1 mm to 20 mm in diameter and may be any color (a white target 1, 2, or 3 mm in size is most commonly used).[2] When testing at the 1-m test distance, the central 30 degrees is three times larger than bowl type perimeters. This allows a defect's shape, size, and density (relative and absolute boundaries of a scotoma) to be studied accurately. If a patient is suspected of being a malingerer or having a hysterical visual field, move the patient from 1 m to 2 m from the screen and double the size of the test object. The diameter of the monocular visual field should double, and the size of the blind spot and any other scotomas will be enlarged, allowing more careful study of those visual field defects (Figure 10-7). If the diameter of the visual field remains the same size, the presence of hysteria or malingering is strongly suspected.

Auto-Plot Tangent Screen

The Auto-Plot Tangent Screen, commonly called an auto-plot (manufactured by Bausch & Lomb), is designed for examining the central and paracentral area (30 degrees) of the visual field (Figure 10-8). The movement of the projected light target is controlled by a handle on a pantograph, which can also mark the recording chart. The auto-plot uses a 1-m screen of unmarked gray vinyl that allows uniformity of target brightness over its entire surface area and enhances target contrast under photopic conditions. Test targets vary in size from 0.5 mm to 15 mm in diameter and may be white, red, green, or blue in color. (A white target 1, 2, or 3 mm in size is most commonly used.) The target may be manipulated to appear and disappear for static testing; however, the auto-plot is primarily used as a kinetic test.

To perform auto-plot testing, the instrument is placed parallel to and at a test distance of 38 inches from the screen on a table 32 inches tall. The accuracy of the set-up may be checked by placing the recording chart in the chart holder and moving the pantograph arm so that the marking pencil is directly over the center of the chart. The target spot should fall directly on the fixation disc located in the center of the screen. The instrument is inexpensive, and the pantograph adds refinement, speed, and mechanical convenience. Because the test objects are projected, they are standardized in size and clarity. The examiner records the results directly on the chart as the test is being performed to ensure accuracy and repeatability. Patient movement is controlled by the chin rest. The major difference between the auto-plot tangent screen and the cloth tangent screen is the auto-plot limitation to one examination distance.

Amsler Grid

The Amsler grid tests the central visual field and consists of a 10-mm square white on black pattern of horizontal and vertical lines forming a square subdivided into a 20 × 20 box grid (Figure 10-9). The pattern covers 20 degrees of the visual field, with each box representing 1 degree.[1] During testing, if required, the patient wears a near correction for the 28- to 30-cm test distance. The paraoptometric occludes the nontested eye and instructs the patient to look at the center fixation point of the grid while the following questions are asked:

"Do you see the white spot in the center of the square chart?"

"Do you see the four corners of the chart?"

"Do you see the four sides of the chart?"

"Do you see the box patterns and are they properly shaped?"

If the patient answers "no" to any of these questions, a replica of the chart is provided and the patient is requested to draw the areas of visual disturbance. The other eye is tested using the same procedure. The Amsler grid may be used by patients at home to monitor daily any progressive

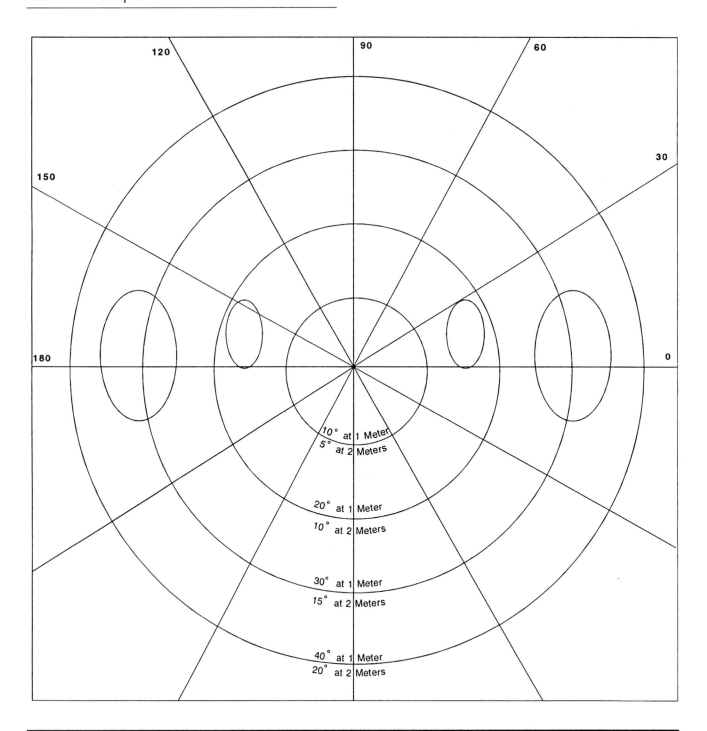

FIGURE 10-7—Visual field measurements at 1- and 2-m test distances.

macular disease. The test is normally used when visual acuity is abnormal or if an ophthalmoscopic examination reveals a defect near the macula.

Arc Perimeter

The arc perimeter consists of a rotatable, semicircular arc of 180–200 degrees (Figure 10-10). It is supported on a stand with a chin rest which keeps the patient's eye in the same position throughout the exam. The surface of the arc is normally black or matte gray with a width of 75 mm and illuminated with a uniform 7 foot-candles. Some arc perimeters have a special target carrier that is wheeled along the arc, whereas others use wand-mounted targets,

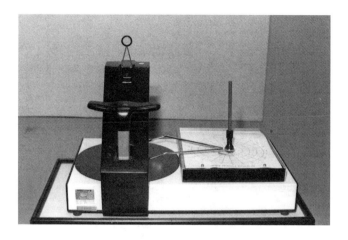

FIGURE 10-8—Auto-Plot Tangent Screen.

such as spherical beads or flat discs. Fixation objects may be white plastic or cardboard discs in a dull finish, with interchangeable sizes from 1 mm up to the same diameter as the width of the arc.[2] Arc perimeters are inexpensive, portable, and simple in design. The entire visual field may be tested,[8] so it is useful in assessing the size (peripheral boundaries) of the visual field. Because of its design, the arc perimeter is unable to plot the central field accurately. Therefore, the accuracy of the instrument's results increases if a tangent screen is used as a supplementary test.

Goldmann Bowl Perimeter

The Goldmann projection perimeter has a hemispherical bowl design (Figure 10-11). It has several advantages over arc perimeters, including that the illumination inside the entire sphere may be controlled, and illumination levels for the targets are variable. Fixation may also be monitored with a viewing telescope during test-

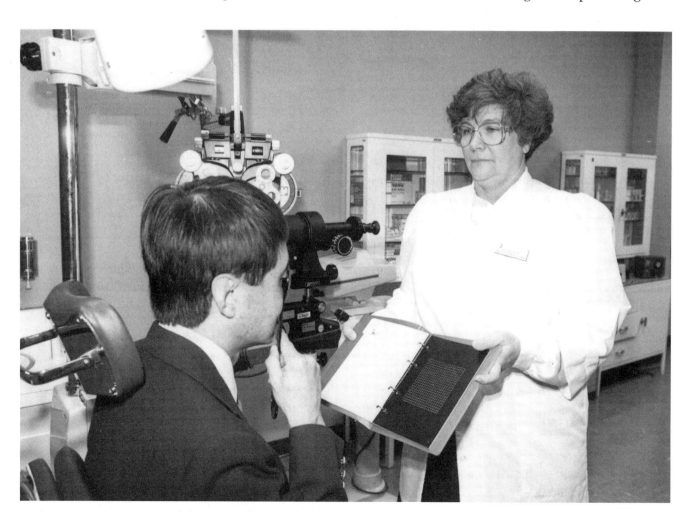

FIGURE 10-9—Visual field testing with Amsler grid charts.

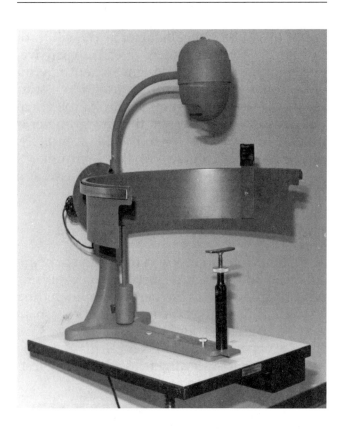

FIGURE 10-10—Arc perimeter.

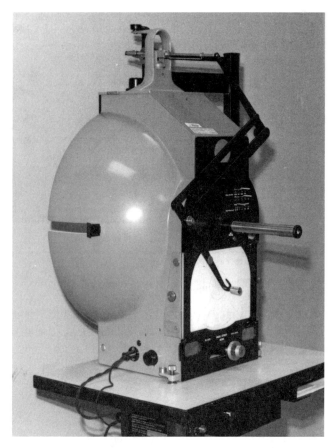

FIGURE 10-11—Goldmann perimeter.

ing. With the Goldmann, central and peripheral visual fields may be evaluated, and testing may be performed by static or kinetic methods.

Automated Perimeters

Most automated visual field analyzers use a bowl display similar to the Goldmann perimeter, which allows accurate testing of both the central and peripheral visual fields (Figure 10-12). Each type of automated visual field analyzer has different test programs but many similar features. Most have programs that not only perform suprathreshold and threshold-related screening strategies, but also full threshold strategies. Many practitioners use a full threshold strategy to obtain qualitative information when early field loss is suspected by screening strategies. Since the exact operating procedure for automated perimetry varies from one type of instrument to another, paraoptometrics should be familiar with their instrument manual.

TESTING PROCEDURES

When performing visual field testing, the patient should be seated comfortably at the required test distance. The fixation point should be directly in front and level with the eye to be tested. The task of concentrating on a fixed spot and responding to a rapid sequence of visual stimuli is not easy. Some patients may become anxious, whereas others may become bored. It is exceedingly important that fixation is maintained during visual field testing. With poor fixation, test results are invalid, as the test stimuli cannot then be correlated with the retinal position. There are several methods used for monitoring fixation, including *direct visualization of the pupil* through a periscope or video monitor; the *corneal reflection system*, which distinguishes between the image of the pupil space and those of surrounding areas; and the *Heijl-Krakau method*, which periodically presents targets within the blind spot that, if the patient is maintaining fixation, should not be seen.

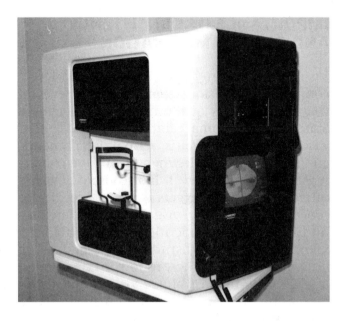

FIGURE 10-12—Humphrey Field Analyzer, an automated visual field tester.

When visual field testing is conducted, the following information should be recorded on the patient's medical record: examiner's name, date of test, patient's name, size and color of test target(s) used, corrected visual acuity, and pupil size. Automated instruments may also require the patient's date of birth and any trial lenses used. The paraoptometric should record comments on the medical record form concerning the patient's cooperation and reliability (e.g., *"Good fixation, good cooperation, etc."*).

Testing procedures for automated instruments are not discussed here. Each instrument has its own operating procedure, which is available to the paraoptometric in the instrument manual. Certain nonautomated instruments, such as the tangent screen, auto-plot, and the arc perimeter, however, have similarities in testing procedures. A recommended procedure that could be used for these instruments is as follows:

1. Occlude the patient's nontested eye. (Note: If an eye patch is used, a piece of gauze under the patch will be more comfortable and reduce the chance of stray light entering the patient's eye, while also preventing the spread of infection between patients.)
2. Explain the test procedure and instruct the patient on how to respond when the target appears and disappears (e.g., say "yes" or tap the instrument table or chair with a pencil or ruler).
3. Show target disappearance to the patient by using a large test target, which is seen in the peripheral field but completely disappears in the physiologic blind spot.
4. Map the blind spot first, from nonseeing to seeing, using a *cross sequence*:
    a. Move the test target into the nonseeing area from one side and instruct the patient to respond when it disappears.
    b. Hold the target steady within the nonseeing area. (The patient should be unable to see the target.)
    c. Reverse the original entry direction of the target, exiting the nonseeing area, while asking the patient to respond when the target reappears (mark #1).
    d. Reverse the direction, asking the patient to respond when the target disappears and then again when it reappears (mark #2).
    e. Position the target midway between the boundaries of marks 1 and 2, and move the target up, asking the patient to respond when the target reappears (mark #3).
    f. Reverse the direction, asking the patient to respond when the target disappears and then again when it reappears (mark #4). (Note: These four movements form a "cross" that evaluates the four sides of the blind spot; Figure 10-13.[9])
5. Next, map the periphery, moving the target from nonseeing to seeing from the periphery toward the center of the visual field.
6. It is recommended that the paraoptometric record the patient's responses after no more than three responses to target presentations along selected radial meridians.
7. When the boundaries of the peripheral visual field have been mapped, test the central visual field by moving the target from seeing to nonseeing.
8. The other eye is tested using steps 1 through 7.

If a scotoma is found during the testing procedure, the paraoptometric may use the cross sequence steps described above to measure the scotoma. These steps will allow the examiner to verify the scotoma's size and position within the visual field.

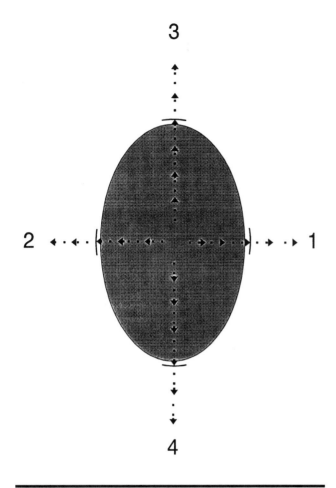

FIGURE 10-13—Cross-sequence examination of the blind spot.

On most of the visual field testing instruments, the test distance is fixed. A fraction is used when recording the results for a specific field test. The numerator is the test target size in millimeters, and the denominator is the test distance in millimeters (e.g., 2/1,000, or a 2-mm test target at a 1,000-mm, or 1-m, test distance).

With all manual and automated instruments for testing the visual field, it is important that the entire screen be evenly illuminated and at the desired intensity level. Each test has a recommended illumination level that should be complied with to ensure accuracy and repeatability of the test. Room lighting will influence the screen-background intensity. Although the background illumination level can be varied in some automated devices, it is always kept constant for the entire examination. Most automated instruments will recalibrate the background intensity when ambient room lighting is changed.

IMPORTANCE OF CONSISTENCY AND PATIENT MOTIVATION

Visual field testing is an important part of a comprehensive vision examination. All seven of the major causes of blindness in the United States (i.e., glaucoma, cataracts, diabetes, other vascular diseases, uveitis, retinal detachments, and senile macular degeneration) have characteristic patterns of defects in the visual field and often show these defects early in the disease process. Additionally, visual field tests are useful to the eye care practitioner in the management of endocrine disturbances, diagnosis of unexplained headaches, follow-up of vascular disease, diagnosis of blurry vision, and documentation of the progression or regression of a disease process.[10]

Since there are so many different reasons for performing visual field testing, there is no "standard" test. A manual technique or automated strategy should be chosen with a specific clinical question in mind to be answered. The paraoptometric should always review specific procedures with the optometrist before administering the test, since individual doctors may have a preferred test procedure method.

By alleviating the patient's discomfort and anxiety, visual field testing may be an enjoyable experience. It is the paraoptometric's responsibility to put the patient at ease to facilitate the collection of quality clinical data. The paraoptometric should never display an expression of dissatisfaction with a patient's performance or any other sign of being in a hurry. Because administering the test repeatedly may become mundane, paraoptometrics should guard against becoming stilted in their responses or exhibiting an indifferent attitude.

REFERENCES

1. Silverstone DE, Hirsch J. Automated Visual Field Testing Application. Norwalk, CT: Appleton-Century-Crofts, 1986.
2. Harrington DO. The Visual Fields: A Textbook and Atlas of Clinical Perimetry (5th ed). St. Louis: Mosby, 1981.
3. Henson DB. Optometric Instrumentation. London: Butterworths, 1983.
4. Leiberman MF, Drake MV. A Simplified Guide to Computerized Perimetry. Thorofare, NJ: Slack, 1987.
5. Bennett AG, Robbitts RB. Clinical Visual Optics. London: Butterworths, 1984.

6. Anderson DR. Perimetry with and without Automation (2nd ed). St. Louis: Mosby, 1987.
7. Whalen WF, Spaeth GL. Computerized Visual Fields, What They Are and How to Use Them. Thorofare, NJ: Slack, 1985.
8. Ellenberger C. Perimetry Principles, Technique and Interpretation. New York: Raven, 1980.
9. Havener WH, Goeckner SL. Introductory Atlas of Perimetry. St. Louis: Mosby, 1972.
10. Tate GW, Lynn JR. Principles of Quantitative Perimetry. New York: Grune and Stratton, 1977.

SUGGESTED READING

Bates SS. Fundamentals for Assisting in Primary Care Optometry. New York: Professional Press/Fairchild, 1983.

Grosvenor TP. Primary Care Optometry: Anomalies of Refraction and Binocular Vision (3rd ed). Boston: Butterworth-Heinemann, 1996.

Stein HA, Slatt BJ. The Ophthalmic Assistant: Fundamentals and Clinical Practice (4th ed). St. Louis: Mosby, 1983.

11 / Contact Lenses

E.S. Bennett and Bruce W. Morgan

PURPOSE AND SCOPE

The contact lens industry is an ever-changing area in health care today, with improvements benefiting thousands of people in the last few years.

In the 1940s, 1950s, and 1960s, improvements in contact lens designs were frequently made but usually consisted of making rigid lenses of polymethylmethacrylate (PMMA) smaller, thinner, and steeper in an effort to make a more comfortable lens by enabling more oxygen to reach the cornea via the tears. With the introduction of soft hydrogel (water-absorbing) lenses in the 1970s, the contact lens industry changed dramatically. Many potential patients who had been afraid to undergo the adaptation process common to PMMA lens wearers were attracted by the initial comfort achieved by hydrogel lenses. The initial success of soft lenses also attracted large corporations to invest in the contact lens industry, and technological improvements in lens materials and design were many and varied throughout the 1970s. The number of chemists solely responsible for working with differing lens polymers increased significantly during this time period.

The impact of new sophisticated bifocal designs, extended-wear and disposable lenses, and rigid oxygen-permeable materials has been both significant and exciting. These innovations have enabled a wide segment of the population to enjoy the benefits of good vision, initial comfort, and a satisfactory corneal oxygen environment. The new developments in contact lens technology have, however, made the roles of the practitioner and paraoptometric more, not less, complicated. There are new modification techniques, special verification equipment and procedures, and an increased emphasis on patient education. This chapter discusses conventional and specialty lens designs to help make the paraoptometric more knowledgeable and productive in an ever-changing industry. It also discusses lens designs in generic terms, since manufacturers are constantly developing new products. For information on specific lens types and parameters, paraoptometrics are encouraged to consult with laboratory representatives and to read professional contact lens journals.

PREFITTING EVALUATION

When a patient interested in wearing contact lenses enters the office, no evaluation may be made without a thorough prefitting assessment of the feasibility of this person as a possible contact lens wearer. A thorough case history is necessary, as well as several testing procedures to evaluate the patient's ocular health. Even if all of the refractive and ocular health testing results in a very suitable candidate, several questions remain to be answered: Is the patient very motivated for contact lens wear? Does this person appear to have good hygienic habits? What is the best contact lens for this patient?

Case History

Obtaining a complete history of the patient's general and ocular health is important in determining the patient's ability to wear contact lenses successfully. The history allows one to assess the motivation of the patient, as well as possibly to determine the lens of choice. Time may be spent answering patient questions and alleviating fears about wearing contact lenses that may be present. The paraoptometric may be invaluable in obtaining information and putting a patient at ease during the case history.

Why is the patient interested in contact lenses? The answer to this question could be a most important factor in determining whether a successful contact lens fit will be obtained. Young, active people (e.g., teenagers) are usually good candidates, as are moderate to high myopes who prefer the cosmetic and visual advantages of contact lenses. In many athletic endeavors and occupations, spectacles may be in the way, easily knocked off the face, or obstructive to good peripheral vision, or they may fog up because of a continuous change of atmospheric environment. In addition, aphakia and certain pathological conditions, such as keratoconus, benefit from the spherical, uniform refracting surface provided by a rigid contact lens.

If a patient desires contact lenses because of encouragement by a member of the family or a friend, his or her motivation may be low and the chances of success reduced. In addition, if the importance of contact lenses is underplayed in the patient's mind, and the realization of the time and money necessary to care properly for the lenses is not emphasized, the patient may quickly become disappointed and discontinue wear.

If the patient is female, special considerations must be taken into account. It is not recommended that a patient be fit with lenses during pregnancy, especially during the first trimester, because of the possibility of corneal swelling, which might adversely affect the lens fit and tolerance. In addition, it is important to know whether the patient is currently taking birth control medication, since this may affect corneal tissue in a similar fashion to pregnancy. It should also be determined whether the patient soon plans to begin or discontinue use of the birth control pill because this could affect the tear film and cornea, causing the patient to alter contact lens wearing time.

Is the patient a chronic allergy sufferer? If so, are antihistamines used to help relieve the problem? If this is the case, the patient may not be a good candidate. If allowed to wear contact lenses, the patient should be warned that dryness and lens awareness may be present and lens wear may need to be restricted or discontinued during the period of antihistamine use.

A patient's occupation, hobbies, and particular visual requirements may indicate possible problems or need for a specific lens type. Patients persistently exposed to airborne foreign matter, chemicals, or other industrial or environmental hazards may not be suitable for contact lenses or may require special protective spectacles or goggles to wear in such environments.

Patients with cosmetically noticeable strabismus ("crossed eye" or "lazy eye") may experience more eyestrain, leading to headaches and disillusion with contact lenses. The reason for this is that lateral prism, frequently incorporated into spectacle prescriptions to help keep the eyes better aligned and functioning together, cannot be incorporated into a contact lens. Vertical prism, however, can be included in the contact lens prescription.

The examiner must know how long the patient has worn spectacles. The longer spectacles have been worn, the more the patient is used to that mode of vision correction and the more time it may take to adjust to a different type of correction. In addition, the patient must be asked whether contact lenses have been worn in the past. If so, why were they discontinued? Finally, does the patient plan to move in the next 3 months? If so, the practitioner may refuse to fit the patient or may refer the patient to another practitioner to complete follow-up care.

Lid and Pupil Considerations

The *palpebral aperture*, or the separation of the lid margins between blinks with normal relaxed distance gaze, may be measured with a millimeter rule or interpupillary stick. The rule is placed vertically near the patient's eye, with fixation over the examiner's shoulder at a distant object.

The average fissure size is 9–10 mm. The position of the upper lid margin to the lower limbus with the patient relaxed and looking straight ahead should be noted in the patient's record.

The visible iris diameter is the distance from the nasal limbus to the temporal limbus and

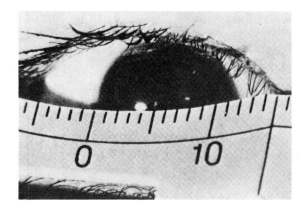

FIGURE 11-1—Determination of the visible iris diameter.

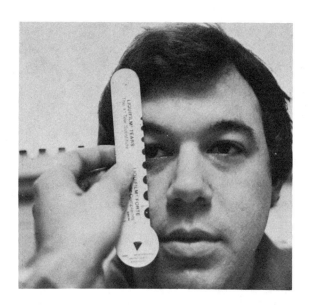

FIGURE 11-2—Pupil diameter measurement.

constitutes the lateral diameter of the iris. With the patient fixating straight ahead, a millimeter rule is angled toward the iris as demonstrated in Figure 11-1. A normal reading is between 10.5 and 12.5 mm. The diameter of the pupil in normal and dim illumination must also be recorded. This may be performed using the same method as was used for determining the visible iris diameter (Figure 11-2).

All of these tests will be useful in arriving at a final lens design. Pupil size determination is invaluable in determining lens diameter and the optical zone diameter. These must be large enough to enable the patient to see well both in daylight conditions (when the pupil is constricted) and in darkness (when the pupil enlarges or dilates).

Blink Rate and Type

Determining the rate of blinking may be accomplished quite easily by counting the number of blinks made by the patient in a minute. The procedure should be performed without the patient's knowledge, or the results could be affected. Patients should be aware that blink rate before fitting may be useful as a baseline value with which to compare values obtained after lens wear has begun. A blink rate of 10–15 times per minute is considered normal.

Does the patient blink completely or partially? As the case history is being performed, observation of whether each blink is a complete blink, a partial blink (lids do not completely cover the cornea), or even a flutter blink (lids cover only approximately half of the corneal surface on blinking) should be performed. If the blink is not full, the cornea will tend to dry, or desiccate, in the exposed areas that are not being relubricated by the tear film during the blink process. A baseline evaluation is needed, since the contact lenses themselves may inhibit the blink. It is important to note whether the blink is incomplete because of the lens, the natural blinking process, or both.

Corneal Sensitivity

Corneal sensitivity may be checked quickly by gently holding the lids apart and touching a wisp of wet sterile cotton wool or swab onto the cornea from one side so that its approach is not seen by the patient.

A normal blink response should result from both central and peripheral corneal touch. If this does not occur, the cornea is abnormal. Abnormal response is a frequent manifestation of long-term PMMA contact lens wear.

Tear Film Evaluation

The tear film should remain uniform over the corneal surface for a minimum of 10–15 seconds after a normal blink. If it quickly breaks up and becomes discontinuous, the outer layer of

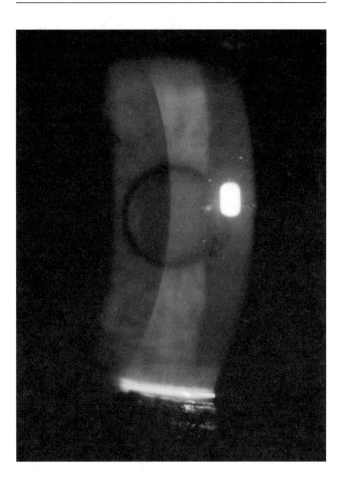

FIGURE 11-3—Dry spots in the precorneal tear film.

the cornea will become drier and susceptible to injury. A short break-up time indicates a problem with the mucoid layer of the tear film.

Tear film quality is best observed by applying fluorescein above or below the cornea and immediately observing the cornea with the slit lamp, using the cobalt blue light and the largest possible circular aperture to illuminate the entire cornea.

The patient is instructed to blink completely and then hold the eye wide open. True dry spots show up as black areas within the fluorescein-covered corneal surface and are consistent and repeatable (Figure 11-3). These are an indication of corneal damage or of some past or current problem.

A few isolated dry areas may occur within seconds. This can be misleading if the rest of the tear film remains normal for 10 seconds or more. The important value to note is the number of seconds it takes for the first dry spot to appear; this is then followed by break-up of the rest of the tear film. A stopwatch can be used to assess the time interval accurately. A reading of 6–9 seconds is borderline, but the patient is still a candidate for contact lens wear. The patient should be informed that "dry eyes" may restrict wearing time. Tear break-up time of 5 seconds or less should be a contraindication to contact lens wear. Low break-up times are indicative of pathologic dry eye conditions in which a mucus deficiency exists. Tear break-up time will usually decrease after contact lens wear. This testing should not be performed immediately following tonometry.

Tear film quality may also be evaluated by inspecting the tear film with a slit lamp and noting whether either or both debris and mascara or other particles of makeup are present. If so, the patient will have to be educated accordingly.

In addition to tear quality, an adequate tear supply or quantity should be present. This may be evaluated by using either Schirmer tear strips or the Phenol Red Cotton Thread test.

For the Schirmer test, the patient should be seated comfortably and told that this procedure measures the amount of tears produced and that it will not be painful but may be mildly irritating. The test itself consists of filter paper strips, 5 mm in width, that are folded 5 mm from one end. The short end is rounded and inserted into the inferior conjunctival sac, which is displaced laterally to avoid contact with the cornea; otherwise, reflex tearing will occur. After 5 minutes, the exposed length of moistened filter paper is measured to the fold. A reading of 15–20 mm in 5 minutes is considered normal, whereas a reading lower than 10 mm (or 6 mm if the shorter 1-minute test is performed) is indicative of a dry eye.[1] Both eyes should be tested at the same time. If a low value is obtained, the strip tends to adhere to the lower lid, so care must be taken in removing the strip. The test may be performed after insertion of an anesthetic for greater patient comfort.

The Phenol Red Cotton Thread test, developed in Japan,[2] was recently introduced in the United States. This is a long (70 mm) cotton thread that is presoaked in phenol red dye and is used similar to the Schirmer test (Figure 11-4). The benefits of this test include better initial comfort, a shorter (15 seconds) test time, greater validity, and no need for an anesthetic.[3]

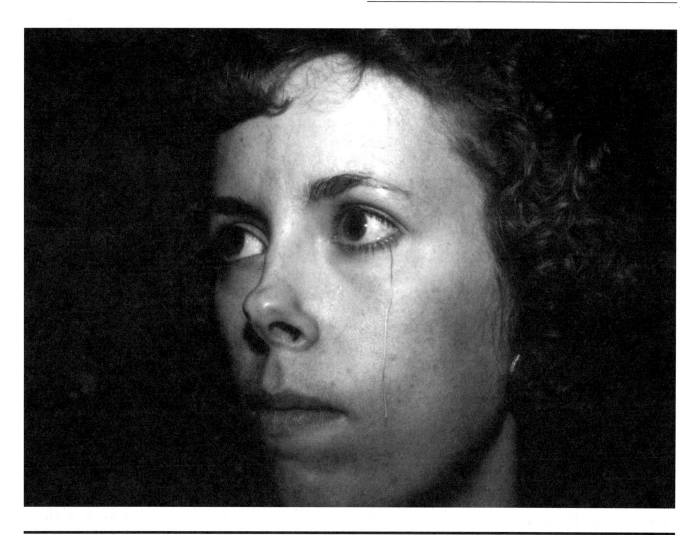
FIGURE 11-4—The Phenol Red Cotton Thread test.

Corneal Evaluation

A thorough corneal evaluation is needed to determine whether a patient is a viable contact lens candidate. After the standard illumination examination, the patient's cornea should be stained with fluorescein. Fluorescein sodium is used in fluorescein-impregnated strips and stains dry or irregular areas of the cornea, which show up as bright areas of green when the cobalt blue filter of the slit lamp is used because damaged cells will absorb the fluorescein. Fluorescein strips should be moistened with a sterile irrigating solution such as Blinx or saline and applied to the upper or lower conjunctiva. To be most effective, only a small drop of solution should be used on the strip, and excess solution should be shaken off before touching it to the eye. It is important that the patient look up or down from the fluorescein strip, because if the cornea comes into contact with the strip, the result will be irritation to the cornea and discomfort to the patient.

Fluorescein dye will not absorb into a PMMA or a rigid gas-permeable lens, but it can temporarily discolor a soft lens. Consequently, if a fluorescein evaluation is performed before a potential soft lens fitting, each eye must be flushed out several times with a sterile irrigating solution while the patient, with his her head tilted back, holds a tissue up near the eye to absorb excess fluid.

Lids

Both the upper and the lower lids should be evaluated as to their appearance. Previous contact lens wearers may have raised areas on the underside of the lids called *papillae*; these are

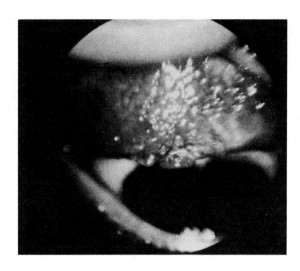

FIGURE 11-5—Nonuniform cobblestone appearance grade 2 papillary hypertrophy of the upper lid.

commonly caused by irritation from the lens edge, reactions to lens surface coating, or an allergic reaction to the solution regimen. Papillae may also be present prior to lens wear. Therefore, the upper lid should be everted and evaluated. A satin appearance of the lid conjunctiva is present when it is devoid of papillae and has a smooth surface. A uniform cobblestone appearance indicates several papillae are present per millimeter of conjunctiva. Usually they are congregated near the tarsal fold and become larger at the nasal and lateral junctions.

A nonuniform cobblestone appearance (NUCA) of the lids would be represented by one to three papillae per millimeter of lid conjunctiva, with the majority of the lid surface being affected. The lid illustrated in Figure 11-5 has a NUCA 2 papillae classification, and the patient would not make a suitable candidate for conventional soft contact lens wear.

In giant papillary conjunctivitis (GPC), the papillae are usually greater than 1 mm in size and are located in all five zones.

The ease with which the upper lid can be everted is an indication of lid tension. A lid that everts quite easily is a loose lid, and this is not a beneficial characteristic for contact lens wearers. Patients with loose lids will have difficulty lifting the lens up on the blink and may experience difficulty in lens removal because the interaction of the lid in forcing the lens out of the eye will be minimal. A tight lid, which is difficult to evert, is common in the Asian population. Normal lid tension may be represented by successful lid eversion with the thumb and forefinger of one hand grasping the lid and rolling it over a cotton swab.

Keratometry

The primary function of the keratometer is to measure the radius of curvature of the central portion of the anterior or front surface of the cornea. Although the keratometer has the disadvantage of supplying information only about the central cornea, it provides a starting point as to the curvature of the trial lens used in the initial fitting process. Keratometry was discussed in depth in Chapter 9.

In addition, the amount of corneal astigmatism may be determined with the proper use of the keratometer. For example, if the keratometer readings (K readings) are 43.00 @ 180 and 44.25 @ 090, the patient has –1.25 D of corneal cylinder at axis 180. Average corneal curvatures are in the range of 42.00 D to 46.00 D. Flat corneas in the 41.00 D or less category may be difficult to fit with a rigid lens, since the lens tends to drop inferiorly. Any distortion of the mire images should be recorded on the preliminary evaluation form (Figure 11-6). Peripheral corneal curvature information may be obtained from an autokeratometer or preferably a corneal modeling system (Figure 11-7).

Hygiene

The hygienic habits of the patient must be considered, especially if soft lenses are chosen. Is the patient slovenly or neatly groomed? How clean are the patient's hands, fingernails, and lashes? Is it believed that the patient will adequately care for the lenses? This is an important consideration, since soft lenses must be properly cared for on a daily basis. Dirt and other foreign matter on the hands or lashes may easily be transferred to a soft lens. Not only does this result in a dirty lens, but also an allergic or inflammatory reaction to the foreign substance on the lens may occur.

Summary

The optometrist can make a proper determination of the patient's viability as a candidate for

UMSL

Preliminary Evaluation for Contact Lenses

University of Missouri-Saint Louis
School of Optometry

Name _____ D.O.B. _____ M F File # _____ Date _____
   Last   First   M.I.
Home Address _____ Phone _____ _____
                                                      Home   Business

History and Contraindications (Please check appropriate boxes.)

Reasons for Contact Lenses	Medical History	Additional Information	Medication
☐ Cosmetic	☐ Allergies		☐ Diuretic
☐ Inconvenience of glasses	☐ Sinusitis		☐ Dilantin
☐ Sports and recreation	☐ Dryness of mouth, eyes, or mucous membranes		☐ Tranquilizers
☐ Occupation	☐ Convulsions/epilepsy		☐ Antihistamines
☐ Other:	☐ Fainting spells		☐ Birth control pills
	☐ Diabetic		☐ Other:
	☐ Pregnant		
	☐ Psychiatric Treatment		
	☐ Thyroid imbalance		

Do you plan to be in the St. Louis area for at least 6 months? Yes ☐ No ☐
Have you worn contact lenses before? Yes ☐ No ☐
If yes, what was the reason for discontinuing _____

O.D.	O.S.
Keratometry _____ / _____	Keratometry _____ / _____
Corneal Cyl. _____ Axis _____	Corneal Cyl. _____ Axis _____
Subjective _____ VA 20/___	Subjective _____ VA 20/___
Cal. Res. Astig. _____	Cal. Res. Astig. _____
Lid-Cornea Relationship ◯	Lid-Cornea Relationship ◯

Slip Lamp Observations

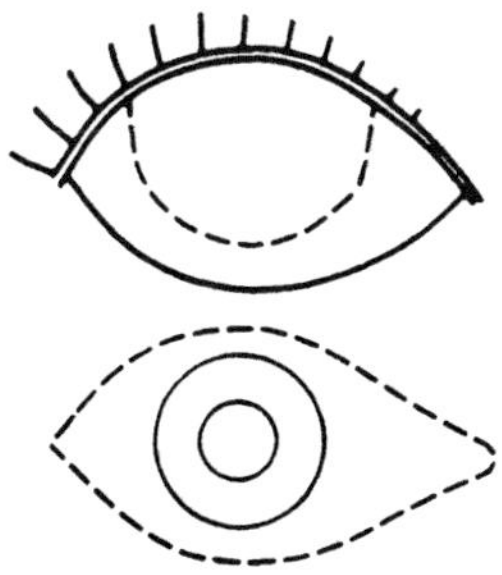

Blepharitis
Bulbar injection
Bulbar edema
Corneal striae
Corneal edema
Corneal staining
Corneal vasculature
Limbal injection
Keratitis
Pinguecula
Pterygium
Uveitis

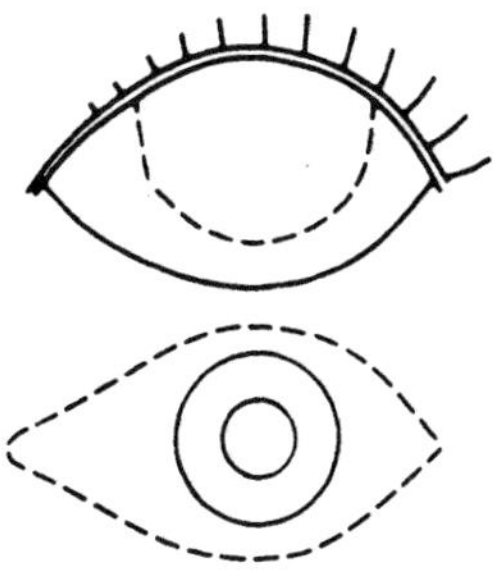

Grade: 0 1 2 3   Tarsal Conjunctival Abnormalities   Grade: 0 1 2 3

Binocular vision status far/near _____ / _____

		O.D.	O.S.
TBUT (sec)			
Schirmer (mm/min)		___/___	___/___
Pachometry (mm)			

Diameter (mm)			Lid Tension	
	Fissure	Cornea	Pupil	Tight ☐
O.D.			/	Loose ☐
O.S.			/	Medium ☐

Additional tests (specify):

Iris Color _____   Blink Rate/Type: O.D. _____
                                        O.S. _____

Motivation: High ☐ Moderate ☐ Slight ☐

Suitability: Yes ☐ No ☐

If no, specify _____

Student Intern _____
Supervising Clinician _____

12 82 UMSL 650

FIGURE 11-6—A preliminary evaluation form for a potential contact lens patient.

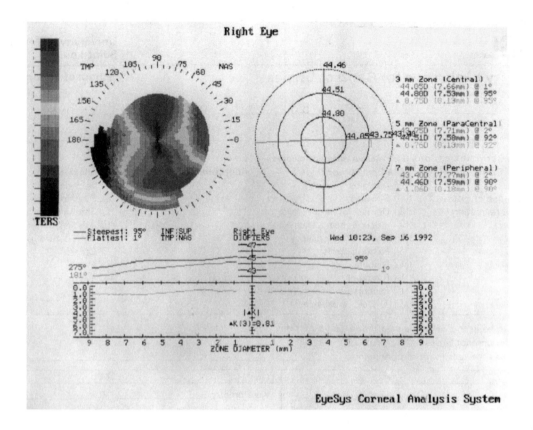

FIGURE 11-7—A corneal topography map (EYESYS, Houston, TX).

contact lenses only after completing the prefitting evaluation. All of the prefitting data may be included in a form similar to the one shown in Figure 11-6. If the patient is a good candidate for contact lenses, the optometrist must then consider the available options, which are discussed in the following sections.

RIGID LENSES

Basic Principles

Rigid gas-permeable (RGP) lens materials provide oxygen to the cornea by direct transmission through the lens material. RGP lenses attempt to maximize oxygen permeability and transmission while maintaining a rigid structure to correct corneal astigmatism. *Permeability* is defined as the ability of the material to allow oxygen to pass through it and is commonly referred to as Dk. Higher permeability is obtained when the molecular sieve, or the spacing between the molecules of the plastic, is such that oxygen can easily diffuse through it. Transmission indicates how much oxygen actually passes through the lens or is transmitted to the cornea. The thinner an oxygen-permeable lens is, the more oxygen that will reach the cornea. It is referred to as Dk/L, where L is the thickness value.

RGP lens design is extremely important to patient success with contact lens wear. Overall diameter, optical zone diameter, back vertex power, base curve radius, peripheral curves, edge and center thickness, and tint should be considered with designing a rigid lens.

Overall Diameter

The length of the lens from one edge to the other is the overall diameter (OAD). Arbitrarily, the lenses may be placed in three categories: When lens diameter is greater than 9.2 mm, the lens is usually considered large; when between 8.5 and 9.2 mm, it is a relatively common diameter; and when less than 8.5 mm, it is usually considered small. Most rigid lenses have diameters between 8.8 and 9.8 mm.

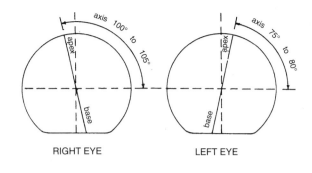

FIGURE 11-8—A contact lens with an inferior truncation.

The overall diameter is usually larger with flat corneas and large pupils; large palpebral fissures (position of the lid margins in relation to the cornea with straight-ahead gaze); and loose lids, where the effect of the lid forces on the lens position is minimal.

Occasionally, in special lens designs, a portion of the lens is removed, producing different diameters in the horizontal and vertical meridians. Such a procedure is termed *truncation*, and two meridians are used to describe the lens diameters of a truncated lens (Figure 11-8).

Optical Zone Diameter

Optical zone diameter (OZD) is the central area of the lens that corrects the patient's vision. It must be larger in size than the patient's pupil because it must cover the pupil during eye movements, blinking, and dim illumination. Otherwise, the patient will complain of ghost images or flare. This phenomenon of blurring or scattering of light most commonly occurs in low-illumination conditions, as in night driving or at the movies, when the pupil enlarges.

Back Vertex Power

Normally, the back lens surface is used as the reference point for the corrective power of the lens, and therefore the term *back vertex power* (BVP) is used. The BVP to be ordered depends on the over-refraction of the trial lens, the tear film, and the vertex distance allowance.

When patients wear spectacles to alleviate their refractive error, the lenses are usually 9–15 mm in front of the corneal apex. This separation is called the *vertex distance*. Since a contact lens is positioned at the corneal apex (center), the effective power of the prescription requires changes with the position of the lens in front of the eye. The effect is significant only for refractive errors of 4 D or greater, and more plus power is necessary in the contact lens. The vertex distance allowance is given in Table 11-1.

Base Curve Radius

The *base curve radius* (BCR) is the back central region of the lens and is important in obtaining a proper lens-to-cornea fitting relationship. Its value is usually very similar to the flatter K reading. For instance, if the K readings were 42.00 D at 180 and 43.00 D at 090, the desired lens is usually 42.00 D or 42.25 D in BCR; however, the BCR also depends on the optical zone lens design and the anatomy of the patient's cornea and lids. A larger optical zone necessitates a flatter base curve to approximate the flattening of the cornea. It is typically provided in either diopters or millimeters (Table 11-2).

The BCR is important in determining the final lens power. If the patient's flatter K reading is 45.00 D or 7.50 mm, the trial lens has a 45.25 D or 7.46-mm base curve radius and has –2.00 D corrective power, and the patient's refractive error is equal to –3.00 DS (diopter sphere), what will be the resultant contact lens power? Since the patient's refractive error is –3.00 D, a –1.00 D over-refraction would be predicted. In addition, the trial lens is –0.25 D *steeper* than "K," which creates a plus tear film layer, and an additional –0.25 D is necessary to correct this. Therefore, the final lens power should be equal to

```
−   2.00   (trial lens)
+  −1.00   (over-refraction)
+  −0.25   (to correct for steeper trial lens)
−   3.25 D
```

Peripheral Curves

Most rigid lenses are designed to have a minimum of two peripheral curves in addition to the base curve. These curves in the peripheral zone are always longer in radius, or flatter, than the base curve. If two peripheral curves are used, the lens is a *tricurve* design. The intermediate or secondary curve will be steeper than the peripheral curve and flatter than the base curve (Figure 11-9).

TABLE 11-1. Vertex distance chart at 12 mm

For plus read left				For minus read right			
−	+	−	+	−	+	−	+
5.37	5.00	9.75	8.75	14.75	12.50	20.25	16.25
5.62	5.25	10.12	9.00	15.00	12.75	20.75	16.50
5.87	5.50	10.25	9.25	15.37	13.00	21.00	16.75
6.12	5.75	10.75	9.50	15.75	13.25	21.50	17.00
6.50	6.00	11.00	9.75	16.00	13.50	21.87	17.25
6.75	6.25	11.37	10.00	16.37	13.75	22.25	17.50
7.00	6.50	11.75	10.25	16.75	14.00	22.75	17.75
7.37	6.75	12.00	10.50	17.12	14.25	23.00	18.00
7.62	7.00	12.37	10.75	17.50	14.50	23.50	18.25
8.00	7.25	12.75	11.00	17.87	14.75	23.87	18.50
8.25	7.50	13.00	11.25	18.25	15.00	24.25	18.75
8.50	7.75	13.37	11.50	18.62	15.25	24.75	19.00
8.87	8.00	13.75	11.75	19.00	15.50	25.00	19.25
9.12	8.25	14.00	12.00	19.37	15.75	25.50	19.50
9.50	8.50	14.25	12.25	19.87	16.00	26.00	19.75

TABLE 11-2. Keratometer diopter conversion to millimeters

Curvature (diopters)	Convex radius (mm)	Curvature (diopters)	Convex radius (mm)	Curvature (diopters)	Convex radius (mm)	Curvature (diopters)	Convex radius (mm)
60.00	5.63	54.37	6.21	48.87	6.91	43.37	7.78
59.87	5.64	54.25	6.22	48.75	6.92	43.25	7.80
59.75	5.65	54.12	6.24	48.62	6.95	43.12	7.83
59.62	5.66	54.00	6.25	48.50	6.96	43.00	7.85
59.50	5.67	53.87	6.26	48.37	6.98	42.87	7.87
59.37	5.68	53.75	6.28	48.25	7.00	42.75	7.90
59.25	5.70	53.62	6.29	48.12	7.01	42.62	7.92
59.12	5.71	53.50	6.31	48.00	7.03	42.50	7.94
59.00	5.72	53.37	6.32	47.87	7.05	42.37	7.97
58.87	5.73	53.25	6.34	47.75	7.07	42.25	7.99
58.87	5.75	53.12	6.35	47.62	7.09	42.12	8.01
58.62	5.76	53.00	6.37	47.50	7.11	42.00	8.04
58.50	5.77	52.87	6.38	47.37	7.12	41.87	8.06
58.37	5.78	52.75	6.40	47.25	7.14	41.75	8.08
58.25	5.79	52.62	6.41	47.12	7.16	41.62	8.11

The function of the peripheral curves is to contour or align with the peripheral cornea, which flattens as it progresses away from the apex. This enables an exchange of tear fluid under the lens with each blink and thus acts in preventing corneal swelling and patient discomfort. This portion of the lens is not used for correcting a patient's refractive error.

Although there is much variance in determining peripheral curve radii, the secondary or intermediate curve is usually about 1 mm flatter than the base curve. The peripheral curve is 2 mm flatter than the intermediate curve or 3 mm flatter than the base curve. If three peripheral curves are desired, the secondary curve may be approximately 0.8–1.0 mm flatter than the

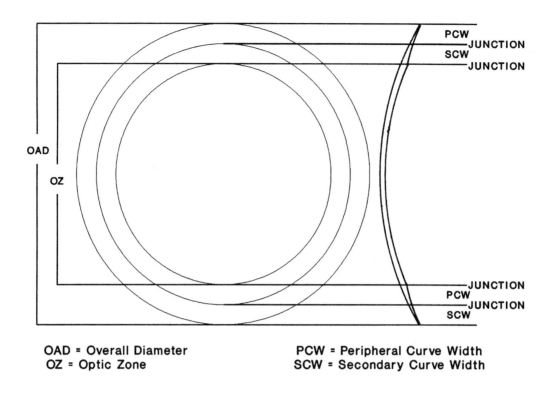

FIGURE 11-9—A tricurve contact lens design. (Redrawn by Catherine Muhr.)

base curve, the intermediate curve may be approximately 1.0–1.4 mm flatter than the first peripheral curve, and the peripheral curve will be anywhere from 1.4 to 2.0 mm flatter than the intermediate curve. In the following example of a rigid lens design, the radius is listed first followed by the width in parentheses:

Base curve = 7.70 mm

Secondary curve = 8.50 (0.3 mm)

Intermediate curve = 9.70 (0.2 mm)

Peripheral curve = 11.40 (0.2 mm)

The widths of the peripheral curves are usually fairly equal but may vary considerably. The width of the outside or peripheral curve is often called the *peripheral bevel*. Aspheric peripheral curves, where there is a gradual flattening from the base curve junction to the edge, are another option that is commonly used.

Since applying the peripheral curves to a lens results in sharp junctions between each curve, a light, medium, or heavy blend is usually recommended to smooth these junctions and create a more even tear flow into the central cornea. This is discussed further in the section on modification.

Edge and Center Thickness

The thickness of the edge and of the geometric center of the lens are usually different values. Both are important in determining how a lens will position on the cornea.

A lens that causes parallel light rays to diverge is termed a *minus lens* and corrects myopic, or nearsighted, patients. A lens that causes parallel light rays to converge is termed a *plus lens* and corrects hyperopic, or farsighted, patients. Thickness increases progressively from center to edge of a minus lens and decreases progressively from center to edge of a plus lens (Figure 11-10).

Center thickness for minus lenses usually ranges from 0.10 mm to 0.19 mm. Center thickness for plus lenses ranges from 0.20 mm to 0.30 mm, although high plus corrections for aphakic patients may be as thick as 0.50 mm or more. If the lens is thicker than desired, it is likely to decenter inferiorly due to the increased lens mass.

The gap between the upper lid and the conjunctiva is approximately 0.08 mm; therefore, a

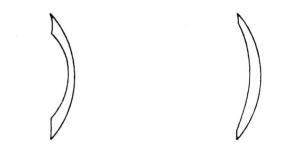

FIGURE 11-10—Minus and plus contact lens designs.

lens that has an edge thickness slightly larger than this amount would be desirable in order to have the lid exert pressure on the lens for the purpose of recentration after the blink. A thick edge, however, may be irritating to the patient and also interfere with the normal blink process. A thin edge may not be grabbed by the lid, and the lens will position inferiorly on the cornea. Therefore, a minus lenticular edge design is recommended for all low minus (e.g., <−1.50 D) and plus lens powers to achieve better lens centration and patient comfort. Consequently, a high minus power lens may have to be thinned at the edge (e.g., >−5.00) to fit properly or be manufactured in a plus lenticular.

Tint

The patient should be informed that the primary purpose for a tinted lens is to identify it easily in case or when it is misplaced. Usually a light or number one blue tint is ordered. Since the tint is through the lens, any patient who has a large difference in refractive error between the two eyes will run the risk of having one lens (the more hyperopic or plus lens) being much darker than the other, causing more of a "shading" effect over the eye since the lens is thicker. When this difference is present, the laboratory should be informed to match the tints as evenly as possible.

Contact Lens Order Form

Once the rigid lens design has been decided on, the order must be written up, phoned in to the appropriate laboratory, and placed with the patient's records. An order should include the following dimensions: BCR, OAD, OZD, power, secondary curve radius and width, peripheral curve(s) radius (radii) and width(s), blend, center thickness, special edge design (if appropriate), tint, and type of material. If a dot is desired for the right lens for purposes of differentiating it from the left lens, this preference should be included. A typical order form is shown in Figure 11-11.

RIGID LENS MATERIALS

Polymethylmethacrylate

PMMA is a transparent plastic that was first considered for contact lens use in the late 1930s. It is lightweight and ease to fabricate. The first PMMA lenses were called scleral lenses because they were extremely large (larger than the cornea) and were fitted with a relatively large, fluid-filled space between the lens and the cornea, therefore vaulting the cornea.

In the late 1940s, the first all-plastic PMMA corneal contact lens was developed. This lens was much smaller than the scleral lens and rested on the cornea. It was somewhat larger and flatter than present lenses and was a monocurve, or one-curve, design. Peripheral curves were introduced a few years later, and bicurve and tricurve lens designs became popular. Small or microcorneal lenses were the next design advance, becoming the lens of choice for many practitioners in the 1960s and 1970s. With more of the cornea exposed to atmospheric oxygen, and with more tear exchange with blinking allowed, corneal edema (swelling or clouding) was lessened and wearing time increased.

The primary problem with the standard rigid PMMA lenses has been persistent corneal edema (in the form of a central corneal haze) due to insufficient oxygen supply to the cornea. PMMA does not allow the passage of oxygen through the material, and consequently, PMMA lenses rely entirely on the tear pump (tear exchange under the lens through blinking), which is usually unable to supply enough oxygen to the central cornea to prevent central corneal clouding (CCC). Therefore, PMMA lenses are not generally a lens of choice in the 1990s, and they have almost totally been replaced by RGP lenses.

UMSL — University of Missouri-Saint Louis

Contact Lens Order Form
School of Optometry

Patient John Thompson
Intern
Laboratory Firestone
Rigid ___ Soft ___ Original Order (date) ___
Daytime Phone #
Appointment Date

	Specifications Ordered O.D.	O.S.	Specifications Verified O.D.	O.S.
Date				
B.C.R.	7.89	7.81		
S.C.R./W	8.90/.3	8.80/.3		
I.C.R./W				
P.C.R./W	10.90/.3	10.80/.3		
O.Z.D.	8.0	8.0		
Dia.	9.2	9.2		
Power	-2.50	-3.00		
C.T.	.16	.15		
Blend	Med	Med		
Tint	blue	blue		

Dot O.D. ☐ Verified by
Additional Information Fluoroperm 30

☐ Accepted ☐ Rejected ☐ Returned for Credit Date returned
Reason for return/reorder
Supervising Clinician BW Morgan O.D.
Rev 1/88 UMSL-653

FIGURE 11-11—A representative rigid contact lens order form.

Silicone/Acrylate

The first successful RGP lens materials were the silicone/acrylate (S/A) lenses. Introduced in 1979, these materials essentially contain four ingredients: (1) methylmethacrylate, (2) silicone, (3) wettability agents, and (4) cross-linking agents. The silicone provides oxygen through the lens via diffusion, methacrylate is the plastic, wettability agents enhance the surface wettability, and cross-linking agents improve the machining capability and overall stability of the lens. The latter two ingredients are necessary due to the poor wetting capabilities, softness, and flexibility of silicone. These lens materials dominated the RGP market in the early to mid 1980s; however, due to the dryness of the materials and the introduction of fluoro-silicone/acrylate materials, the use of S/A lens materials has declined in recent years.

Fluoro-Silicone/Acrylate

The addition of fluorine (known for its nonstick properties in Teflon-coated cooking materials) to S/A lens materials created fluoro-silicone/acrylate (F-S/A). This material has enhanced surface wettability because fluorine enhances the affinity of the tear film mucin for the front surface of the lens. Higher oxygen permeability lenses were also possible because the silicone content could be increased and because fluorine provides some oxygen permeability via solubility. F-S/A lens materials may be divided into low Dk and high Dk. Low Dk lenses are defined as having a Dk between 25 and 50. These are U.S. Food and Drug Adminstration (FDA) approved for daily wear and are typically the "workhorse" of RGPs used today. Some manufacturers produce this material with an ultraviolet absorber. This is an important benefit as we learn more about the harmful effects of

TABLE 11-3. *Fluoro-silicone/acrylate rigid gas-permeable lens materials*

Lens name	Dk	Manufacturer
Fluorex 300	30	GT Labs (Chicago, IL)
Fluoroperm 30	30	Paragon Vision Sciences (Mesa, AZ)
SGP III	43	Permeable Technologies (Morganville, NJ)
Boston RxD/Envision	45	Polymer Technology Corp. (Boston, MA)
Fluorex 500	50	GT Labs (Chicago, IL)
Fluoroperm 60	60	Paragon Vision Sciences (Mesa, AZ)
Boston Equalens	64	Polymer Technology Corp. (Boston, MA)
Fluorex 700	70	GT Labs (Chicago, IL)
Fluoroperm 92	92	Paragon Vision Sciences (Mesa, AZ)

sunlight on the eye, and particularly the crystalline lens. Polymer Technology Corp. (Boston, MA) manufactures a lens in an aspheric design known as the Envision lens. The advantage of this and similar designs is the ability to have better alignment of lens to cornea. In addition, there are fewer parameters (i.e., base curve radius and overall diameter); therefore, the design is less complicated, and the possibility exists for having an in-office fitting inventory of this design. Most RGP candidates would most benefit from a low Dk F-S/A lens material. This includes myopic patients, patients with borderline dry eye, and those needing a refit from a PMMA or low Dk S/A lens material (e.g., these individuals typically experience warpage and wettability problems if refit into high Dk F-S/A lenses).

High Dk (e.g., >50) F-S/A lens materials are available, most of which are FDA-approved for extended wear. These materials are more advantageous than hydrogel lenses for extended wear due to higher oxygen permeability and oxygen resulting from the tear pump; in addition, the smaller diameter of the lens eliminates limbal compression, and the surface wettability results in a lower incidence of GPC (lid inflammation) than is present with soft lenses. High Dk F-S/A lenses are recommended for patients desiring flexible (occasional) or extended-wear lenses, hyperopes (e.g., the greater center thicknesses impede oxygen delivery), and individuals who have a high oxygen demand. A partial list of available F-S/A lens materials is provided in Table 11-3.

SoftPerm

Styrene-based materials were introduced in the 1980s because of such benefits as a low specific gravity and good flexural resistance.[4] These materials have been incorporated into the center of a material that cross-links or molecularly bonds an outer hydrophilic skirt with the RGP center material. This lens is called the SoftPerm lens. It has a rigid center (8.0 mm with a 7.0-mm optical zone and one peripheral curve). The outer skirt of the SoftPerm is a hema-based hydrogel with an approximate water content of 25%. The overall diameter of this lens material is 14.3 mm. The primary benefits of the SoftPerm lens are initial comfort, astigmatic correction, and good centration. The latter benefit is especially important to patients having irregular corneas as a result of keratoconus, trauma, or other causes because a rigid lens may not center properly and a hydrogel lens will most likely not provide adequate vision. The problems with the SoftPerm lens include the cost, edema from a tight-fitting relationship, tearing at the junction between the soft and rigid portions, limited parameter availability, flexure, and difficulty in lens removal. The latter problem may be minimized by instructing patients to apply a few drops of saline or rewetting drops in the eye before removing the lens; the lens may then be removed either by gently pinching the lower section and removing it like a hydrogel or moving it onto the sclera and pinching it off.

Silicone Elastomer

Silicone elastomer lenses were introduced in the 1980s. This lens provides the wearer with the benefits of outstanding oxygen permeability (Dk = 340). The greatest problem with this material is the poor wetting characteristics of silicone, although surface modifications to this material have been somewhat successful in providing at least short-term wettability. The Silsoft lens is currently available in a range of aphakic powers. Although the lenses may last only 6 months when worn on an extended-wear basis, the excellent oxygen transmission, enhanced ease of handling versus a larger hydrogel lens, and better initial comfort than that of RGPs make it the preferred option for the pediatric aphakic patient.

PROGRESS EVALUATION AND SYMPTOMATOLOGY

The following procedures should be performed during a progress evaluation. The paraoptometric may not perform all procedures, but he or she should be familiar with them.

Case History

When a rigid lens patient enters the office for a progress evaluation, a thorough case history is a necessity. How many hours has the patient been wearing the lenses before entering the office? How many hours per day are the lenses generally worn? Are any problems present that need to be evaluated? Table 11-4 lists common patient complaints, possible causes, and methods of treatment.

Visual Acuity with Lenses On

Evaluate visual acuity with the lenses on. If it is reduced, possible causes are warpage (e.g., the lenses will have toric base curve radii when verified with the radiuscope), flexure (e.g., the lens is bending during the blink process and therefore inadequately correcting the patient's astigmatism). This is diagnosed by performing keratometry over the lenses which result in toric readings), or surface deposition.

Over-Refraction

When performing retinoscopy, is the reflex clear? Does the patient's vision improve with either adding or decreasing power as found by refracting with the lenses on? If plus is found on the over-refraction, the lens power should be verified with a lensometer because it is possible that the patient accidentally added minus power if, in fact, an abrasive cleaner was being used.[5]

Slit Lamp Examination with Lenses On

How are the lenses positioned? Are they centering centrally or superior-centrally, or are they decentering laterally or inferiorally? Do they tuck underneath the upper lid? Two to three millimeters of lens movement is considered normal. Does the optic zone adequately cover the pupil in dim illumination? This may be observed by moving the slit lamp beam away from the central cornea and observing the enlarged pupil. What does the fluorescein pattern look like? Be sure to record areas of bearing and pooling, which is where the lens touches or stands away from the cornea.

Slit Lamp Examination with Lenses Off

Slit lamp examination with lenses off is probably the most important test of all, especially in long-term PMMA wearers, who in many cases have suffered many years from low-level corneal anoxia, or oxygen deprivation.

CCC should be evaluated initially, since this phenomenon, if present, tends to subside gradually on lens removal. If a patient complains that vision is blurred through spectacles once the contact lenses have been removed, CCC should be suspected. It appears as a central, circular, gray area that is best seen with sclerotic scatter (when the slit lamp beam is focused at the limbus, which is the conjunctiva-corneal junction, and the microscope is focused in the

TABLE 11-4. "Dirty dozen" patient symptoms of rigid lens wear

Symptom	Cause(s)	Result	Treatment
Sudden pain (one eye only)	Foreign body sensation	Superficial spiral-like stain	Decrease lens wear for a minimum of 3 days
	Abrasion		
	Rough edge	Dense arcuate peripheral stain	Polish edge or replace lens if chipped
Dryness	Small lens		
	Inferior lens		Large flat lens, thin edge (CN)
	Thick edge	3-and-9 staining	Blinking exercises
	Poor blinking		Decrease wearing time
	Poor tear quality/quantity		
	Use of antihistamines/changes in hormonal balance	Diffuse punctate stain	Decrease wearing time
	Failure to use solutions (burning)		Use solutions
Burning	Dryness due to:		
	Above causes	Lid edema	Blend curves
	Bearing/poor venting	and	Alter lens wear during work
	Environment	Conjunctival infection	
	Insufficient sleep		
Gritty feeling	Lid inflammation	Lid infection and grade 2–3 papillary hypertrophy	Decrease wearing time
	Rough edge	Arcuate stain	Polish lens edge
Blur when reading	Infrequent blinking	3-and-9 staining	Emphasize proper blinking
	Uncorrected or residual cylinder	Conjunctival infection	Refit
	Decentered lens	Lens film	
Fogging	"Scratched" lens		
	Viscous tear film	Lens film	Clean and polish
	Poor blinking		
	Steep lens?		Refit
Fluctuating blur	Flare (small decentered lens)	Portion of optical zone outside pupil	Larger lens
	Scratched lens	Film that temporarily clears after blink	Clean and polish
	Residual cylinder	Noticed on over-refraction	Refit
Itching	Solution reaction		
	Allergic reaction to mucoproteinaceous deposits on the lens surface	Lids infected and inflamed	Change solutions More rigid cleaning regimen
Discomfort after several hours of wear	Flat lens	Mechanical (central) abrasion	Decrease wear until staining has resolved
	Dramatic increase in wearing time	Overwear abrasion	
Sudden blur	One eye only: decenter lens		
	Both eyes: switched lenses		
Dull headache (after several hours' wear)	Accommodative/convergence fatigue		Exercises, breaks
	Uncorrected residual cylinder/flexing		Equivalent sphere, front-surface toric or thicker lens
Psychological	Patient is "over-reactor"		Psychological

Source: Reprinted with permission from ES Bennett, R Grohe. Rigid Gas Permeable Contact Lenses. New York: Professional/Fairchild, 1986;217.

corneal plane being studied). Spectacle blur of 15–30 minutes is usually representative of grade 1 CCC (a diffuse haze over most of the cornea), 30–90 minutes is usually representative of grade 2 CCC (a central haze with diffuse borders), and 90 minutes or more usually indicates grade 3 CCC (a dense central haze).

Fluorescein should be instilled to evaluate the corneal integrity. The dye will stain any irritated areas of the cornea. Central corneal staining could be a result of overwearing the lenses or the lens bearing on the cornea, but it is usually the result of a tight fit. Peripheral corneal staining is usually a result of corneal desiccation, and irregular lacy or etched zigzag line staining is representative of dust or any other foreign body that becomes trapped between the contact lens and the cornea.

The blood vessels at the limbus should be evaluated to see whether any encroachment of these vessels into the cornea is taking place. This condition is called *neovascularization* and is the result of oxygen deprivation. If the condition is present and lens wear is not decreased or discontinued, the blood vessels will encroach further onto the corneal surface toward the pupil, and scarring of the cornea could occur. In addition, any redness of the conjunctiva should be noted, and the lids should be evaluated.

Postrefraction

Has the refraction changed since the initial examination? If the corneas are edematous, the patient may be unable to achieve a clear end point. If 20/20 or better acuity is obtained, it may be with an increased myopic refraction.

Keratometry

Have the corneal curvatures steepened, flattened, or changed in astigmatism since the prefitting examination? Are the keratometer mires clear or distorted? Distorted mires may be caused by a flat lens bearing on the cornea, by corneal scarring, or by corneal warpage syndrome. Corneal warpage syndrome is a condition experienced by many long-term PMMA lens wearers in which the cornea becomes distorted over time. Much controversy exists as to the cause, but the condition could be a result of either or both mechanical pressure of the lens against the cornea and a change in fitting relationship because of low levels of anoxia. Patients experiencing this condition show distorted keratometer mires and usually an inability to see better than 20/30 or 20/40 on postrefraction. It stands to reason that this same problem could occur with RGP lens wearers after long-term wear if the lens-to-cornea fitting relationship is poor.

Evaluation Form

All of the clinical results described above should be recorded on a form similar to that given in Figure 11-12. In addition, the diagnosis, any modifications performed, recommended treatment, instructions to the patient, and any reminders of the time of the next visit should also be recorded.

SPECIAL LENS DESIGNS

Front Surface Toric Lenses

The amount of astigmatism possessed by both the anterior surface of the cornea and the spectacle refraction is usually quite similar. Since a spherical rigid contact lens corrects in full the amount of anterior corneal astigmatism, patients will usually obtain excellent vision through these lenses. Since the spectacle astigmatism also includes the effects of the posterior cornea and the crystalline lens (lenticular astigmatism), however, some patients may have more than a small discrepancy between the corneal toricity and the refractive astigmatism. If the difference, or residual astigmatism, is greater than 0.75 D, an anterior or front surface toric lens could be recommended to improve the quality of vision.

For instance, if the patient's spectacle correction is –2.00 –2.00 x 180 and the corneal curvature readings are 43.00 @ 180 and 44.00 @ 090, the amount of residual astigmatism will equal:

$$\begin{array}{r} -2.00 \times 180 \text{ spectacles} \\ - -1.00 \times 180 \text{ cornea} \\ \hline -1.00 \times 180 \text{ residual} \end{array}$$

FIGURE 11-12—A representative contact lens progress evaluation form.

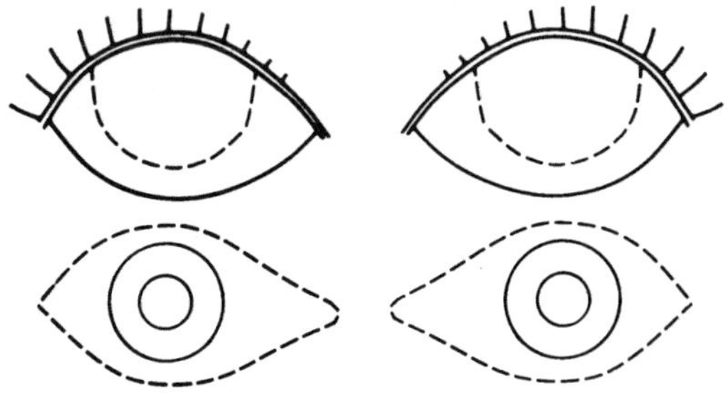

Toric Peripheral Curve, Toric Base Curve, and Bitoric Lens Designs

Patients who show 2.50 D or more of corneal astigmatism as demonstrated via keratometry are good candidates for a special posterior lens design. A spherical lens has a tendency to decenter or ride eccentrically on a highly toric cornea because of the inability of the lens to align properly with the cornea. If the lens was manufactured in either or both a toric base curve and toric peripheral curve design, better alignment is obtained. Another indication for special posterior lens designs is in cases in which a spherical lens is unable to correct all of the corneal cylinder. This problem sometimes is encountered with thin RGP designs, which tend to flex somewhat on the cornea.

Toric peripheral curve lenses have one primary spherical back curve with two different peripheral curves on the back. In this design, the optic zone is elliptical, with the short axis of the ellipse being along the flatter curve (Figure 11-13).

A *toric base curve lens* is a back surface toric lens. It has two different curves on the back with a spherical front curve.

A *bitoric lens* is designed with two different curves on the back and two different curves on the front. The front surface toricity is necessary to correct any astigmatism present that is not corrected by the back surface toric design, which in fact often induces some astigmatism as a result of the different refractive indices between the lens and the cornea.

Bifocal Lenses

In the past 20–25 years, many rigid bifocal lens designs have been introduced on the market. These have included concentric (annular) designs, several designs resembling spectacle bifocal lenses, and aspheric or progressive addition lenses.

Annular Bifocals/Simultaneous Vision Design

Annular bifocal designs have a central distance optic zone surrounded by a single annular near zone, providing correction for distance and near at the same time to the patient. The often-used design obtains its two refractive powers by different back or posterior surface optic zone curvatures. The distance zone curvature is steeper than the near zone curvature (Figure 11-14).

Among the advantages of concentric or annular bifocals are the absence of prism, a center thickness similar to a conventional lens, and a simple manufacturing process. The disadvantages of simultaneous-vision-design lenses are that one out-of-focus image is present at all times, and the snug fit may cause physiologic problems such as corneal hypoxia. Halos and flare with blur in low illumination occur regularly.

Translating Segmented Bifocals

Translating segmented bifocals are usually manufactured by fusing two plastics of different refractive index together, with the bifocal segment resembling one of the various segments found in spectacle lenses or a crescent shape. To ensure that the near segment represents the lower portion of the lens when on the cornea, prism ballast is added so that the heavier mass around the base of the lens positions itself downward by gravity. Truncation of the bottom edge is also used, but usually in conjunction with prism. If properly fitted, when the patient looks straight ahead, good distance vision is achieved; when viewing downward for near work, the lenses are pushed upward and the patient is looking through the inferior near zone. The benefits of fusing a higher-index near lens material into the distance lens button (or carrier) are both the creation of a thinner lens and the elimination of "image jump" (jumping of the image when viewing from one distance to another—a common problem in one-piece RGP bifocal designs). Since RGP lens materials are softer than PMMA, they are difficult to fuse. The first FDA-approved fused bifocal design was the Fluoroperm Fused Bifocal (Paragon Vision Sciences, Mesa, AZ), which is available in an average diameter of 9.4 mm (horizontal)/9.0 mm (vertical) (Figure 11-15). A popular one-piece RGP bifocal with monocentric optics (i.e., eliminates image jump) is the Tangent Streak (Fused Kontacts, Kansas City, MO) (Figure 11-16). Both the Fluoroperm Fused and Tangent Streak bifocal designs are typically fitted flatter than "K" and incorporate between 1.75 and 2.50 D.

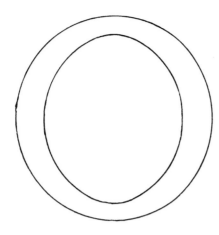

FIGURE 11-13—An elliptical optical zone diameter with the application of toric peripheral curves.

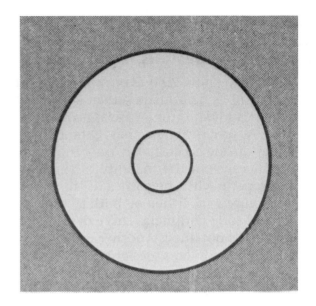

FIGURE 11-14—An annular or concentric contact lens bifocal.

The advantages of these designs include a fairly large reading segment and the ability to manufacture toric lens designs. The disadvantages include an inferior decentered lens because of prism ballast, corneal clouding, truncation rotating laterally (usually nasally), and the need to fit a large (usually greater than 9 mm) diameter lens. Nevertheless, this form of bifocal lens design is quite often the lens of choice and is an effective use of the alternating vision concept. With the use of RGP materials, the physiologic problems of corneal clouding could be reduced.

Aspheric Progressive Addition Lenses

Another approach to the simultaneous vision design is the use of a lens with an aspheric back design. Aspheric posterior flattening of the lens provides plus refractive power toward the periphery of the pupil area. This lens shows promise as design and manufacturing techniques are improved. There is some compromise in vision, however, because of the small distance vision zone, and there are patient complaints of flare and halos, especially at night.

Trifocal Lens Designs

Trifocal rigid contact lenses are also available. The example shown in Figure 11-17 has a small intermediate segment that has half the refractive power of the near addition.

FLEXIBLE LENSES

Flexible lenses consist primarily of hydrogels and silicone materials. Hydrogel lenses are made from a type of plastic polymer that absorbs and binds water into its molecular structure. They are often referred to as "soft" lenses. Instead of molding the cornea as rigid lenses do, flexible lenses conform to the cornea and therefore correct very little, if any, corneal astigmatism.

History

The idea of a soft contact lens is probably as old as the idea of a contact lens in general. Because of the difficulty in finding a suitable soft lens material, however, it was not until the late 1950s that the first soft lens was manufactured. It was invented by Otto Wichterle, a Czechoslovakian polymer chemist who was interested in developing a material that would have optimum compatibility with living tissue. It would possess shape, stability, and a softness similar to that of the soft surrounding tissue.

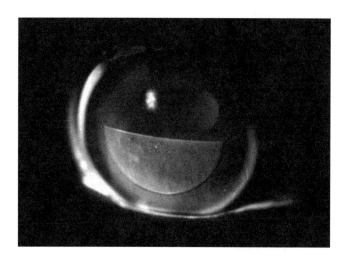

FIGURE 11-15—The Fluoroperm Fused Bifocal (Paragon Vision Sciences, Mesa, AZ).

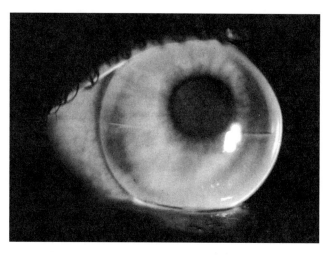

FIGURE 11-16—The Tangent Streak Bifocal (Fused Kontacts, Kansas City, MO).

Early success with animals prompted Professor Wichterle to attempt to persuade specialists in the domain of optics to adopt this invention, but they regarded the idea of an optical device made of rubbery material as ridiculous. After several years of unsuccessful efforts, he took the initiative and manufactured more than 5,500 lenses in a 6-month period and eventually persuaded eye care practitioners to use them. The results are now history. One of the first companies to invest in this material was Bausch & Lomb (Rochester, NY). The introduction of the Bausch & Lomb Soflens to the American market in 1971 marked the first of many soft lenses to be approved by the FDA. Since that time, soft lenses have been manufactured that can provide astigmatic correction; be worn overnight; be disposed of daily; and provide regular replacement, color enhancement, and presbyopic correction. Soft lenses account for approximately 80% of all contact lenses worn in the United States.[6]

Manufacturing Techniques

Spin Cast

The spin-casting technique is accomplished by placing a small quantity of the hydrogel plastic on a flat platform that can be spun. As the rate

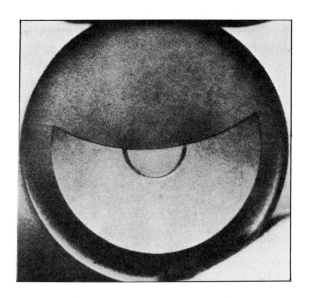

FIGURE 11-17—A trifocal rigid lens.

of spinning is increased, centrifugal force causes the material to move toward the periphery, resulting in the formation of a flat film. If the material is now placed in a curved bowl instead of a flat platform and the bowl is spun, it assumes the proper shape for a correcting lens. A slower spin speed will produce a flatter curve, and a faster spin speed will produce a steeper curve. The lens is hydrated, freeing it of the mold, and then extracted of impurities by boiling at 190°F.

Lathe Cut

Almost all of the soft lenses used in the United Stated today are manufactured from a lathe, much in the same manner as PMMA lenses. In fact, they can be machined and polished in much the same way as PMMA, except that the polishing compounds must be modified to work effectively. The material must be kept dry and any excess moisture withdrawn.

The lens is hydrated in saline and boiled. As the lens hydrates, every dimension of the lens changes, and the manufacturer must apply correction factors in order to predict the final dimensions after hydration. The lens must be manufactured so that it has a shorter base curve radius, a smaller diameter, and a greater power than the final lens. Therefore, quality control with soft lenses may be less stringent than with rigid lenses because of these dimensional changes. Reproducibility has improved over time because of improvements in manufacturing techniques.

Any lens that has been manufactured in the rigid lens design may be duplicated in a lathe-cut hydrogel lens. Therefore, a wider variety of the lathe-cut lens designs may be created with the lathe-cut technique than by spin casting.

Cast-Molding

The simplest and least expensive method of production is cast-molding. Material is injected into a mold with anterior and posterior curved surfaces. Multiple molds may be used to produce large quantities of lenses at one time. Reproducibility is typically quite good, and this has been a very successful method of disposable lens manufacture.

Lens Design and Uses
Daily Wear

Most of the flexible lenses on the market are meant to be worn during the waking hours only or for a maximum of 12–16 hours. Overnight wear of these lenses may result in corneal edema, insult, and possibly a red-eye reaction.

Extended wear is discussed in this chapter in the section on extended-wear lenses.

Chemistry

Soft hydrogel lenses are composed of polymers capable of absorbing a substantial amount of water. A polymer is a macromolecule made up of many repeating units or monomers. The chemical structure of hydrogel lenses is very similar to rigid PMMA lenses, except that a hydrophilic (water-absorbing) group will form part of the monomers of this kind of polymer.

Water-soluble substances (substances that can pass through water) may enter a hydrogel lens if they are smaller than the areas of interconnecting spaces in the plastic. These areas or spaces in hydrogels are full of water. The average diameter of the spaces increases as the water content in the hydrogel increases. Most water-soluble drugs, such as steroids and antibiotics, can diffuse in and out of any hydrogel lens with relative ease. This holds true also for preservatives, metabolites (urea, glucose, and lactic acid), and electrolytes (sodium chloride). Substances of larger dimensions, such as proteins, viruses, and bacteria, cannot penetrate intact hydrogel contact lenses. Contamination of hydrogel lenses by proteinaceous deposits and bacteria usually occurs only on the surface of the lenses. These substances can penetrate deeply into pinholes, cracks, and other defects of deteriorated hydrogel lenses.

Because hydrogel lenses are classified as medical devices by the FDA in the United States, each newly developed hydrogel lens has an additional nonproprietary name as do drugs. This name is not capitalized. The stem *-filcon* has been adopted for all new polymers used in hydrogel lenses. Examples include deltafilcon, crofilcon, and vifilcon.

The oxygen transmission of hydrogel lenses appears to be quite good. Naturally, the thicker the lens, the less oxygen that will be transmitted. The oxygen permeability (i.e., Dk) of most of these lenses is comparable to the rigid oxygen-permeable lenses on the market today. The transmission will decrease whenever the lenses acquire a proteinaceous film or any type of coating appears on the front surface, or if the lens dehydrates (i.e., on a dry eye). Oxygen reaches the cornea almost totally as a result of passing through the lens and only minimally, if at all, because of a tear pump.

Advantages and Disadvantages: Patient Selection

Advantages of hydrogel lenses include the following:

- Good initial comfort
- Reduced adaptation time when compared to rigid lenses
- Easy removal of lenses
- Availability in opaque tints
- Ability for some designs to be worn on a planned replacement or even daily disposable basis
- Rare dislocation of the lens onto the sclera
- Rare ejection of the lens from the eye
- Rare occurrence of flare
- Ability to wear lenses on a part-time basis

Disadvantages include the following:

- Poor visual acuity because of uncorrected astigmatism (if spherical design or rotated soft toric lens)
- Fluctuating visual acuity because of deposit formation
- Greater risk of ocular infection
- The possibility of an allergic reaction to the preservatives in the disinfecting solution or to the deposits on the lens surface
- Fragility of the material
- Short lens life
- Difficulty in verifying

A new patient who is able to obtain good vision with a soft lens (comparable to the vision achieved through spectacles) and is motivated to wear contact lenses but concerned about comfort is a good candidate, since the initial comfort obtained with these lenses will be a desirable characteristic. A former RGP patient who was never satisfied with the comfort of the old lenses is another good candidate. Since soft lenses do not correct spectacle astigmatism, if a patient has very little refractive astigmatism but much more corneal astigmatism (i.e., –0.25 x 180 refractive; –1.25 x 180 corneal), his or her vision will most likely be better through a soft lens than through a rigid one. Patients whose vision is blurred more than one line from that obtained through spectacles, satisfied rigid lens wearers, and those exhibiting poor hygiene are not good candidates for these lenses.

Tints

There are three types of tints available in hydrogel contact lenses: light blue handling or visibility tint, tints that enhance eye color, and tints that change the present eye color (i.e., opaque tints).[7] Unless unavailable in the desired soft lens material, all patients being fitted in a soft lens material should be provided with a visibility tint due to the difficulty in locating a lens that may have been displaced during handling. All patients should be informed about the availability of color enhancing and opaque lenses because the interest in these lenses is growing dramatically. Notably, the opaque lenses that can change any iris color, even brown eyes to blue, have been very successful. These lenses may also greatly help in the cosmesis of patients who have experienced ocular trauma or other similar ocular disfigurement.

Fitting and Follow-Up Care

Fitting, case history, and follow-up care are performed in much the same way as for rigid lenses. If a patient seems to be a good candidate for hydrogel lenses, the same prefitting tests are performed as for rigid lenses, with one notable exception. Fluorescein should not be instilled before soft lens insertion because these lenses can absorb the fluorescein dye and temporarily change color. Fluorescein should be instilled either at the time of the general ocular health examination or after the soft lens fitting has been completed. A patient should not insert the lenses until a minimum of 1 hour after fluorescein has been used unless the fluorescein is thoroughly rinsed out of the eyes, in which case, 10–15 minutes should be sufficient. Since fluorescein is extremely important in assessing corneal integrity, some patients may not desire to wait this long before reinserting their lenses. Such a patient should place a tissue on the cheek immediately below the eye to be rinsed out, and several drops of a sterile ophthalmic irrigating solution should be instilled into the eye. The patient should then blot the excess fluid from the eyes, paying particular attention to the nasal canthus, where the dye tends to accumulate. This procedure should be performed three times per eye, and by the third rinsing no green dye should be visible on the tissue. To be safe, lenses should be inserted a minimum of 10 minutes after rinsing is completed.

Soft lenses vary greatly in base curve radius and diameter. The lenses are quite large, usually ranging from 13.5 mm to 15.5 mm in size, and therefore they tend to overlap the cornea and extend onto the sclera while tucking underneath both the upper and the lower lids in most cases. Lenses are usually classified as high–water-content lenses (70–80% water), mid–water-content lenses (50–65% water), and low–water content designs (45% water and less). Thick lenses tend to move more on the cornea than ultrathins, which have a tendency to adhere to the cornea because they avoid the lifting effect of the upper lid. Soft lenses may also be cut in an ultrathin design. Soft lenses, in the majority of cases, have a standard OZD and peripheral curve radius and width for each lens design; therefore, only a limited number of specifications need to be given on the order form (Figure 11-18).

On a follow-up examination, a thorough case history similar to the one given to rigid lens patients should be administered. Slight or moderate lens awareness could be a result of dryness, excessive lens movement, lid inflammation, or corneal insult. If unilateral pain is experienced, the lens should be examined closely for tears or nicks. Itching is usually a result of a mild allergic reaction to the solution preservatives or to substances or pathogens adhering to the front surface of the lens.

The lens should be assessed on the eyes to determine whether they move any less than at the time of fitting, and whether there are any deposits or coating on the lenses. Discoloration may be evaluated by observing the lenses against a white background (e.g., paper or tabletop). Deposits are viewed better by removing and drying the lens and viewing with a 10× reticule magnifier. All test results and patient instructions should be documented on the appropriate form.

Special Designs

Toric Lenses

The biggest disadvantage of spherical soft lenses has always been their inability to correct refractive astigmatism. Since a large portion of the ametropic patient population is astigmatic, many patients either accepted the blurred images they were seeing through their soft lenses or were contraindicated as hydrogel patients. Manufacturers realized that a toric hydrogel lens was a definite need, but their development was quite slow in comparison to spherical soft lenses because of several factors. One problem was the inability to produce a stable, reproducible lens design. Second, a toric lens needs to remain stabilized on the eye, and since the effect of the upper lid may be such that the lens tends to rotate away from the desired position, blurred vision was a problem. In the last 10 years, however, numerous high-quality, reproducible soft toric lenses have been introduced. Extended-wear and planned replacement torics have also become available.

STABILIZATION

Toric soft lenses differ from spherical lenses by incorporating a necessary stabilizing mechanism into the lens design. Common stabilization techniques include prism ballast, truncation, and changing the edge design.

- Prism ballast. The incorporation of prism into the lens causes the thicker, heavier part of the lens to rotate with the prism in the down (vertical) position and maintain rotational stability.
- Truncation. A lower-edge truncation along the prism base may enhance stability of

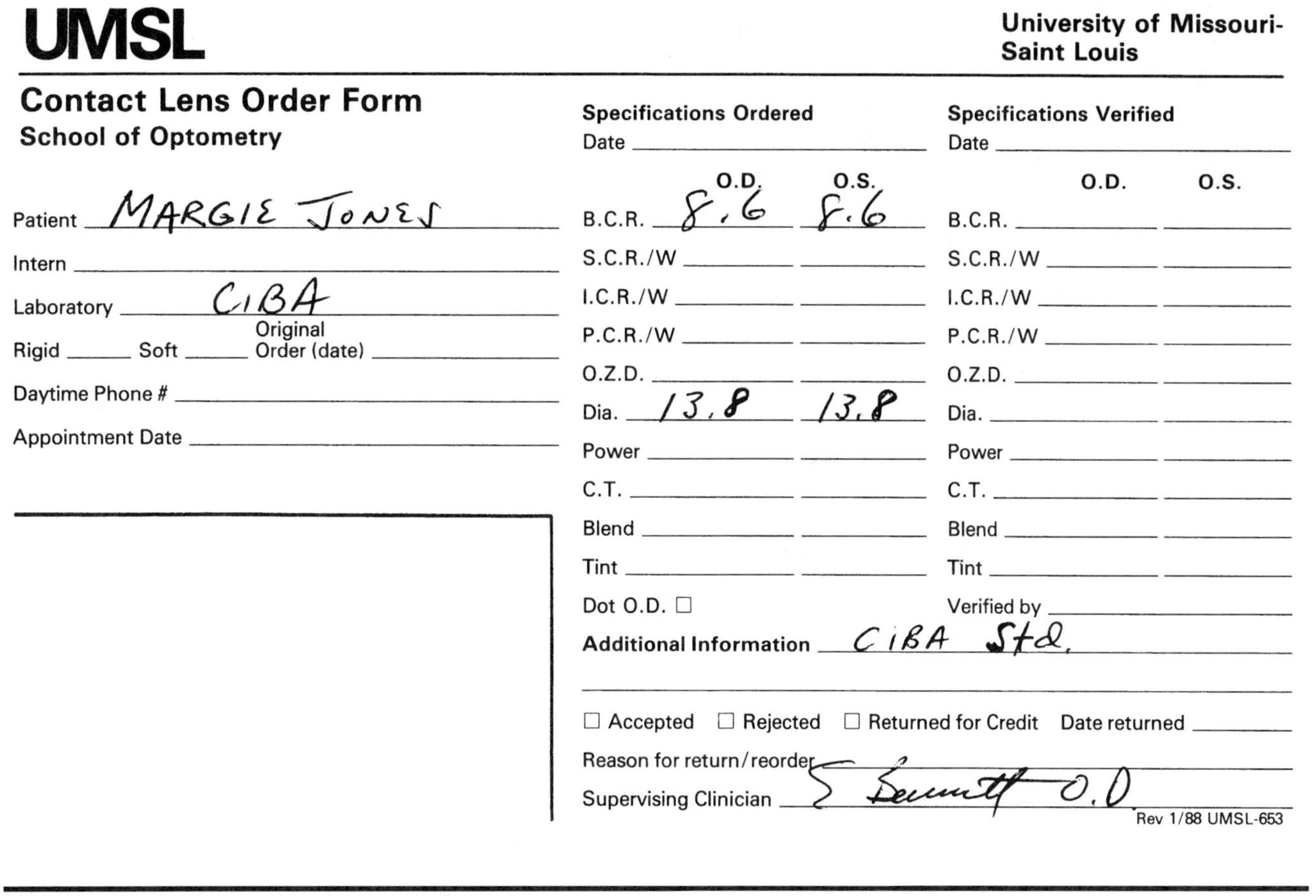

UMSL

University of Missouri-Saint Louis

Contact Lens Order Form
School of Optometry

Patient MARGIE JONES

Intern

Laboratory CIBA

Rigid ____ Soft ____ Original Order (date) ____

Daytime Phone #

Appointment Date

Specifications Ordered	O.D.	O.S.	Specifications Verified	O.D.	O.S.
Date			Date		
B.C.R.	8.6	8.6	B.C.R.		
S.C.R./W			S.C.R./W		
I.C.R./W			I.C.R./W		
P.C.R./W			P.C.R./W		
O.Z.D.			O.Z.D.		
Dia.	13.8	13.8	Dia.		
Power			Power		
C.T.			C.T.		
Blend			Blend		
Tint			Tint		
Dot O.D. ☐			Verified by		

Additional Information CIBA Std.

☐ Accepted ☐ Rejected ☐ Returned for Credit Date returned

Reason for return/reorder

Supervising Clinician S Bennett O.D.

Rev 1/88 UMSL-653

FIGURE 11-18—A representative soft lens order form.

the lens by allowing the lower truncation to conform to the lower lid margin or for large diameters to "lock" into the lower conjunctiva (Figure 11-19). A lower-edge truncation in soft lenses is rarely uncomfortable and does not often compromise physiologically or mechanically the inferior portion of the cornea, conjunctiva, or lid. This combination prevents the lens from incorrectly locating on the eye so that the axis of the cylinder component is correctly aligned for the patient's astigmatism. Truncation and prism ballast may be used in combination to enhance stability further.

- Alteration of edge design. If the edge of the lens is designed such that it is much thicker on one side than on the other, the thick edge should stabilize inferiorly. Therefore, the need for prism ballast is eliminated, and the lens may be manufactured much thinner and may consequently be worn more comfortably in many cases. One such method is termed dynamic stabilization. The thin zones at the top and the bottom are covered by the lids and the thicker center positions horizontally between the lids. The periballasted design differs from prism ballast lenses in that it has no prism in the optical portion of the lens, only in the periphery. The lens is fabricated by removing the superior portion of a high minus lenticular carrier; therefore, center thickness may be reduced and improved optical quality achieved.

ANGLE OF ROTATION DETERMINATION

The inferior portion of the lens may rotate away from the vertical position either because of the effect of the lids during the blink reflex

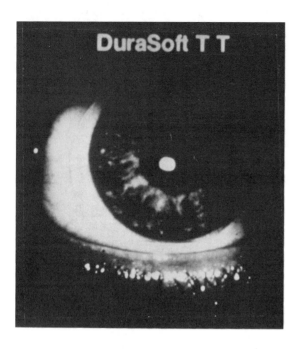

FIGURE 11-19—A truncated soft toric contact lens.

or because of the cylinder power and axis. In addition, larger, thicker, less hydrated lenses will be less likely to rotate because it is more difficult for the lids to exert an effect. When rotation is apparent, there are several methods of determining the actual amount.

- *Trial frame method.* The trial frame is placed on the patient's face, with care being taken to align the brow bar in the horizontal plane. A clear plastic rule or an inscribed disc placed in the trial frame cell can be used to determine the position of the lens by reading from the trial frame axis scale.

- *Reticule.* The slit lamp beam of a biomicroscope source may be rotated to align with dots marked on the lens. A protractor reticule (an eyepiece for the slit lamp with a degree scale incorporated into it) may be positioned in the microscope eyepiece for direct axis reading.

- *Estimation.* One can acquire an ability to estimate the angle of rotation of the lens accurately by observing any deviation of the base of the lens from the vertical. An easy mistake for the beginner is underestimating the amount of rotation. It is beneficial always to have a mental image of a 90-degree section of the lens from vertical to horizontal and to know how many degrees the lens seems to rotate with respect to 90 degrees.

The actual axis may be determined by using the LARS (*l*eft *a*dd, *r*ight *s*ubtract) principle. Observe the location of the identification mark (or markings) on the lens. Several different types of identification marks are used, including an inferior round dot at 6 o'clock, laser marks 20 or 30 degrees apart, or a "pagoda-like" design[8] (Figure 11-20). If the identification mark (or the central laser mark) has rotated 10 degrees to the observer's right, 10 degrees should be subtracted from the patient's refractive axis to obtain the axis of the soft toric lens to be ordered (Figure 11-21). For example, if the refraction is –2.00 –1.00 x 180, the axis to be ordered would be 180 – 10 = 170. Conversely, if the lens rotates 10 degrees to the observer's left, the lens to be ordered will be 180 degrees + 10 degrees = 190 degrees.

CANDIDATES FOR SOFT TORIC LENSES

Candidates for soft toric lenses include the following:

- Patients who desire soft lens comfort or who are unable to wear hard lenses comfortably

- Motivated patients who have 0.75–2.00 D of with-the-rule astigmatism (i.e., refractive cylinder [axis between 160 and 020] or against-the rule astigmatism [axis between 070 and 110])

- Patients having much more refractive than corneal astigmatism (therefore, vision should be blurred through a rigid lens)

THOSE WHO ARE NOT CANDIDATES FOR SOFT TORIC LENSES

Patients who are not candidates for soft toric lenses include the following:

- Those who have rotational problems at time of fitting

- Patients with oblique astigmatism

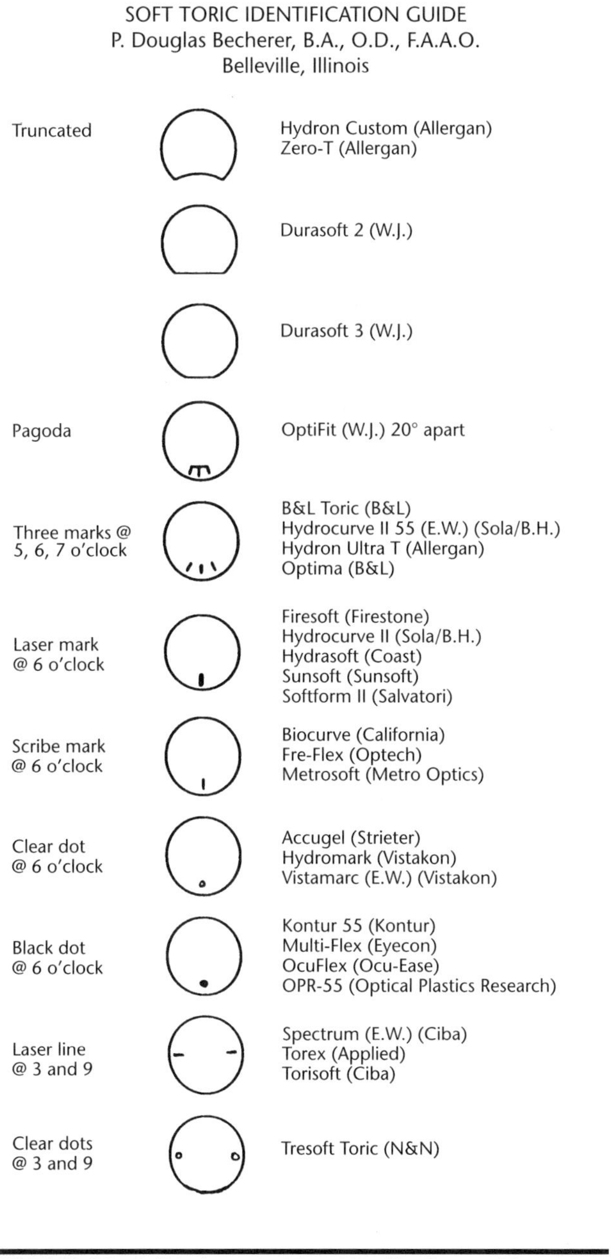

SOFT TORIC IDENTIFICATION GUIDE
P. Douglas Becherer, B.A., O.D., F.A.A.O.
Belleville, Illinois

Marking	Lenses
Truncated	Hydron Custom (Allergan) Zero-T (Allergan)
	Durasoft 2 (W.J.)
	Durasoft 3 (W.J.)
Pagoda	OptiFit (W.J.) 20° apart
Three marks @ 5, 6, 7 o'clock	B&L Toric (B&L) Hydrocurve II 55 (E.W.) (Sola/B.H.) Hydron Ultra T (Allergan) Optima (B&L)
Laser mark @ 6 o'clock	Firesoft (Firestone) Hydrocurve II (Sola/B.H.) Hydrasoft (Coast) Sunsoft (Sunsoft) Softform II (Salvatori)
Scribe mark @ 6 o'clock	Biocurve (California) Fre-Flex (Optech) Metrosoft (Metro Optics)
Clear dot @ 6 o'clock	Accugel (Strieter) Hydromark (Vistakon) Vistamarc (E.W.) (Vistakon)
Black dot @ 6 o'clock	Kontur 55 (Kontur) Multi-Flex (Eyecon) OcuFlex (Ocu-Ease) OPR-55 (Optical Plastics Research)
Laser line @ 3 and 9	Spectrum (E.W.) (Ciba) Torex (Applied) Torisoft (Ciba)
Clear dots @ 3 and 9	Tresoft Toric (N&N)

FIGURE 11-20—Soft toric contact lens identification markings.

- Those who have greater than 2.00 D of refractive astigmatism unless patient motivation is high, RGP lenses have resulted in failure, or both

SUMMARY

The problems with toric hydrogel lenses include the possibility of lens rotation, which may cause vision compromise and frequently results in an increased number of lens exchanges and more chair time. The cost of these lenses is higher, the delivery time slower, and the quality control poorer than with spherical lens designs. Thinner lenses, however, have reduced the likelihood of edema as well as increased patient comfort. In addition, the cost of the most recently introduced lens designs is not as high as that for previous designs. As available lens parameters are increasing and quality control is improving, this mode of lens wear will continue to become more popular.

Presbyopic Correction

The soft lens industry has progressed to the point where more and more presbyopes are enjoying the comfort and vision they achieve with soft lenses. Because bifocal soft lenses are still in a stage of infancy, many practitioners have elected to use the monovision mode of fitting.

MONOVISION

Fitting single-vision contact lenses for the presbyope by correcting one eye for distance and the other eye for near is a method that has been used for years with rigid lens wearers and is a frequently used option for soft lens wearers. The major advantage of monovision is the elimination of reliance on special lens designs (prism ballasted, crescent, or aspherical). Being spherical soft lenses, the fitting and care is essentially identical to that of any other soft lens. The principal disadvantage is that this method will blur one eye for distance tasks, and consequently, binocularity or the use of both eyes together will be compromised. Therefore, in most cases the dominant eye is fit with the distance lens. Although this may be of assistance, the monovision patient may encounter interference with many normal activities, such as driving a car, participating in sports, and any other tasks that require binocularity and stereopsis.

What should be considered when determining eligible monovision patients?

- Occupations that demand either or both good acuity and depth perception for long periods of time are contraindicated. People who do not have an intense near demand, such as most industrial workers, housewives,

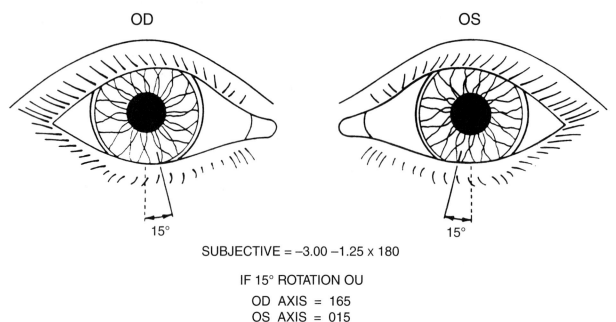

FIGURE 11-21—The LARS (left add, right subtract) principle.

and indoor office workers, however, are good candidates.

- Patients who are unwilling to wear conventional bifocal spectacles or contact lenses and would be able to accept some visual compromise are candidates.

- Single-vision soft contact lens patients who are incipient presbyopes would also qualify. Some of these individuals undoubtedly would only need to change one lens.

Considerations for determining the eye corrected for near should include the following:

- Using the nondominant eye
- The eye with the more poorly corrected acuity at distance
- The eye with the greater plus to blur finding
- The eye with the lesser near addition requirement

By using these specifics as criteria for selecting the near vision eye, you can better ensure patient adaption to monovision.

With absolute presbyopes, the distance eye may be slightly overplussed and the near eye underplussed (if vision is not significantly compromised) to lessen the anisometropia and better equalize the images seen by the two eyes. For driving, it is preferable to fit the left eye with the near lens so that road signs and the rear and right-hand outside mirror will be seen clearly. Another possibility consists of a driving prescription to wear over monovision contact lenses when critical distance binocularity is required. This consists of a plano spectacle lens over the distance eye and the proper lens over the nondominant eye to restore good distance visual acuity. This has been found to be beneficial for nighttime driving but not necessarily for daytime.[9]

The advantages of monovision include the following:

- It is less time-consuming than special bifocal lens designs.
- It is less expensive than other presbyopic corrections.
- Only one eye requires change for present soft contact lens wearers.
- Single-vision lenses may be more acceptable physiologically than bifocal lenses.

Disadvantages include the following:

- There is an effect on depth perception and binocularity.
- There is a possible loss of balance.
- Vision is blurred.

The bottom line for patients who are going to be fit with the monovision method is that a sufficient amount of time should be spent educating them as to the blur received, the adjustment time necessary for learning to change fixation alternately (it could take as long as 4 weeks), and the problems associated with driving and other critical distance tasks.

SOFT BIFOCAL LENSES

Several types of soft lens bifocals were introduced in the United States in 1982. These lenses varied in their design, but the methods of near addition were similar to rigid lens designs. Proper centration and limited movement (less than 1.5 mm) are critical to achieving a successful fit.

Soft bifocal lenses are indicated for the following:

- Highly motivated patients who desire the cosmetic benefits of soft bifocals over spectacles
- Previous soft contact lens wearers
- Those with mild to moderate presbyopia (most lens designs are targeted toward mild to moderate presbyopes, with a few exceptions.)

Contraindications of soft bifocal lenses include the following:

- Excessive near demand
- Critical, demanding attitude
- Successful monovision patient

The role of the paraoptometric in educating presbyopic patients is critical. Patients should not be given high expectations or more than likely they will be disappointed. Both the positives and the negatives must be communicated. There is an adaptation period with these lenses just as with bifocal spectacles, and the patients must adjust their eyes to determine the best acuity for near and distance. Acuity at near should improve after adaptation. Patients must be warned about the effects of dim illumination. The pupils will dilate, and a ghost image may be seen. Night driving especially could be affected by this problem; halos around headlights will be seen. Fortunately, the pupils constrict as the approaching car nears; nevertheless, it is recommended that every bifocal soft lenses wearer be a passenger the first time the lenses are worn in the evening to experience these changes.

EXTENDED-WEAR LENSES

Extended-wear refers to day and night (i.e., during sleep) wear of contact lenses that are removed at regular intervals for cleaning and disinfection. Several soft and RGP lens materials are FDA approved for up to 7 days extended wear. Because of the greater risk of eye infection due to insufficient oxygen transmission, surface contamination, and so forth, however, these lenses are most often prescribed for either occasional extended wear (i.e., typically 2–3 days at a time) or even daily wear for patients in need of higher oxygen transmission. Beyond 24 hours, the length of time lenses are to be worn before removal is up to the practitioner and the patient.

The essential difference between wearing a lens overnight and removing it before going to sleep is the rest and repair given to the cornea. Even at the reduced oxygen level present during sleep, the cornea is usually capable of repairing the day's oxygen deprivation and traumatic stress from a well-fitted lens of either the rigid or daily wear soft variety. When this repair period is delayed by keeping either of these types of lenses on the eye overnight, the recovery of a distressed cornea cannot, in most wearers, occur at a satisfactory rate. A lens to be worn on an extended-wear basis must transmit more oxygen than a daily wear lens because a lens that can transmit sufficient oxygen with the open eye may be totally inadequate with the closed eye.

When soft lenses first came on the market in 1971, the concept of overnight or extended wear began to surface. Although the water content of these lenses did permit some oxygen transmission, it usually was not enough to allow extended wear on most patients.

The soft lens industry then began to urge its polymer chemists to develop high–water-content lenses that could satisfy patients' need for continuous overnight wear. FDA approval was granted for aphakic extended-wear lenses in 1979. With further development of extended-wear lenses for myopia and, to a lesser extent, hyperopia in the form of ultrathin and standard thickness higher-water hydrogels, soft silicone lenses, and RGP lenses for overnight wear, it appears that many patients are eligible to choose extended-wear as their mode of lens wear.

Indications

There are many patients for whom an extended-wear lens is the most suitable, if not the only, form of visual correction; these include aphakics, medical patients for whom the lens can be used as a bandage, children, and myopic patients.

Aphakics

This is perhaps the most important group of candidates for extended-wear because of the large number of potential patients and their great difficulty with lens handling. These patients have benefited tremendously from the availability of extended-wear lenses.

Medical Patients

In medical cases (e.g., patient with bullous keratopathy, dystrophy, recurrent erosion), the extended-wear soft lens has been shown to be superior to other makeshift methods when used as a bandage. Being a rather large lens, it blankets the cornea, retaining its moisture and protecting its surface. Because the extended-wear lens is well tolerated, it provides an effective, and in many cases pain-relieving, cover for the eye.

Children

Aphakic and anisometropic (having a large refractive error difference between the two eyes) children may benefit from extended-wear lenses. The pediatric aphakic need to use extended-wear lenses is greater than in adult aphakics because most pediatric surgeons are reluctant to implant an intraocular lens in an infant or small child and because children may have difficulty handling lenses. Extended-wear lenses are handled less often than daily-wear lenses and can be handled by the parent or the guardian.

Myopic Patients

With myopic patients, the prime motivating factor appears to be one of obtaining a feeling of normalcy. Individuals would be able to see the clock immediately on awakening as well as the surrounding environment. In addition, they would be able to reduce the frequent handling and care required of daily wear lenses. With extended-wear, however, comes increased responsibility from both the practitioner's viewpoint and the patient's. Frequent, thorough eye and lens evaluations need to be performed at the first sign of redness, irritation, or blurred vision out of the ordinary. If these symptoms occur, the lenses should be removed; this should be followed by a visit to the contact lens practitioner as soon as possible. Either or both corneal edema and insult as well as red-eye reactions are more of a risk with extended wear than with daily lens wearers, and potential extended-wear patients should be informed of this possibility before initiating overnight wear.

Contraindications

Some reasons for not selecting a patient for extended wear may include the following:

- Any obvious contraindication to soft lenses also negates their use for extended wear, including corneal compromise, ocular allergy, edema, and decreased visual acuity.
- There is low to moderate hyperopia in some cases because of the increased thickness of plus powered lenses.
- Some patients are unable to remove lenses in an emergency.
- An unmotivated or uncooperative patient may not meet scheduled follow-up appointments and may fail to clean and disinfect the lenses periodically.
- A patient who does not seem interested in his or her appearance is likely to have an attitude that will also affect lens care.
- Very young patients who are wearing their first myopic correction should not be considered for extended-wear lenses. To earn the luxury of extended-wear, the young patient should be familiar with daily wear lenses in order to learn good lens hygiene and appreciate the subtleties of contact lens wear.

Types of Extended-Wear Lenses

An adequate oxygen supply to the cornea is critical for maintaining good ocular health with extended-wear lenses. Extended-wear lenses can meet this requirement in one of three ways: by means of a high–water-content lens, since there is a direct relationship between gas permeability and water content for any given material; by making the lenses as thin as possible, because of the further relationship between oxygen flow and lens thickness; and finally, by using a nonhydrogel lens that is oxygen permeable.

Extended-wear lenses include high–, medium–, and low–water-content soft lenses, silicone lenses, and high Dk RGPs. Paraoptometrics may learn about different lens types and their parameters by reading professional journals and material supplied by manufacturers and laboratory representatives.

High–Water-Content Lenses

These lenses contain 70% water or more. High–water content hydrogels tend to have lower mechanical strength because of the higher water-to-plastic ratio, which increases lens fragility. When reduced wearing time is indicated, thus increasing the frequency with which the lens is handled, the increased fragility may cause excessive breakage. Consequently, these lenses are generally made thicker to offset this disadvantage. In addition, because of the large spaces or pore diameters, many molecules of substances such as hormones and small enzymes that cannot penetrate low–water content lenses will enter into extended-wear materials.

Other problems related to high–water content soft lenses include the fact that they deteriorate with age more rapidly than do those with a lower water content. The lenses also tend to dehydrate during wear, which may cause the lens to steepen and minimize movement, consequently increasing the amount of debris trapped underneath the lens and possibly triggering a red-eye reaction.

Reproductivity has also been a problem because these lenses are more difficult to manufacture and the material is more susceptible to variation from one batch to another.

Medium–Water Content Lenses

The lesser oxygen permeability of a medium–water content lens is more than compensated for by a much thinner lens design allowing comparable oxygen transmission. Many of the same disadvantages present with high–water content lenses are evident in this group, through generally to a lesser extent. These lenses, as a group, appear to provide the greatest amount of oxygen transmission of the three hydrogel groups.

Low–Water Content Lenses

A low–water content lens should transmit approximately the same amount of oxygen as their high–water content counterparts if manufactured in an ultrathin design. The center thickness of these lenses is typically 0.035 mm in myopic powers.

The advantages of a thin low–water content lens are increased comfort because of a thin-edge design, a tendency to absorb less debris, longer lens life, less dehydration, and the ability to enzymatically clean them. Disadvantages include lens fragility because of the extremely thin center thickness and, in some designs, an absence of lens movement because of a thin-edge design.

Silicone Elastomer Lenses

Perhaps the only material to meet the oxygen requirement of the cornea in both the open and closed eye state is the 340 Dk nonhydrogel Silsoft silicone lens. The material is much stronger than hydrogel and resists splitting. It can withstand rougher handling than the hydrogel lens and has "memory," or the ability to return to its original shape after being flexed by one's fingers.

Silicone materials have traditionally experienced problems with wettability, and consequently, rapid build-up of protein and lipid deposits limits lens life. Because of these difficulties, combined with the high cost of manufacturing, the silicone elastomer lens is only produced for the aphakic patient.

Rigid Gas-Permeable Lenses

There are numerous high Dk (i.e., >50) S/A and F-S/A RGP lens materials available for extended wear. These materials have the benefits of increased oxygen transmission, good surface wettability, good tear exchange, and absence of limbal compression versus their soft counterparts. The impact of RGP extended wear has been minimal, however. This is a result of such factors as the introduction of disposable soft lenses, a more conservative practitioner approach toward extended wear in general, and the presence of some complications, although these are rarer than with soft lenses. These complications include adherence, vascularized limbal keratitis, and warpage-induced decreased visual acuity.

DISPOSABLE AND PLANNED REPLACEMENT LENSES

In 1987, the first disposable soft contact lens was introduced in the United States with the primary purpose of weekly extended wear followed by disposal. Since that time, disposable lenses have acquired other applications and wearing schedules. Technically, disposability infers one application and then discarding. In the contact lens industry, however, disposable lenses have been defined as extended-wear lenses being discarded every week and daily-wear lenses being discarded every 2 weeks. A daily disposable lens that is discarded every day is also now available. "Planned" or "programmed" replacement refers to replacing lenses on a schedule from monthly to every 6 months.

Benefits

Disposable and planned replacement lenses have numerous advantages over conventional extended-wear lenses. The primary benefit of disposable lenses is a reduction in surface deposit–related complications such as GPC and red-eye reactions. Therefore, this concept is ideal for most patients who tend to develop deposits on their lenses more readily. The presence of moderate to severe papillary hypertrophy may necessitate a daily wear disposable or planned replacement regimen. Other benefits of always wearing relatively new, clean lenses include consistent quality of vision via minimal lens discoloration and spoilage, and better long-term comfort.[10]

Each disposable lens is packaged sterile; therefore, there is a reduced opportunity for contaminants because they are more likely to adhere to coated lenses. With sterile packaging and infrequent lens handling, the probability of office visits related to lens complications, notably from lens aging, will be reduced.

Disposable lenses have also been used for therapeutic purposes, such as with corneal abrasion and recurrent erosion patients to increase comfort, drug delivery time, and wound healing.

Disposable lenses are usually supplied to the patient in either a four- or six-pack form. Therefore, if a lens tears or becomes contaminated, the patient is likely to have a replacement on hand. In addition, it is easier to monitor compliance with disposable lens patients than with conventional extended-wear lens patients because disposable lens patients may require office visits on a regular basis to obtain their next supply of lenses. The patient may then be scheduled for a follow-up visit.

Other rather controversial advantages are convenience and less cost. The majority of patients fitted with the disposable concept do not use surfactant cleaners, enzymes, or disinfecting systems. They simply apply comfort drops on awakening, at bedtime, and as needed, and may use nonpreserved saline to rinse the contact lens before insertion. This eliminates the opportunity for solution confusion complications and for preservative sensitivity. Also, there is less money spent on solutions and less time with the care regimen, which benefits the frequent traveler. Many practitioners believe a solution regimen should be prescribed with these lenses, accompanied by regular cleaning, however. In addition, the patient may not desire (or the practitioner may not recommend) 7-day extended wear. Therefore, removal for disinfection purposes is necessary.

Problems

There are possible problems associated with the disposable system as well. The patient may be tempted not to use any care regimen; therefore, lens contamination may become problematic. Patient compliance with the scheduled lens replacement plan could also be a potential problem, and lenses may be worn for a longer than desired period of time (e.g., 2 weeks instead of 1 week). In addition, by dispensing lenses in a four- or six-pack form, the practitioner does not evaluate every lens on the patient's eye and, although the reproducibility is generally quite good, it is not guaranteed; therefore, the fitting relationship may be affected. Likewise, the possibility of a defective lens is present.[11]

Whereas regular replacement minimizes complications present with deposited lenses, it does not increase oxygen transmission, especially if the lenses are worn for extended wear. In fact, if a tight-fitting relationship exists, the amount of oxygen may actually be decreased. Recent studies have concluded that the relative risk of ulcerative keratitis with extended wear of disposable lenses is four and one-half to seven times greater than with conventional extended wear.[12, 13] Therefore, it must be understood and emphasized to patients that these lenses do not provide greater oxygen transmission and that asymptomatic complications, particularly from oxygen deprivation, may occur.

Implementation

As a result of the large number of lenses involved in these programs, especially with the introduction of daily disposables, and the increase in popularity of frequent lens replacement, it is important to have a good system for successfully implementing these lenses into the practice. All staff members should have a good understanding of the benefits, fees, follow-up schedule, care, and so forth of these lenses. Typically, extended-wear disposable lens patients are provided with a 3-month supply and are evaluated (after the initial follow-up care has been completed) either every 3 or 6 months. In the latter case, patients are either shipped lenses at the 3- and 9-month intervals, or they simply return to the office for their lenses only.

It is important for the office to control inventory carefully because of both space limitations and patient satisfaction. Once a 3-month supply has been dispensed to the patient, this should be deleted from the inventory and the lenses either immediately replaced or a system used such that they are ordered shortly before the next 3-month visit.

The fee structure of disposable lenses should emphasize professional services. In addition, a fee structure may be available to patients that breaks down the cost of disposable lenses versus traditional extended wear such that they can observe that a large difference in cost is not typically present, especially when the reduced solution cost is considered. This, in combination with the other aforementioned benefits, may make disposable and planned replacement lenses a very attractive option for patients.

LENS CARE AND HANDLING

This may be the most important section in this chapter. If the patient fails to understand instructions related to lens care and handling, discouragement and possible failure may result. Proper and thorough patient education may significantly increase the number of happy and successful contact lens patients in the office.

Rigid Lens Solutions

It is important for eye solutions to be

- Sterile and stable
- Self-sterilizing if in multidose form
- Harmless if instilled undiluted
- Unreactive on lens materials for which they were designed
- Compatible with other solutions used for the same material

The general components of solutions include salts, buffers, viscosity-increasing materials, surface-active compounds, and preservatives.

Wetting and Soaking Solutions

Most solutions for RGP lenses combine the function of wetting and soaking into one solution. The principal functions of a wetting and soaking solution include the following:

- Acting as a lubricant between surfaces of the lens and the surfaces of the cornea and the lids, therefore minimizing discomfort to the patient during the initial insertion of the lenses and their subsequent wearing. This, in turn, encourages the prolonged wearing of lenses.
- Encouraging even distribution of tears over the lens, thereby improving the optical performance.
- Acting as a mechanical buffer between the lens and the finger during the act of lens insertion, thus preventing lens contamination. This same buffer action prevents discomfort and possible corneal insult should the lens be inserted too rapidly.
- Disinfecting the lens. Sources of microorganisms may include fingers, dirty lenses, and contaminated solutions.

- Maintaining the lens in a hydrated state, an important consideration with gas-permeable lenses, which contain up to 2% water.
- Preventing storage case scratches that may occur to the surface of the lens, loosening the adhesion of any accumulated mucus.

All RGP lenses are relatively hydrophobic (water-repelling). This is natural with all plastic and even more characteristic of RGP lenses because of the silicone added. Wetting and soaking agents are able to convert the dry plastic surface into a more hydrophilic (water-loving) one that will spread the fluid over the lens surface. For purposes of optical clarity, it is important that the tears spread evenly over the surface of the lens. Most RGP contact lens solutions use polyvinyl alcohol as their wetting agent, which possesses several properties favorable to rigid contact lens wear.

Saliva is not recommended as a suitable wetting agent. Microorganisms could enter the eye if the cornea were injured and saliva were between the lens and the eye.

Cleaning Solutions

When the lens is removed from the cornea, it will be covered with ocular secretions containing oils, mucus, crystalline deposits, and so forth. These contaminants must be removed before storing the lens. It is insufficient to clean the lens with water. Not only do the deposits adhere tenaciously to the surface, but also oil and mucus, which are not soluble in water, are not adequately removed by rinsing or by storage in the soaking solution. Some type of detergent should be used, such as that found in RGP lens cleaning solutions.

Commercially available cleaners come in many forms, including gels, liquids, and slightly abrasive cleaners, and vary in their suitability and effectiveness. In addition, systems are available for thorough cleaning via friction. Included in this category is the Hydra-Mat II by PBH (San Diego, CA) (Figure 11-22). Never allow the patient to resort to household products to clean lenses. These products may cause problems for the wearer, such as redness and irritation, as well as damage to the lens.

Fine abrasives such as calamine lotion and some silver polishes may be rubbed on the lens-

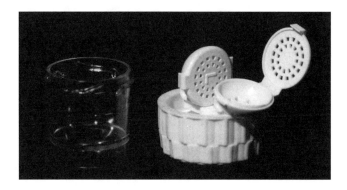

FIGURE 11-22—The Hydra-Mat II (PBH, San Diego, CA).

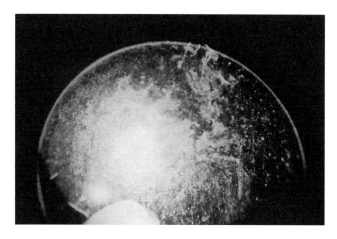

FIGURE 11-23—Ocular lubricants can rinse surface debris off of a rigid gas-permeable lens.

es without scratching them but may certainly compromise RGP lenses and should not be used. Kerosene and lighter fluid also should not be used. Alcohol should never be used, because it damages the surfaces of some types of plastic lenses. Acetone can dissolve a lens.

The lens should be cleaned in the palm of the hand using the "pinky" finger to move the lens. Several drops of cleaning solution are applied and both sides of the lens are rubbed gently in a *back and forth motion*. A circular motion may change the power of the lens in the minus direction, particularly if an abrasive cleaner is used.[14] The lens is then rinsed in tap water or saline until it is "squeaky" clean. It is now ready to be placed in a wetting/soaking solution for storage. *Note that tap water is not recommended as a rinsing agent immediately before inserting the lens in the eye due to an increased risk of microbial infection.*

Multipurpose Solutions

There are many solutions on the market today that combine two or more functions. Use of combination wetting/soaking solutions for gas-permeable lenses has the advantages of keeping the lens hydrated while in the case and enhancing wettability.

Lubricants and Artificial Tears

Ocular lubricants have the advantages of rewetting the lens while on the eye and rinsing debris off the surface (Figure 11-23). All are short-acting because they need good spreading properties if used as a tear substitute, but they should also have a high enough viscosity to form a thick film if they are to be used as cushioning agents. If they are too viscous, the patient experiences blurred vision.

Preservatives

Preservatives used in RGP lens solutions include benzalkonium chloride (BAK), chlorhexidine, thimerosol, ethylenediamine tetra acetate (EDTA), benzyl alcohol, and polyaminopropyl biguanide (PAPB). BAK, which is widely used as a preservative in ophthalmic medications, kills a wide spectrum of bacteria and fungi. It is normally used at a level of 0.004%. At a higher percentage it tends to produce ocular irritation, but it is used in soaking and cleaning solutions at 0.01% under the premise that it will be rinsed off prior to lens insertion. It is not used with soft lenses because evidence shows that the plastic binds with the preservative and actually concentrates it, which may potentially result in a severe allergic reaction. The effectiveness of BAK is enhanced, especially against *Pseudomonas*, when used in combination with EDTA, allowing a lower concentration than otherwise necessary. Pure benzoyl alcohol possesses certain characteristics that are regarded as ideal for an ophthalmic preservative. It is water-soluble and exhibits negligible binding to the surface of RGP lenses. PAPB has replaced chlorhexidine as a preservative in one of the RGP care systems because it exhibits greater antimicrobial effectiveness. Thimerosal and chlorhexadine are discussed in more detail when considering soft

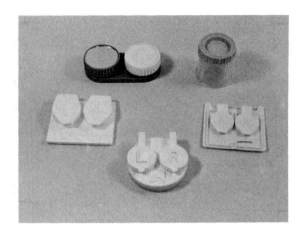

FIGURE 11-24—Several different types of cases for use with rigid gas-permeable lenses.

lenses in the section on cold (chemical) disinfection. Chlorhexadine, in particular, is used in several RGP lens solutions because of its rapid kill time and compatibility with silicone-based materials.

Lens Cases

A wide variety of lens cases are available. Some are shown in Figure 11-24. It is important that the case does not leak, is deep-welled to hold sufficient solution, has enough contrast for clear lenses to be seen when stored, and allows easy differentiation of the left and right lenses. Many manufacturers are developing hard lens cases with ridges on the bottom of the wells for good contrast and easy removal. The more flexible superpermeable lens materials may adhere to a smooth-walled case if placed convex side up.

Lens Insertion and Removal

Patients should be taught insertion and removal procedures either at the time of fitting or at the time of dispensing. If the patient can successfully apply and remove the lenses a minimum of two times, he or she should be competent enough to leave the office with the lenses.

One of the keys to successful education of patients on application and removal procedures is continual encouragement and complimenting in an effort to relax patients and ease anxiety. Having a foreign body on the eye is an entirely new and strange phenomenon for anyone.

Before inserting the lens, the patient should wash and dry his or her hands and wet the lens with the prescribed wetting agent. At that time, one of two methods of application should be explained to the patient. The following instructions are written in the second person as the paraoptometric would address the patient.[14]

Insertion Method 1

1. Place the lens on the moistened tip of the first or second finger of the dominant hand.
2. Position head down, wrist bent slightly *forward,* and the finger 2 or 3 inches in front of the eye and pointed straight at it.
3. Look down; lift the upper lid with the forefinger of the other hand and press it up and back under the bony margin of the brow.
4. Look ahead; pull down the lower lid with the thumb and press it against the lower bone margin (Figure 11-25). Do not let the thumb slip down onto the cheek.
5. Closing the other eye if preferred, look directly "through" the lens and advance it to the eye until it stops.
6. Remove lens finger.
7. Release the *lower lid first*; look down; then slowly let the upper lid down over the lens.

Insertion Method 2

1. Place the lens on the moistened tip of the middle finger of the dominant hand.
2. Look down; pull up the top lid with the middle finger of the *other* hand and press it against the bony margin of the top brow.
3. Look ahead; pull down the lower lid with the first or third finger of the "lens" hand.
4. Continue, following steps 5 to 7 in Method 1.

Several methods may be taught for lens removal, including the following[14]:

Removal Method 1

1. Bend the head over the table, and look *straight ahead*, at a target if preferred. The eyes should be opened as wide as possible.
2. Place the fingertip of your index finger at the outer corner of the eye.

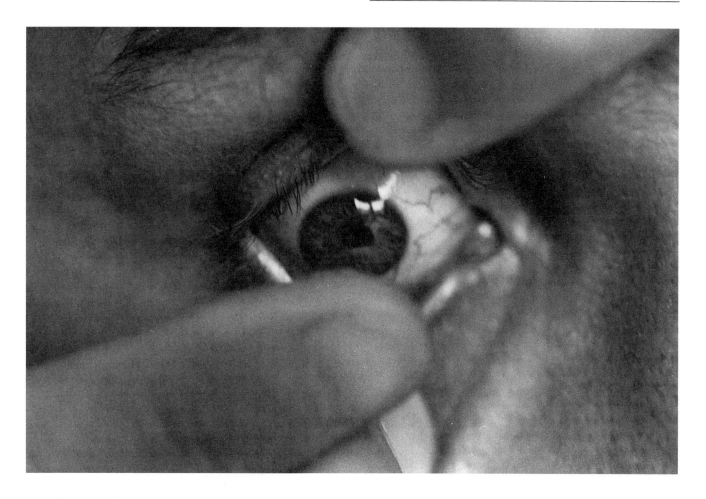

FIGURE 11-25—Proper lid retraction for insertion of a rigid gas-permeable lens.

3. Pull the lids laterally toward the ear, blink, and catch the lens in the other hand held close under the eye (Figure 11-26).

HELPFUL GUIDELINES

- The lid margins must clear the top and bottom of the lens until the blink.

- When blinking, flick the lid only. Do not press hard on the eye.

- Do not pull too hard or let the fingertip slip off the junction of the lid.

- Do not release pressure on the lid junction until the blink is completed.

- Do not rest the other fingers of the hand on the cheek near the eye.

- If the lens does not come out with the first blink, relax, *reposition eye and finger, and repeat.*

Removal Method 2

The same result may be achieved using both hands for a more forceful ejection.

1. Position the middle and index fingers of the same hand over the lower lid.
2. Hold the upper lid up with the middle and index fingers of the opposite hand.
3. As in method 1, pull the lids laterally and, while blinking, the lens is ejected (Figure 11-27).

Removal Method 3

1. Use the middle and forefinger of each hand to pull the lids apart. For the right eye, the fingers of the right hand should be placed well up on the lower lashes to exert control on the lid, and the fingers of the left hand should be placed well down over the lashes of the upper lid for the same reason. The

250 Chapter 11

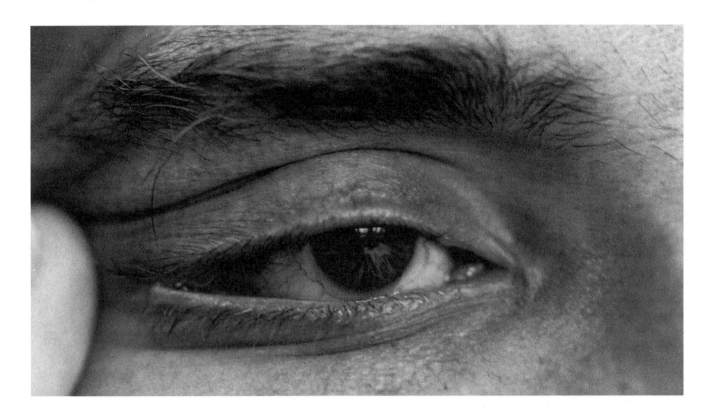

FIGURE 11-26—Pulling the lids laterally for removal of a rigid gas-permeable lens.

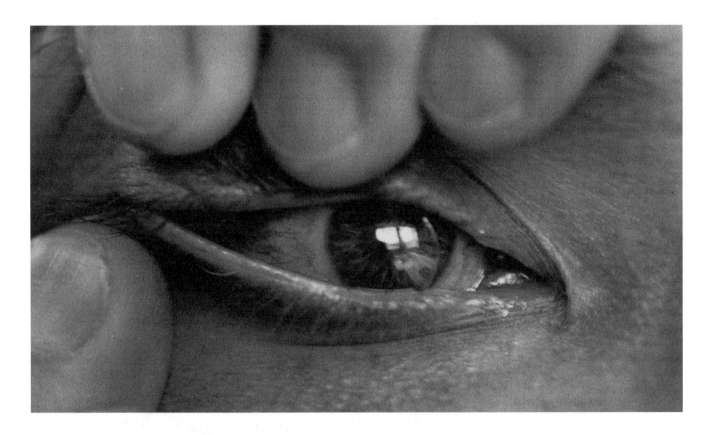

FIGURE 11-27—Using both hands for removal of a rigid gas-permeable lens.

opposite approach would be used for the other eye.
2. With your fingers, press the lid margins back (slight pressure against the eye), exposing as much of the eye as possible.
3. Then, push the lids vertically toward each other. The lens should become dislodged, adhering to the lashes.

If difficulty is experienced with the removal during the instruction period, a DMV suction cup may be used for removal of the lens to save any further time loss and psychological trauma to the patient. Whether the patient should be allowed to use a DMV at home is controversial. If it is decided to allow the patient to use one, mention must be made of the corneal insult that may occur if the cornea and not the lens is in contact with the DMV.

Recentering

The patient must know how to recenter a lens if it displaces off the central cornea. This may be a traumatic event if it occurs away from the office without instruction beforehand. The patient must be told that the lens may be left on the white of the eye for several hours without injury or discomfort, and in any case, it *cannot slip behind the eye*. Three methods for recentering the lens may be explained to the patient.

Recentering Method 1

1. Lean over a table with the face parallel to it.
2. With the middle finger of each hand on the center of the lid margins, gently pull the lids off the eyeball.
3. Look in all directions as far as possible. When the lens slides onto the cornea (the clear part of the eye), look straight down, releasing the *lower* and then the upper lid.

If the lens positions itself out of sight under the top lid, hold the head erect, pull the lid well up off the eyeball, look down as far as possible, and move the eye from side to side until the lens slides down into view. If movement seems difficult, flood the area with drops of saline.

Recentering Method 2

1. Locate the lens by inspection in a mirror.
2. Turn the eye in a direction opposite to the lens position.
3. With the fingertip, press the lid margin gently against the white of the eye beyond the lens edge and slide it onto the cornea (Figure 11-28).

Recentering Method 3

1. Immobilize the lens with the fingertips on the lid margins.
2. Slowly move the eye so that the cornea slides under the lens.

Patients should leave the office with written instructions explaining the above procedures, as well as whom to call and the appropriate phone number(s) if an emergency arises.

Patient Instructions

An important duty for the paraoptometric is patient education. Often, not enough time is spent in this area. The following is a list of helpful reminders that patients should be told of at the time of dispensing. This is by no means a comprehensive list.[14] These reminders should be told to the patient as well as given in written form to reinforce what has already been said.

1. Normal adaptive symptoms
   a. Tearing is the natural response of eyes that are not used to having foreign objects on them; it will subside rapidly as wearing time increases.
   b. Minor irritation is a tickling or awareness sensation, which gradually disappears with wear, that may cause mild discomfort on upward gaze due to the lens coming in contact with the upper lid.
   c. Intermittent blurry vision is usually attributable to excess tears.
   d. The eyes are sensitive to light (photophobic), when outside on a sunny day.
   e. The eyes suffer minor irritation from wind, smoke, and dust.
   f. The eyes are mildly red (injected) from minor irritation.

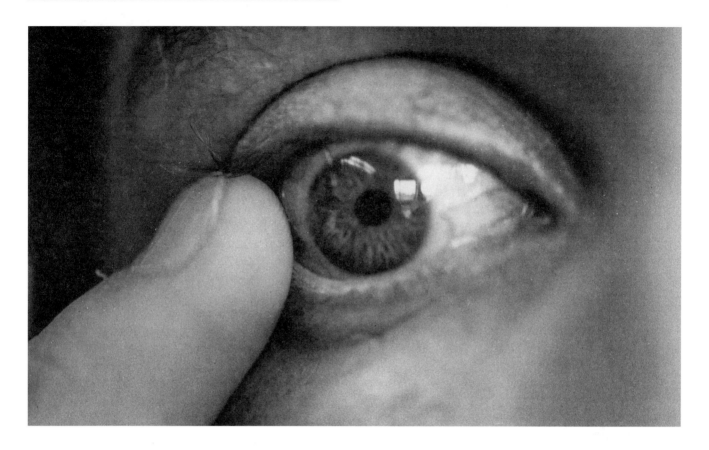

FIGURE 11-28—Recentering a rigid gas-permeable lens.

2. Abnormal adaptive symptoms
   a. Sudden pain or burning that is greater than minor irritation is abnormal. If a sudden sharp pain is felt, it can be from dirt or a lash under the lens. Remove, clean, and reinsert lens.
   b. You experience a severe or persistent haze or halo seen around lights.
   c. You experience severe redness or irritation.
   d. You experience blurry vision through spectacles for more than an hour after removal of lenses.
3. Do not overwear your lenses. Your cornea is living tissue and needs oxygen to remain transparent. The oxygen comes from the air and dissolves in the film of tears covering the cornea; it is then taken up by the surface of the cornea. If the lenses are overworn or there is an inadequate flow of tears under your contact lens, the cornea will suffer from swelling and possible corneal injury.
4. Because your contact lens prescription is not identical to your spectacle prescription, your vision may be somewhat *blurred* through your spectacles. If this blurring is excessive and lasts more than an hour, it probably means the corneas are not receiving an adequate amount of oxygen. If this occurs, call the office for an appointment.
5. Always have a current pair of spectacles to use when taking a break from contact lens wear. Spectacles are essential if, for some reason, contact lens wear has to be discontinued. If spectacles are not currently owned, you should be prescribed a pair after all-day wear has been established with the contact lenses.
6. If you must discontinue contact lens wear for more than 1 day (because of abrasion, lost lens, or some other reason), it is important to build your wearing time back up *gradually* to all-day wear. A wearing sched-

ule of 4 hours the first day, increasing 1 hour per day afterward, is recommended. If full-time wear is reinitiated immediately, the risk of injury to the cornea is increased dramatically. A good rule to follow to increase wearing time is not to wear lenses for more than 2 hours longer than on the day before.

7. After adaptation is complete, your lenses may still bother you in the morning, in smog, and in smoke-filled rooms. Colds, hayfever, and other illnesses may also affect comfort. Alcohol and certain medications may upset the metabolism of the eye and cause irritation if contact lenses are worn.

8. It is important to wait a minimum of 30 minutes after waking to insert your lenses and to remove them a minimum of 30 minutes before going to sleep.

9. Saliva should not be used as a wetting agent. Many microorganisms live in the mouth, and a potential eye infection is not worth the risk.

10. Lenses may easily be scratched or lost. If the lens is dropped on the floor or another surface, dampen either your fingertip or a cotton swab with wetting solution and pick it up. If it does not come up, gently slide a piece of paper under the lens to avoid dragging it against a hard surface. In addition, use of a soft tissue when handling the lenses and storage overnight in soaking solution will prevent scratches. If you experience a film over your lenses that clears temporarily after blinking or see scratches on the lens surface, the lenses need to be professionally cleaned and polished. The lense scratches can be polished out only so often before the lenses are permanently damaged, however. To prevent loss, be sure not to insert and remove lenses over an open sink drain. In addition, if at all possible, do not remove a lens while outdoors.

11. Be near a mirror or hard surface when inserting and removing lenses. In addition, make sure your hands are clean and free of creams or other substances that could irritate the eyes.

12. It would be to your benefit to purchase a second pair of lenses. If a lens is lost or broken, you'll be able to maintain full-time wear without interruption.

13. You may want to purchase insurance for the lenses.

14. Never bend or squeeze your lenses when handling them; never leave them near any heat, since they may become distorted.

15. Cosmetics should be put on after the lenses have been inserted, and the use of glittery eye shadow and waterproof mascara should be avoided because the large particle size may be very irritating to the eyes. During the initial fitting and training sessions, patients should avoid wearing eye makeup. It may run and smear, get on the fingers, on the lens, and into the eye. When trapped under the lens, cosmetics may cause discomfort. A soft pencil, water-based liquid, or water-soluble, cake-type eyeliner may be used safely. The highly waterproof types of eyeliner, however, should be avoided, since a flake from this type may easily become lodged under the lens. If flaking occurs, a lesser amount or another type should be used. Eyeliner should not be applied to the inner margin of the lid.

Any cream or oil that is used on the face or hands may be transferred to the contact lenses, causing discomfort and blurred vision. Be sure to apply these substances *after* inserting the lenses. The use of hair spray may cause problems by coating the lenses. Use hair spray *before* inserting lenses to eliminate this problem. Avoid wearing lenses while hair spray or other aerosols linger in the air.

Some women's eyes become uncomfortable with contact lens wear during menstrual periods, pregnancy, or menopause. Fluid retention produced by hormonal changes in the body may cause the cornea to swell and change shape. The result is an ill-fitting lens. For these reasons, if a woman starts to take or stops taking birth control pills or becomes pregnant, she should advise her eye care practitioner.

16. Rigid gas-permeable lenses require special care and must be handled very carefully. Although these lenses are flexible, it is not advisable to bend or flex the lenses between your fingers. Such treatment could cause the lens to warp or change shape, and that, in turn, would result in blurred

TABLE 11-5. Contact lens wearing schedule

Day	Hours on	Hour off	Hours on
1	___	___	___
2	___	___	___
3	___	___	___
4	___	___	___
5	___	___	___
6	___	___	___
7	___	___	___
8	___	___	___
9	___	___	___
10	___	___	___
11	___	___	___
12	___	___	___
13	___	___	___
14	___	___	___

vision and a possible change in the fit of the lens to the eye. In addition, these lenses break if flexed excessively.

Be sure not to invert a lens during handling. These lenses can possibly turn inside out if handled roughly during cleaning, while being picked up off the floor or other hard surface, or if placed upside down in the contact lens case. If you experience discomfort and blurred vision on insertion, more than likely you have inverted the lens.

It is extremely important to keep the lenses in a moist, wet state when they are not being worn. This is accomplished by soaking them in the recommended solution when they are in the lens case.

17. The contact lens storage case should be cleaned periodically and replaced when necessary. Use soap and warm water. Rinse well and let dry before using.
18. After the initial contant lens fitting, dispensing, and follow-up, you should have regular contact lens evaluations to assure proper lens fit and corneal health.
19. In general, it is recommended that you schedule your progress evaluations, wearing your lenses for a minimum of 4 hours before the scheduled examination time (Table 11-5).

Soft Lens Care and Handling

Disinfection Regimens

Thorough disinfection of soft lenses is more important than in the case of rigid lenses because the water content of these lenses makes them porous and renders them easily contaminated by bacteria and other microorganisms. This is especially true with high–water-content (70% and greater) soft lenses. Chemicals, pollutants from the air, dirt from the air or hands, and tear substances can easily penetrate the matrix of these lenses, possibly resulting in an eye infection. Regular cleaning and disinfection of soft lenses keeps them free of these pathogenic organisms and minimizes the possibility of ocular sensitivity reactions. Lenses may be disinfected by using heat or thermal disinfection, cold or chemical disinfection, or hydrogen peroxide. Paraoptometrics are encouraged to read the instructions provided with each solution, since constant improvements and innovations are being made.

HEAT DISINFECTION

The use of heat is a very effective but little used method of killing microorganisms and disinfecting the lenses. The higher the temperature, the less time needed for disinfection. The disinfection process is usually completed in less than

30 minutes. It is a relatively simple procedure for a patient to perform, as it consists only of placing the case (with the lenses and proper solution enclosed) into the unit, which is plugged into a nearby outlet, and turning the unit on. When the red indicator light shuts off, the disinfection cycle is complete, but the patient should wait at least another 15 minutes to allow the unit to cool down before removing the case. Heat disinfection has the advantages over cold disinfection of fewer allergic reactions, quick and thorough disinfection, and lower cost to the patient over the long term. The disadvantages include a shorter lens life because of the possibility of boiling mucoproteinous deposits into the lens and the inconvenience for travelers who are unable to find an electrical outlet. Although heat disinfection is effective, the disadvantages have caused practitioners to use forms of cold disinfection in recent times.

Unpreserved salines are typically used with heat disinfection for wetting, rinsing, and soaking. These include single-dose packaged saline; aerosol cans, which eliminate the problem of contamination; and saline in various sized containers that must be used within a certain time frame. Homemade saline from salt tablets is no longer used because of its association with microbial infection; salt tablets are no longer available on the market.

COLD (CHEMICAL) DISINFECTION

This method is easier than heat disinfection. As with rigid lenses, the soft lenses are removed and stored (usually overnight) in a disinfecting solution. Although the chemical system is more convenient, is simpler, and increases lens life by not boiling deposits onto the lens surface, it is more expensive over the long term, takes 4–6 hours to disinfect a lens, and causes toxic and allergic reactions in some patients.

Preservatives used in chemical disinfection include thimerosal, chlorhexadine, EDTA, Dymed, and Polyquad. The first two are worth noting for possible complications that may occur with their use. Thimerosal is a mercury-containing compound commonly used in a concentration of 0.001%. In chemical disinfection regimens, it has been effective, but it can cause a mild allergic reaction in mercury-sensitive patients; these patients experience redness, burning, and itching. Chlorhexadine in a concentration of 0.005% is commonly used in conjunction with thimerosal. It is more effective and faster than thimerosal, but it is also more toxic; therefore, its use with soft lenses has decreased in recent years. The introduction of Dymed and Polyquad has greatly increased the use of chemical disinfection due to their low toxicity and decreased allergic effects on the patient. When a patient does experience an allergic reaction to the chemical disinfection regimen, a switch to hydrogen peroxide or heat disinfection and unpreserved saline is recommended.

HYDROGEN PEROXIDE

The following is the FDA-approved method of soft lens disinfection using hydrogen peroxide as the disinfecting agent. The lenses are first soaked in a 3% hydrogen peroxide solution for the indicated period of time. Commercially available hydrogen peroxide is not recommended, since it may be incompatible with the lens. Then, by the use of a catalytic disk, a neutralizing solution, or a neutralizing tablet, the acidic pH produced by the hydrogen peroxide is neutralized.

Advantages of hydrogen peroxide include its ability to clean the lens while it disinfects, the elimination of the thimerosal and chlorhexadine toxicity, and the fact that no electricity is needed. The disadvantages include increased expense, possible patient error resulting in an intraocular toxicity reaction, and inconvenience because of the several steps involved in the disinfection process. FDA approval of a one-step process, however, has made hydrogen peroxide a useful and beneficial disinfection method that is easier for patients to follow and is less expensive than other modes of lens disinfection.

Cleaning

The lifespan of soft lenses is limited because of their brittleness and the accumulation on the surface of matter from tear film, such as proteins, lipids, and other debris that may decrease the patient's vision. Examples of coated lenses are shown in Figures 11-29 and 11-30.

Surfactant cleaners are recommended for use on a daily basis; they contain soaps and detergents to help remove oils, makeup, lipids, and some proteins from the lens surface. Surfactant cleaners are applied to the surface of the lens with a rubbing

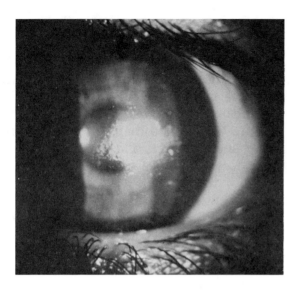

FIGURE 11-29—A mucoprotein-coated soft lens.

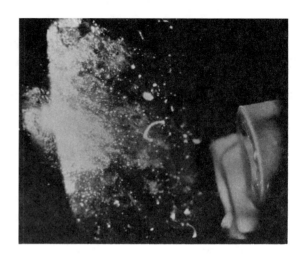

FIGURE 11-30—A soft lens with lipid contamination.

action. These cleaners may prevent the binding of proteins onto the surface by heat disinfection. Many solutions on the market may be used for heat and chemical disinfection. Although many procedures have been used, perhaps the most effective method has the patient, with washed hands, hold the lens in the palm and use the middle or index finger of the other hand to rub the front and back surfaces of the lens firmly in a back and forth motion after a few drops of the surface cleaner have been applied. Rubbing for 30 seconds on each surface should be performed. The patient must be told that it is friction that cleans the lenses and not more application of a cleaner. The cleaner should be thoroughly washed off the lens before disinfection or insertion, since it can be very irritating if the lens comes into contact with the eye because of the preservative concentration.

An enzymatic cleaner has often been used in tandem with the surfactant cleaner because of its ability to remove denatured proteins and other materials from the lens surface and prolong lens life. The enzyme cleaner is used by placing an enzyme tablet in the indicated amount of distilled water or saline, where it will dissolve, and then placing the lens into the solution for a minimum of 15 minutes or 2 hours, depending on lens material and manufacturer's recommendations (although it is often performed as an overnight procedure). Individual vials are provided for storing the lenses. This procedure is not done *instead* of disinfection, and the lenses should be disinfected after enzymatic and surfactant cleaning. The Ultrazyme enzyme tablet (Allergan Optical, Irvine, CA) may be used directly with the hydrogen peroxide solution, thus eliminating a step with this method of disinfection. The enzyme cleaner may be used once a week or every other week as the need arises. If used more often than once a week, it may not provide any more assistance and in fact may decrease the surface quality. If coating is a frequent problem, one alternative is to increase the concentration of the enzyme by filling the vial only three-fourths full with distilled water or saline and using this regimen on a weekly basis. The enzyme cleaner may bind in the matrix of higher–water-content lenses and therefore cause the patient to experience a severe allergic reaction. Thus, when dispensing a soft contact lens to a patient, prior knowledge of whether the enzyme regimen is compatible with it is a requirement.

Soft Contact Lens Cases

Soft contact lens cases must be both durable and deeply welled to hold a sufficient amount of solution to keep the lens in the hydrated state (Figure 11-31). The case should be cleaned with soap and water and rinsed with saline at least once a week.

Insertion and Removal

With both rigid and soft lenses, it is beneficial for the paraoptometric to demonstrate insertion and removal procedures initially on a new

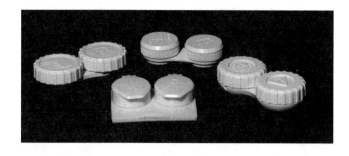

FIGURE 11-31—Representative soft contact lens cases.

patient. In addition, if the patient experiences repeated failure in lens-handling procedures, the paraoptometric should once again insert and remove the lenses on the patient both to reinforce these procedures and to decrease any possible anxiety. If the patient is not successful during the allotted time period for training, extra time should be used or the patient rescheduled as soon as possible for a return visit. It is extremely important that the patient believes in the eventual success of this endeavor. Although lens removal is usually a more difficult procedure for rigid lens patients to learn, inserting the large soft lenses is more difficult for a new soft lens patient to master. Emphasis on pulling the lids back to have a wide palpebral aperture is a necessity. Whereas a patient with an 11-mm palpebral aperture should be able to handle a 13.5-mm diameter soft lens easily, a patient with a 9-mm palpebral aperture would probably be contraindicated for a 15-mm soft lens. In addition, patients with short, thick fingers tend to have difficulty with large soft lenses. The following (or similar) insertion and removal instructions should be given orally and in written form to the patient.

INSERTING LENSES

Initially, you should insert and remove lenses over a cloth or paper towel spread on a table. Relaxation is the secret of success in this learning process. Use a mirror if it helps, but learn to do without it. When pulling the lids apart the finger should be placed *directly on the lid margin at the lashes* and at a point halfway between the corners of the eye.[14]

Before handling your lenses, always wash and rinse your hands thoroughly. A mild, noncosmetic soap should be used because those containing complexion creams, deodorants, or perfumes leave a film on the hands that may be transferred to the lenses and cause eye irritation. Dry your hands with a clean lint-free towel, or shake off the excess water and let your hands air dry.

Before handling your lenses, avoid oily substances such as hand creams, lotions, or cosmetics. Fingernails should be trimmed, especially on the fingers handling the lenses. Long fingernails may be hazardous when handling lenses and during their insertion and removal.

For your insertion and removal routine, always start with the right lens so as not to place the lens on the wrong eye.

Insertion Method 1

1. Remove the right lens from the storage container.
2. Place it in the palm of the hand, and rinse with rinsing solution. Always inspect your lenses for foreign particles, tears, or other damage before placing them on your eyes. The lens should be moist, clear, clean, and intact.
3. Grasp the lens gently and place it on the index finger of the inserting hand. Check to make sure the lens is not inside out. Because of the flexible nature of soft lenses, they may often become inverted (turned inside out). To determine whether a lens is inside out, look at the concave side up on the index finger and examine the profile. In the correct position, the edges will turn in (Figure 11-32). If it is inside out, the edges tend to flare out (Figure 11-33).
4. Secure the upper lashes against the brow with the opposite hand. Secure the lower lid to the cheekbone, with the middle finger of the hand holding the lens. The lids must be separated as much as possible to allow room for the lens to contact the cornea (clear part of the eye) without touching the lids or lashes.
5. Slowly bring the lens toward your eye while looking "through" the lens and finger, and gently place the lens squarely on the cornea (Figure 11-34).
6. Slowly release the lower lid, then the upper lid, and then blink a few times. If the lens tends to stick to the finger instead of to the cornea, lift the lens from the finger, wipe

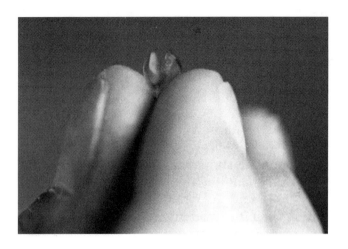

FIGURE 11-32—The correct position of the edges when the lens is right side out.

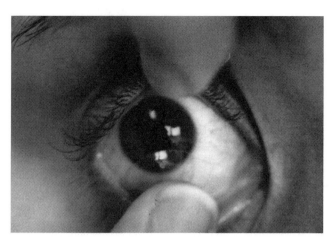

FIGURE 11-34—Proper insertion of a soft lens.

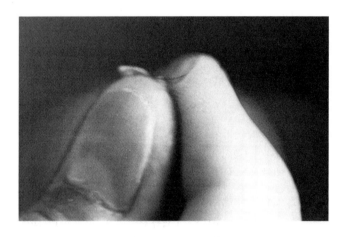

FIGURE 11-33—The position of the lens edges when the lens is inverted.

any excess saline off the finger tip and proceed as before.
7. Repeat the procedure for the left lens.

Discard the solution in the storage container so that fresh solution may be used in the evening. If the lenses are uncomfortable, tend to fold on the eye, or move more than usual, or if vision is blurred after insertion, please check whether

- The lens has been properly cleaned and, if cleaned, thoroughly rinsed;
- The lens is inside out;
- The lens is torn. Many times a lens defect that takes the appearance of a scratch is actually a tear. Check the edge as well as the center portion of the lens. If a tear is suspected and discomfort is experienced, do *not* wear the lens. Contact the office for an appointment. Most tears occur because of rough handling, fingernails, chipping by the storage case, or drying out of the lens.

If everything is in order and irritation and blur continue, call for assistance.

Insertion Method 2
1. Lift the lens carefully from the storage case.
2. Place the rinsed lens on the index finger of your preferred hand.
3. Inspect the lens for foreign particles or defects and see whether it is right-side out.
4. Hold the lower lid down with the middle finger of the same hand and look up.
5. Place the lens on the lower white part of your eye and remove trapped air by applying gentle pressure.
6. Look down to position the lens on the eye and slowly release the lower lid. Blink a few times to ensure that the lens is centered, free of trapped air, provides good vision, and is comfortable.
7. Follow the same procedure for the left eye.

NOTE: If necessary, the upper lid may be held with the other hand. The middle finger is used to grasp the lid at the lid margin and raise it against the brow.

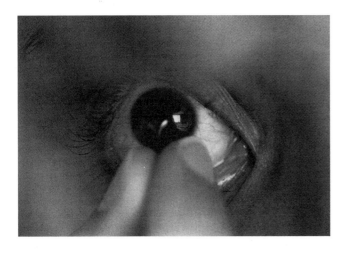

FIGURE 11-35—Pinching a soft lens directly off of the eye.

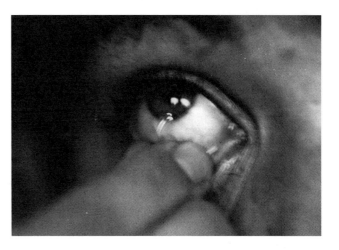

FIGURE 11-36—Removal of the soft lens off of the inferior conjunctiva.

REMOVING THE LENSES
Removal Method 1

1. Wash and dry hands thoroughly.
2. Pull down the lower lid with the middle finger of your preferred hand. Gently pinch the lens off of the white part of the eye using the thumb and index finger; be careful not to use the fingernails (Figure 11-35).
3. Reverse hand positions for the left eye.

Removal Method 2

1. Make sure the lens is centered (your vision will be clear if it is).
2. Pull down the lower lid with the middle finger of your preferred hand.
3. With the tip of your index finger (same hand), lightly touch the bottom edge of the lens. If necessary, use a mirror to assist you.
4. While looking up, slide the lens down onto the white part of the eye.
5. Then, *gently* pinch the lens off of the white part of the eye using your thumb and index finger; be careful not to use your fingernails (Figure 11-36).

After removal, do not squeeze the lens between the thumb and index finger to avoid the lens edges sticking together. If the lens edges do stick together, place the lens in the palm of your hand and soak it thoroughly with saline. Gently roll the lens with your index finger in the palm of your hand in a back-and-forth motion. If gentle rubbing does not separate the lens edges, soak the lens in saline solution until it resumes normal shape.

Patient Education

As explained in detail in the section on flexible lenses, many possible symptoms and related complaints are possible because of the softness of the material used in soft lenses. Many possible complaints will be avoided if the paraoptometric gives adequate patient education at the time of dispensing. As with rigid lenses, the following instructions should be given to the patient in both oral and written form.

1. *Cleaning lenses.* After removal, place a few drops of cleaning solution on the lens in the palm of your hand. Rub the lens thoroughly for 10–20 seconds with the index finger, being careful not to contact the lens with your fingernail. Do not rub the lens if it folds in half. Do one side of the lens and then the other. Rinse the lens with rinsing solution and place it in the storage case, making sure the lens is completely covered with the appropriate disinfecting solution. Change the disinfection solution daily.
2. *Lens storage and disinfection.* The disinfecting storage solution prescribed is a recommended antibacterial system that will keep your lens free of contamination only if fresh solution is used daily and if lenses are

properly cleaned and rinsed before overnight storage. Periodically check your solution's expiration date to guard against adverse effects and ensure proper hygiene of your lenses.
3. *Hydration.* Soft lenses must always be in a hydrated (wet) form. If for some reason the lens is dropped and allowed to dehydrate (dry), it will not be ruined; however, it will become brittle and could break easily when handled. Place the lens back into the proper storage solution for a minimum of 1 hour to allow the lens to return to a soft, flexible state.
4. *Water.* Fresh water or tap water contains impurities that could eventually discolor and ruin a soft lens. Do not use water as a wetting, rinsing, or storing solution. You may shower while wearing your lenses, but be careful not to get soap or shampoo into your eyes.
5. *Eye drops.* Eye drops or other eye medications or solutions intended for rigid contact lenses must **not** be used by wearers of soft lenses. If used, medications or preservatives will be absorbed by your lenses and serious damage to either or both the lenses and eyes could result.
6. *Blurring of vision.* If vision blurs while you are wearing your lenses, it is usually because of drying of the lenses; it should clear up after blinking several times while you move the eyes back and forth. Instilling a few drops of your prescribed saline or comfort drops will also help; if it does not, make sure that your lenses are in the proper eyes. If the blur persists, call for assistance.
7. *Spectacles.* Always have a current pair of spectacles to wear when taking a break from contact lens wear. Spectacles are essential when lenses are torn or lost, or when lens wear must be discontinued because of an eye infection.
8. *Sports wear.* Soft lenses may be worn for sporting and athletic activities and are superior to rigid contact lenses for such activities because they are not easily dislodged from the eyes.
9. *Swimming.* Soft lenses may be worn during swimming if care is taken on insertion and removal. Recent studies have shown that the lenses will not absorb significant amounts of microorganisms or chlorine if worn while swimming; although the possibility for absorption exists, the occurrence is rare. If you wear lenses while swimming, do not attempt to remove them for at least 30 minutes after swimming because the water will usually cause lenses to adhere strongly to the eye. If they do not move freely after 30 minutes, call the office and arrange for assistance.
10. *Eye makeup and hair sprays.* If eye makeup or hair sprays come into contact with your soft lenses, they may cause severe eye irritation by coming in contact with your eye, or they may permanently destroy the lenses through absorption. (For more information, see the discussion of cosmetics in the section on rigid lens care and handling.)
11. *Sleeping with contacts.* Unless your lenses are the type prescribed for extended wear, do not sleep with your lenses on. If you have forgotten to remove them, on waking check to see whether the lenses move freely on the eye. If they do, remove them for the day; if they do not move, place a few drops of your rinsing solution on the eye. After a few moments they should move freely and be removed. If, after a few moments, they do not move, call the office and arrange for assistance.
12. *Contact lens case.* The storage case should be cleaned periodically and replaced when necessary. Use soap and warm water. Rinse well and let air dry before refilling with the prescribed storage solution.
13. *Pain, discomfort, and redness.* If these symptoms occur, remove lenses, clean and rinse them, and put them back on. If symptoms persist, remove lenses and telephone the office for an appointment.

The wearing schedule for the soft lens patient may be similar in design to that for the hard lens form. Some practitioners prefer to build up soft lens patients' wearing time at a faster rate than that for rigid lens patients because of limited adaptation symptoms.

In conclusion, the exact instructions vary from office to office, according to the preference of the optometrist. In all cases, however, the patient must be aware of what constitute the proper solutions, the way to handle the lenses competently and the reason for correct handling, and possible complications and pitfalls of lens wear.

VERIFICATION

Accurate verification of the parameters and surface quality of contact lenses is one of the most important duties of a paraoptometric working with contact lenses. The procedures are not difficult to perform, but it is essential that no shortcuts be taken when verifying hard, soft, or RGP lenses.

Rigid Lenses
Power

The back vertex power may be easily determined by using a lensometer. The lens should be cleaned and dried with a lint-free tissue, the eyepiece focused for the examiner, and the lens placed against the lens stop with the convex surface facing away from the lens stop as with a spectacle lens. The contact lens should be mounted on a contact lens holder, if available. If a holder is not available, the lens should be held between the thumb and index finger, with care being taken not to apply any pressure that would temporarily warp the lens. A warped lens would cause a blurred or toric image (two separately focused images, e.g., one at –2.50 D and the other at –3.25 D), thus giving the paraoptometric a false reading. The lens must be well centered against the lens stop; otherwise, the lens may appear to contain a prismatic element. To ensure proper adhesion and centration, a drop of water may be placed on the lens stop prior to lens placement against the stop. If the target does not come into sharp focus, it is an indication of either or both poor optics and poor surface quality of the contact lens. The front vertex power of a contact lens should be verified for high plus (aphakic) lenses.

Base Curve Radius

RADIUSCOPE
The most common method of measuring the base curve of a rigid lens is with a radiuscope

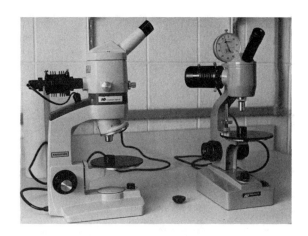

FIGURE 11-37—The AO Radiuscope and Marco Radiusgauge.

(Figure 11-37). The radiuscope is essentially a microscope with a dial gauge attached to read the position of the microscope stage. Some modern radiuscopes have dispensed with the external dial gauge; the radius reading is shown on a scale at one side of the field of view in the microscope (usually calibrated to 0.01 mm).

A suitable lens holder is filled with water or saline. The clean lens is placed centrally on the holder with the convex surface in complete contact with the water. Without the water present, the images formed by reflection at the front surface are as bright as the images formed by the back surfaces, and it then becomes difficult to tell quickly which image is required. Only a small quantity of water should be used; otherwise, the lens will float and may move during measurements. The holder is placed on the radiuscope stage and centered. The radiuscope eyepiece is correctly adjusted. By observation through the radiuscope, the target is imaged on the surface of the lens by moving either the radiuscope and target or the radiuscope stage. The image used by many radiuscopes is in the form of a star pattern (Figure 11-38). When this image is in focus, the dial gauge reading is recorded (or the dial gauge is set to zero). If zero is not used as the starting point, then it should be set on the nearest whole number. That number will be compensated for when taking the final base curve reading (e.g., starting point = + 2.00; end point = 7.50; base curve is 7.50 + 2.00 = 9.50 mm). Before a final image is obtained, a filament will

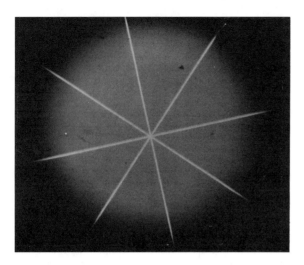

FIGURE 11-38—A star-pattern radiuscope image.

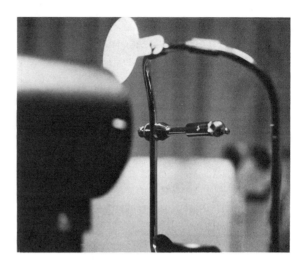

FIGURE 11-40—Using a keratometer to determine the base curve radius.

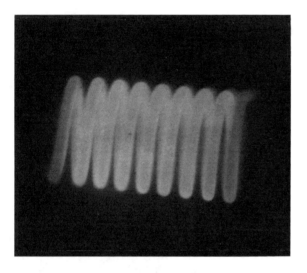

FIGURE 11-39—The filament image that precedes the final star-pattern when determining the base curve radius with a radiuscope.

come into focus (Figure 11-39), and finally another star image, which indicates the end point. If this second star image does not come to a sharp focus, the lens is either warped or toric. If warpage or toricity is present, the two principal meridians are recorded in millimeters of radius. For example, if half the image is in focus at 7.50 mm and the rest of the image is in focus at 7.80 mm, it is recorded as 7.50/7.80.

KERATOMETER

A second method currently used to measure the base curve radius uses a conventional keratometer. The procedure is similar to measuring the curvature of the cornea, but a special lens holder is required. The holder consists of a clamp that mounts it to the headrest of the instrument; a depression to hold the lens; and either a front surface mirror with the lens floating concave side up on a small drop of water or, lacking a mirror, the concave side of the lens facing the instrument (Figure 11-40).

The keratometer is focused on the reflected mires and aligned in the same manner as when measuring the cornea. Alignment of mires and the dioptric power reading on the drum are noted and the power converted to millimeters of radius unless this is already provided on the drum. There is a very small difference in the conversion from diopters to millimeters (commonly 0.12–0.25 D) between corneal and base curve radius readings because a concave and not a convex surface is being measured.

Diameter

Lens diameter may be verified by several methods.

HAND-HELD MAGNIFIER (RETICLE)

A 7–10× hand-held measuring magnifier with a measuring reticle may be used to verify the overall lens diameter. The reticle is held close to the eye, using a distant light source as a background. A clean and dry lens is placed at the zero mark on the reticle scale, and the point where the opposite edge intersects the scale is the lens diameter. The scale is divided into tenths of a millimeter; therefore, the overall diameter can be determined within 0.05 mm.

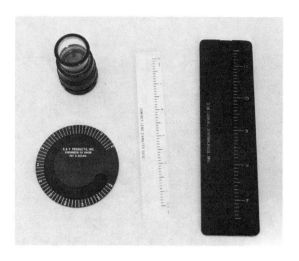

FIGURE 11-41—Slot gauges used for diameter determination.

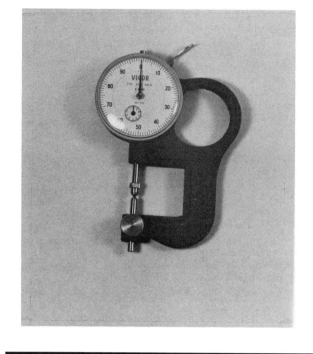

FIGURE 11-42—A contact lens center thickness gauge.

SLOT GAUGES

Various slot gauges (Figure 11-41) may be used to determine diameter. When a lens is unable to slide freely, the diameter at the center of the lens may be read from the external scale. Care must be taken not to exert much pressure when measuring a RGP lens because it can bend and a smaller diameter will therefore be erroneously recorded.

OPTICAL ZONE DIAMETER

The OZD may be measured in the same way as overall diameter by using a hand-held or projection magnifier.

Peripheral Curve Widths

The peripheral curve widths may be measured in the same way as the overall diameter with a hand-held magnifier. Unless the junctions have medium or heavy blends, the widths should be easy to determine. All of the curves plus the optical zone should equal the overall diameter. For instance, for a tricurve lens:

$$OAD = OZD + 2 (SC + PC)$$

If OAD = 9.0 mm, OZD = 7.6 mm, SC = 0.3 mm, and PC = 0.4 mm, then

$$9.0 = 7.6 + 2 (0.3 + 0.4).$$

Peripheral curve radii may be difficult, if not impossible, to verify due to the typical small diameters involved.

Center Thickness

Hand-held thickness gauges or those on small stands calibrated in millimeters are routinely used to measure center thickness (Figure 11-42). They have ball-bearing or rounded pedestals to minimize the possibility of scratching. The thickness at the edge or at the junction between the periphery and the front optical zone in a lenticulated lens may also be determined.

Edge and Surface Evaluation

The edge should always be evaluated before dispensing a lens to the patient. An uncomfortable lens with a rough, sharp, or blunt edge could give a patient a negative attitude toward rigid lenses in general. Every lens that comes into the office ought to be handled with the fingers first, before the use of a projection device. This may be accomplished by placing the lens either between the thumb and forefinger (back surface against the thumb) or with the back surface against the palm of the hand and the forefinger

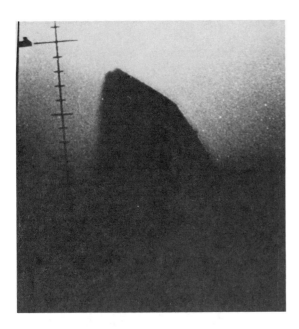

FIGURE 11-43—A blunt rigid lens edge.

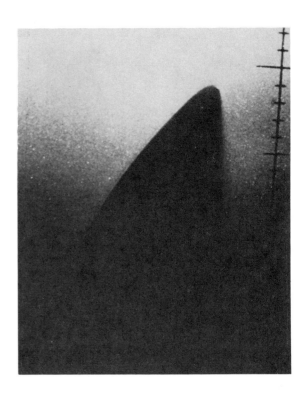

FIGURE 11-44—A representative good rigid lens edge.

pushing the lens across the thumb or palm. If it glides freely, the edge is smooth. If it tends to resist movement or move with force, then the edge is defective.

A projection magnifier is ideal because verification of the edge contour, anterior and posterior smoothness, and surface quality may be examined. A blunt edge is "cut off" at the top (Figure 11-43), a sharp edge is too thin and pointed, and a good edge is usually rounded with the apex in most cases being displaced posteriorly (Figure 11-44).

Prism Ballast Lenses

Many types of bifocal lenses, as well as front surface toric lenses, use prism for stabilization purposes. It is easier and more accurate to determine where the base of the prism is located if the lens is ordered with one dot placed at the prism base of the right lens. The left contact lens is ordered with a dot located at the base also, but in addition, another dot is placed directly opposite the base at the apex.

The base curve is verified as a single-vision lens. To verify power, the lens is put on the lensometer stop with the prism base down. After verification of the sphere power, cylinder, and axis (if present) as with a spectacle lens, the prism is verified by measuring how far the image target is displaced from center, as would be done with spectacle lenses. For example, if the center of the target image is on the 1Δ ring, the contact lens has 1Δ of base down prism.

Toric Base Curves

A back surface toric lens has two different curves on the back instead of one spherical curve. When taking the measurements of a radius warped lens, the maximum base curve reading and the minimum reading should both be used. The difference between these two readings may be multiplied by 1.5 to approximate the desired refractive cylinder. For example,

$$\begin{array}{r} 44.00 \\ -41.00 \\ \hline 3.00 \times 1.5 = 4.50. \end{array}$$

Check the findings on the lensometer. Toric lens designs are more difficult to manufacture than spherical lens designs; the radiuscope and lensometer readings must be compared for accuracy, and the mire images for clarity.

Bifocal Lenses

In addition to determining the amount of prism present in many bifocal lens designs, the near power and seg height must be evaluated. The power may be determined by placing the reading segment over the top of the lensometer; a reduced stop diameter is helpful for this, since the near portion of the lens is relatively small. Another method of obtaining a clear target image (although the clearest image could still be a little blurry) is to mask off the lens stop or the lensometer by putting a piece of masking or drafting tape over the lens stop. Then, with the tip of a pen or pencil, punch a hole approximately 3 mm in diameter. The lens to be verified is placed over the hole with the concave side against the lens stop in such a way that the segment is in focus. In many of the crescent designs, the power determined by the lensometer should equal the desired add power; actually, it is the addition of the distance and the near equal lensometer reading. For example,

$$\begin{array}{r} -4.00 \text{ (distance)} \\ + +2.00 \text{ (near)} \\ \hline -2.00 \text{ (lensometer reading at near)}. \end{array}$$

The size, shape, and position of the addition depend on the lens type. A hand-held magnifier may be used to verify the seg height. To accomplish this, the lens must be placed on the measuring reticle and the distance from the bottom of the lens to the top of the center of the segment measured.

Tolerances

Contact lenses should meet the tolerance standards given in Table 11-6.

Hydrogel Lenses

Paraoptometrics should verify soft lenses in the office. Primarily because of variances in water content, lens parameters printed on soft lens labels may vary from those of the lens. Although the accuracy achieved when verifying soft lenses is compromised when compared to rigid lenses, the verification of soft lenses in the office is not any more sophisticated or significantly more difficult. Five parameters may be measured quite easily.

Power

The back vertex power may be verified while the lens is in the dry or wet state.

BLOTTING TECHNIQUE

Using tweezers, remove the lens from the solution and place it on a lint-free tissue. Both surfaces of the lens are blotted, and the lens is then moved to a dry spot on the tissue and blotted again. This procedure should be repeated, at minimum, two times. Then air dry the lens for 5 seconds and place it with the back surface against the lens stop of the lensometer in the same manner as when verifying a spectacle lens. Evaluate the clarity of the mires. If they are not clear, reblot and remeasure the lens. If they still are not clear, reject the lens. If the mires are clear, record the lens power. The process is repeated two more times; the back vertex power is the average of the three measurements.

WET CELL

Another common method of determining lens power is placing the lens in a wet cell filled with saline. The lens is placed in the wet cell concave or back surface down. The cell is then placed against the lens stop of the lensometer just as with spectacle lenses. The power wheel is turned from greatest to least plus until a clear focus is obtained (Figure 11-45). The reading on the lensometer must be multiplied by the factor provided below to obtain the back vertex power of the hydrogel lens (BVP = lensometer reading × factor ± 0.25 D).[15]

BVP	Factor
0 to –10	4.0
–10	3.5
0 to +10	4.0
+10 to +15	4.5
+15	4.7

Sources of error include slight inaccuracies in the correction factor; lens thickness, base curve, and diameter not being taken into account; and lensometer error (a slight error in the lensometer readings will be magnified by the correction factor). Other devices such as the Tori-Check (General Ophthalmics, Park Ridge, IL) and the Soft Lens Power Check (Optical Science Industries, Spicer, MN) are more expensive, but allow the soft lens

TABLE 11-6. Contact lens tolerance standards

Parameter	Tolerance
Diameter	±0.05 mm
Posterior optic zone diameter	
Light blend	±0.1 mm
Medium-to-heavy blend	±0.2 mm
Base curve radius	±0.025 mm
Secondary, intermediate, peripheral curve width	
Light blend	±0.05 mm
Medium-to-heavy blend	±0.1 mm
Secondary, intermediate, peripheral curve radius	±0.1 mm
Power	
+10.00 D	±0.12 D
>+10.00 D	±0.25 D
Prism power	
+10.00 D	±0.25Δ
>+10.00 D	±0.50Δ
Cylinder power	
<2.00–4.00 D	±0.25 D
2.00–4.00 D	±0.37 D
>4.00 D	±0.50 D
Cylinder axis	±5Δ
Toric base curve radii	
Δr 0.00–0.30 mm	±0.02 mm
Δr 0.21–0.40 mm	±0.03 mm
Δr 0.41–0.60 mm	±0.05 mm
Δr >0.06 mm	±0.07 mm
Bifocal add power	±0.25 D
Center thickness	<±0.02 mm
Edges	As specified
Surface quality	No bubbles, striae, waves inhomogeneities, crazing, pits, scratches, chips, lathe marks or stone marks
Tint	Pigment inert and uniformly distributed

power to be read directly from the lensometer without the use of a conversion factor.

Base Curve Radius

Measurements of the base curve of a soft lens are difficult and inexact. Methods using a template system have gained some popularity.

TEMPLATE MATCHING

The template matching method consists of a series of spherical templates of various radii similar to those used for peripheral curve application. The objective of this method is to obtain a good match between the back surface of the lens and the cornea. The degree of the match is interpreted by the presence or absence of air bubbles under the lens. If the base curve of the lens is flatter than the template, edge standoff will be present and air bubbles will be present peripherally. If the base curve is steeper than the curvature of the template, an air bubble will be present centrally between lens and template.

Center Thickness

Thickness of a soft lens should verify correctly because manufacturers know the swell rate (increase in size) when the dehydrated lens is hydrated. The thickness may be measured with a radiuscope. The lens is blotted dry with a lint-free tissue and placed on the radiuscope platform (Figure 11-46). The radiuscope is focused on the upper surface (concave) of the lens, and

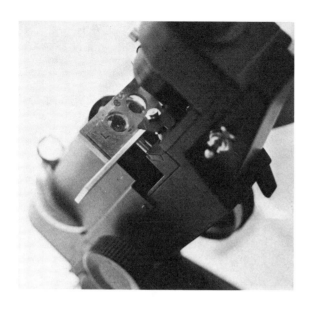

FIGURE 11-45—The use of a wet cell for soft lens power verification.

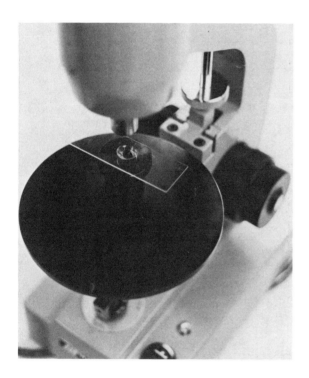

FIGURE 11-46—Determining the center thickness of a soft lens placed on a radiuscope.

the reading is taken. The lens is removed, the platform is focused on, and the reading taken. The thickness of the lens is the difference between the two readings. Because the lens loses water, or dehydrates, the measurements should be made soon after blotting.

Overall Diameter

The overall lens diameter may be determined by placing the lens in a wet cell filled with saline. The cell is then held up to the light with the hand-held magnifier positioned against the wet cell on the side closest to the back surface of the lens.

Surface and Edge Inspection

The surface and edge may be inspected by using the wet cell and hand-held magnifier, a projection magnifier, or tweezers holding the lens in front of a slit lamp biomicroscope (in the plane of the eyes). The last is the best method to detect lens nicks and tears.

RIGID LENS MODIFICATION

The Modification Unit

In-office modification of rigid contact lenses requires very little equipment, and for most modifications, there is only a small time demand for the paraoptometric. An essential piece of equipment is a *spindle unit,* consisting of a small electric motor that may be mounted in a wooden box, below a plastic or metal bowl, or on a counter top (Figures 11-47 and 11-48). The motor may be of either constant speed or variable. The spindle speed should be approximately 1,000 rpm or less when working with the newer, softer materials.[16] Brass, plastic, or diamond-impregnated radius tools may be used for the modification process.

The modification unit should have a splash bowl to prevent water and polish from splashing onto the table and operator. A large contoured bowl is preferred because of the ease in placing the hands and tools near the spindle. A variable speed unit has the advantage of giving the operator the alternative of determining the rate of modification. A number of modification units are available and spindle sizes vary, so the radius tools for one unit may not be compatible for another unit.

Polishing Compounds

Any polishing compound specifically made for RGP contact lenses is effective during the mod-

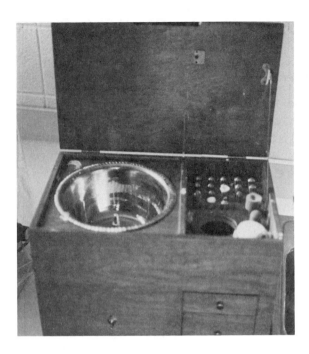

FIGURE 11-47—A large all-in-one variable speed modification unit (Deluxe Modifier from Duffens Contact Lens Co., Indianapolis, IN).

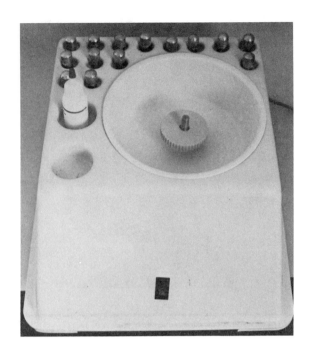

FIGURE 11-48—A one-speed plastic modification unit (Adjustocon from Polychem, Gaithersburg, MD).

ification process. Due to slight differences in viscosity and abrasiveness, however, it is important to become familiar with the particular polishing compound being used because modification times will vary slightly from compound to compound. Silvo, a compound manufactured for polishing silver, was commonly used to make lens modifications of the PMMA material. Silvo is incompatable with RGP lenses because it contains ammonia, which may affect surface wettability.

XPAL polish has been formulated for polishing rigid contact lenses, specifically RGPs. It is supplied as a powder to which water may be added to make up the polishing solution. A contact lens wetting solution or soft lens cleaner may be added to XPAL instead of water to form a more viscous solution so that it will stay on the modification tool longer and create fewer problems with changing lens optics. Premixed solutions are available from most laboratories for use with RGP lenses. These solutions, such as Silo-O2-Care (Polychem, Kensington, MD) and Boston Polish (Polymer Technology Corporation, Boston, MA), are more expensive but tend to reduce the time necessary to perform the indicated modification procedure.

Procedures

Reducing Lens Diameter

Reducing the lens diameter may significantly improve the fit and centration of an RGP contact lens in some cases. This procedure is quite invasive, however, and has been shown to cause microcracks and other lens surface defects in some of the newer, softer RGP materials.[17] Therefore, caution should be exercised when using this procedure, and it should be avoided for all high Dk lens materials. If diameter reduction is performed, careful inspection of the lens surface and edge should be done on completion to rule out defects caused by the procedure.

MOUNTING LENS ON THE TOOL

Many of the procedures used to reduce diameter require proper mounting and centering of the lens on a concave lens holder. This may be accomplished by cutting a small piece of double-faced tape and placing the lens on a concave lens holder. The tape should be pressed down smoothly into the concave top of the holder with the tip of the little finger or with a pencil eraser so that it adheres firmly to the center of the lens holder. The edges of the tape should be folded around the upper rim of the holder so that it adheres well.

The holder should be gripped in one hand, and the lens placed lightly on the tape-covered concave surface with the other hand. The convex surface of the lens should lie within the concave surface of the holder and be centered as well as possible.

The lens holder is kept vertical, and the lens should be rotated slowly between the fingers. If the lens does not appear to be centered, it should be shifted slightly with the fingers while rotating until it appears centered. The holder should be placed on the spindle of the modifying unit and the power switched on for an instant, and then off. As the spindle rotates while slowing down, the lens will appear stationary if centered. Otherwise, the lens edge will show a wobble, and the "high spot" will be readily seen. The lens should be pressed inward gently at this point with the fingernail. When the lens is centered, simply pressing down on the center of the lens with the little finger so that it adheres tightly to the tape will keep the lens securely fixed during future operations.[18]

SWISS FILE OR EMERY BOARD

The shape of the finished lens edge is to a great extent determined by the way the lens is cut down. Thus, the very fine number 6 Swiss file is recommended both to shape and to cut down the lens in the same operation. The lens holder with a well-centered lens mounted on it should be placed on the spindle. The file should be dipped in water and held horizontally, with both hands resting firmly, on the rim of the splash pan (Figure 11-49).

The file is held in position 1, as demonstrated in Figure 11-50. The file should be held lightly against the lens edge and slowly rotated through position 2 until it assumes position 3, approximately 30 degrees past the vertical. The direction of rotation should then be reversed until the file is back at position 1. This back-and-forth rolling motion reduces the diameter of the lens while rounding and shaping the edge at the same time. The file must be kept wet at all times. This technique also gives the lens a

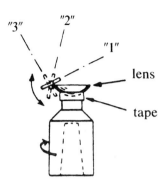

FIGURE 11-49—Shaping the edge and diameter reduction using a file.

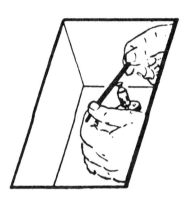

FIGURE 11-50—Proper position of the file for edge shaping and small diameter reduction.

small outside (CN) bevel to reduce lid sensation and aid patient comfort. For a wider outside bevel, as in a high minus lens, the file may be rotated still farther, perhaps 40 or 45 degrees past the vertical position, and then rolled back to the starting position.

Since the lens is rotating clockwise at high speed during the above operation, only moderate pressure of the file on the lens edge is needed to cut down and shape the edge. The amount of diameter reduction depends on the pressure applied and on the thickness of the lens edge. Usually, one back-and-forth rotation of the file will reduce the diameter by 0.05–0.10 mm, and the more gently the file is applied, the smoother the edge will be and the less polishing that will be required. For large reductions in diameters, a coarser file, a number 2 or a number 4, may be used to speed up the operation, and the final cut may be taken with the number 6 file for a smoother finish. Lens diameter may be checked at any time during the operation by removing the lens holder (with the lens still attached) and using a diameter gauge or viewing with a measuring magnifier. With this method, the plus lenses should be left 0.10 mm oversize, and minus lenses 0.05 mm oversize. This excess will be removed in the final polishing of the edge.

Applying Intermediate/Peripheral Curve(s)

PROCESS FOR PERIPHERAL CURVE APPLICATION

To apply a peripheral curve to the lens, cut and attach smoothly a square of waterproof adhesive tape to the surface of the appropriate radius tool or use a precut velveteen pad. The velveteen pad or tape placed on the radius tool should be wet thoroughly with water. Apply the appropriate polishing compound liberally to the wetted pad or tape just before using it, and keep applying it as needed. The polishing compound acts as both an abrasive and a cooling agent.

The tool should be placed on the spindle and the water started. The convex side of the lens should be attached to the suction cup, properly centered, with the fingers held as far down on the suction cup as possible for more control. The lens should be held lightly against the rotating tool. The suction cup should be held at about a 30-degree angle to the vertical, and the whole rim of the lens should be evenly in contact with the covered tool at all times.[19] The suction cup should be turned continuously, slowly, and evenly with the fingers, in a direction opposite to the tool rotation. Since the tool rotates clockwise, the suction cup should be turned counterclockwise. The lens should be lifted away from the covered tool about every 10 or 15 seconds and more polishing compound applied to the covered tool; then the procedure continues.

Instead of having the suction cup at a 30-degree angle to the vertical, an equally effective method places the lens vertical to the holder and rotates the lens in a small figure-eight design (Figure 11-51). If properly performed, this method will minimize the possibility of creating an oval optical zone. When applying a peripheral curve radius using the figure-eight

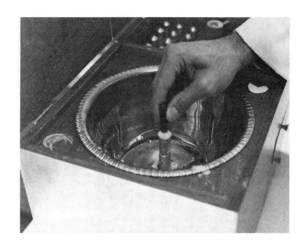

FIGURE 11-51—Application of a peripheral curve using the figure-eight technique.

technique, always place the fingers as far down on the suction cup (toward the lens) as possible.

An alternative method is to use a spinner. The lens is mounted onto the suction cup of the spinner. The lens is then placed on the center of the tool and held initially at a 90-degree angle; once the motor is started, the spinner is tilted to a 45- to 60-degree angle.

The amount of curve applied depends not only on the time that the lens is held against the covered tool and the pressure applied, but also to some extent on the consistency of the polishing compound and the flatness (degree of curvature) of the particular tool as related to the base curve of the lens. A correction must be made to the radius of the tool relative to the thickness of the pad or tape covering it. For example, an 8.30-mm radius tool covered with a 0.20-mm thick pad will generate a curve of 8.50 mm radius.

Practice and experience are necessary for a paraoptometric to determine the length of time needed to produce a curve of desired radius and width. Once proficiency is obtained, records of all lens modifications should be kept, including the curves applied and the time for each curve. This is done to assess improvement as well as to be able to duplicate a lens design accurately if necessary.

The width of the curves applied may be measured in two ways while the lens is still on the lens holder.[18] The first method consists of holding the lens so that a straight-line fluorescent tube can be seen reflected from the lens

TABLE 11-7. Approximate time table for blending junctions on a rigid gas-permeable lens			
Method used	Light blend	Medium blend	Heavy blend
Tape	5 secs	10–30 secs	Until determination of zones difficult
Soft material	5–10 secs	30 secs	Until definite blurred area

surface and tilting the lens so that the reflection is made to pass from the center to the edge of the lens. In this manner the width may be estimated, and after some practice, the estimations may be done quite closely and rapidly. Another method would be coating the entire concave surface of the lens with a black quick-dry ink using a felt-tip marking pen, before generating the curves. A thin coat is applied and allowed to dry before the operations are performed. The amount of coating removed at any stage of the operations indicates the extent of the curve applied.

BLENDING

Once two peripheral curves have been applied, an obvious sharp junction is created between them. This junction may be smoothed out by a process called blending. Blending creates an even tear flow under the lens and by doing so usually causes the lens to move on the eye more than an unblended lens.

The tool selected for blending should have a transition zone that approximates a radius halfway between the two peripheral curves. The tool should be covered with a pad or tape; an allowance for the thickness must be made (usually 0.2 mm for tape and 0.4 mm for pad). The pad or tape on the radius tool should be wet with polishing compound, which should be reapplied frequently. The procedure to be performed is identical to that of a peripheral curve, only the time is significantly shorter.

The suction cup should be held with the centered lens against the rotating tool either vertically, if the figure-eight technique is to be used, or at a 30-degree angle to the vertical, applying pressure to achieve the desired blend.

There are three types of blends possible (Table 11-7). A light blend results in the transition zone still being easily observable with a measuring magnifier and the optical zone and other curves still easily observable. This is sometimes referred to as a *touch blend* since only a few seconds of blending is necessary. A *medium blend* makes the transition zone become less distinct and measurement of the curves more difficult. A *heavy blend* blurs but does not obliterate the transition zone. Measurements for the curves may only be estimated.

To determine the tool needed for making the blend, the following example should be helpful.

$$7.95 = \text{Base curve radius}$$

$$9.20 = \text{Secondary curve radius}$$

$$12.20 = \text{Peripheral curve radius}$$

First blend = 7.95
+ 9.20
17.15 ÷ 2 = 8.57

8.57 Blend radius
− 0.20 Tape
8.37 ~ 8.40 Tool

Second blend = 9.20
12.20
21.40 ÷ 2 = 10.7

10.70 Blend radius
− 0.20 Tape
10.50 Tool

If the radius tool you need is not available, use the next flatter tool.

A process, aptly termed *bull's-eyeing*, can occur when applying or modifying peripheral curves on oxygen-permeable rigid lenses. Since these lenses are generally soft and flexible, very little pressure of the lens against the brass tool

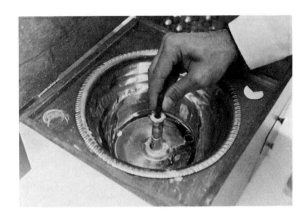

FIGURE 11-52—Application of a CN bevel using a 90-degree cone tool.

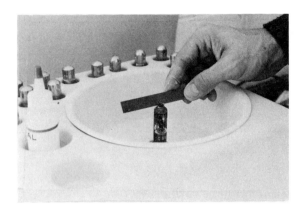

FIGURE 11-53—The use of a moleskin-covered strip for edge shaping.

is required. If too much pressure is applied, roughening or deterioration of the lens periphery may occur and the lens may be ruined.

Edge Shaping and Polishing

Several methods of shaping and polishing the lens edge may be performed. Six of these methods are discussed next.

CN BEVEL

The anterior part of a blunt or thick edge may be thinned by using a CN tool. A 90-degree brass cone tool is most commonly employed (Figure 11-52). The tool is prepared by placing a square of velveteen or adhesive tape with one corner removed into the tool so that it conforms to the tool surface. The lens is mounted against a suction cup by its concave surface and then placed down into the bevel tool so that the convex surface is against the tool. Alternate rocking of the lens laterally and vertically should be performed while the tool is spinning. The lens should be examined every 10–15 seconds until the lens reaches the desired edge thickness. The abrasive tool must be kept moist with the appropriate modifying compound. This is not a polishing procedure as the edge will be quite sharp and somewhat rough after applying a CN bevel.

MOLESKIN-COVERED STRIP

This method is effective for small amounts of diameter reduction and shaping the edge. The moleskin-covered wood strip is moistened with water, and some of the polishing mixture is applied. The strip should be held in the same manner as the fine Swiss file and used in exactly the same way—that is, roll the strip over the edge of the rotating lens, from position 1 to position 3 and then back again (Figure 11-53).[18] Since the wood strip provides a rigid backing to the saturated moleskin, pressure may be applied to the lens edge, influencing its final shape. Therefore, if a greater flattening of the lens edge at its concave side is desired, the wood strip should be held almost parallel to the rim of the lens for a longer period of time, as shown in position 1. If a greater amount of outside (CN) bevel is desired, the wood strip should be held at a considerable angle past the vertical for a longer period of time, as in position 3, thus applying the polishing action to the convex side of the lens circumference.

The total polishing time should be 2–3 minutes, or even slightly longer, since a well-polished edge is of greatest importance in providing maximum comfort to the patient. As an added precaution, an additional method, such as the sponge tool or finger polishing, may be performed.

EDGE-POLISHING TOOL

Using a sponge tool is an effective edge-polishing method. This method, as demonstrated in Figure 11-54, consists of mounting the convex surface of the lens on the suction cup.[19] The sponge tool, which contains a central hole, should be thoroughly moistened with water and placed on the spindle. Turn the polisher

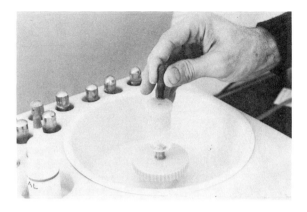

FIGURE 11-54—A central aperture hole for edge shaping.

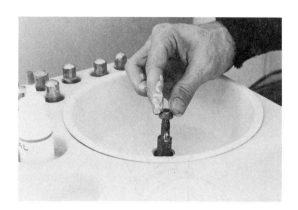

FIGURE 11-55—Finger polishing a rigid lens surface.

motor on first, then moisten the sponge well with polishing compound. To avoid splash, never apply polishing compound unless the tool is spinning.

With the suction cup held vertically, push the lens into the central hole in the sponge. Hold the suction cup vertically and move the lens up and down for 30–60 seconds. Rotate the lens as it moves up and down. The inside surface of the edge is polished as the lens moves down, and the outside surface of the edge is polished as the lens moves up. Keep the sponge wet with polishing compound at all times. A large lens may become lodged in the hole, especially if the lens was loosely adhering to the suction cup. Extended use of this procedure can reduce the diameter of the lens by 0.10–0.20 mm.

FINGER POLISH

The lens should be mounted concave side up on a brass tool containing a suction cup or a brass tool with double-sided tape. The lens must be centered on the tool. While the lens is rotating, polishing compound is applied to the index finger and thumb, which are used as polishing pads by moving the fingers up and down over the lens edge (Figure 11-55). At least 2 minutes of polishing per lens should be performed. Although this is a good final polishing procedure, the edge must have been semipolished before the use of the fingers in order to prevent possible injury. The edge may be inspected with the aid of a projection magnifier.

To remove the lens from the double-faced tape that attached it to the lens holder, rotate the holder slowly with the fingers of one hand while pressing the thumbnail of the other hand gently between the lens and the tape.[20] The lens will be gradually released from the adhesion of the tape until it is entirely free.

Surface Polishing and Power Changes

REMOVING SCRATCHES FROM THE CONCAVE SURFACE

Removing scratches from the concave surface of a lens may be accomplished by attaching the convex surface of the lens to a suction cup, centering it by eye. The lens should be held with light pressure against a rotating spherical tool (sponge with spherical shape) that has been saturated with polish and placed on a motor-driven spindle. A 30-degree angle should be maintained with the vertical, and the lens should be rotated slowly with the fingers, counterclockwise opposite to the spindle rotation direction (Figure 11-56).

The lens should be lifted away from the tool every 10–15 seconds; fresh polish is applied to the tool, and the procedure continues. Scratches in the optical and intermediate/peripheral curve areas(s) will be removed in 30–120 seconds. Protein deposits, however, are more common on the concave surface of the lens, and these are generally removed in the first 30 seconds of this procedure.

Another method uses a concave polishing tool. The convex surface of the lens is mounted on the lens holder. The cone-shaped sponge moistened with water should be placed on the

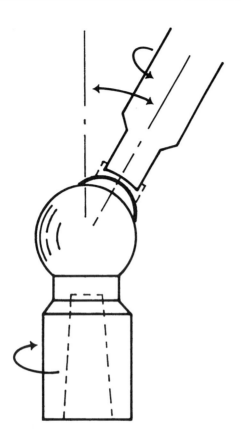

FIGURE 11-56—Polishing the concave surface of a rigid lens edge with the use of a spherical sponge tool.

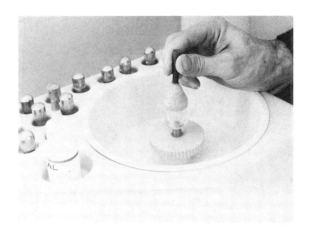

FIGURE 11-57—Polishing the concave surface of a rigid lens with a concave polishing tool.

motor spindle. The motor should be turned on and the sponge moistened well with the polishing compound. The suction cup should be tilted slightly and the lens should be placed just off the center of the sponge (Figure 11-57).[19]

The lens is depressed into the sponge about one-eighth of an inch and the holder rotated 10–15 seconds. When the tool is spinning, the position of the lens and the shape of the sponge form a convex surface matching the concave surface of the lens. The sponge should be kept wet with polishing compound at all times.

REMOVING SCRATCHES FROM THE CONVEX SURFACE

To remove scratches from the convex surface of a lens, the lens is attached to the suction cup, convex side out; centering should be done by eye. A flat sponge tool (convex polishing tool or similar sponge tool) that has been saturated well with water is used. The convex surface polishing tool is placed on the motor-driven spindle.

The polisher motor is turned on first and the sponge is then moistened well with the polishing compound. The suction cup should be tilted slightly (approximately 30 degrees) and the lens placed halfway between the center and the edge of the sponge. The lens is depressed into the sponge about one-eighth of an inch and rotated against the rotation of the tool.[19] After two full rotations, the center of the lens is polished by tapping it gently 10 or 12 times in the center of the rotating tool. The center of the lens should not be held against the tool for more than a second at a time; otherwise a power change will likely occur. Polishing compound is added frequently, and the lens is removed every 15 seconds to examine the front surface and to check power to be sure a change has not occurred (Figure 11-58).

Adding Minus Power

The tools commonly used to change lens power are illustrated in Figure 11-59 and discussed below.

TOEPAD AND SPINNER

The toepad should be mounted on the modification unit; good vertical alignment is a must. The concave surface of the lens is mounted on the spinner, making sure the lens is centered. The spinner should move easily and freely. Water and polishing compound are then applied to the toepad. While the toepad is spinning, the lens should be brought in perpendicular to the toepad. The edge of the lens is touched to an area approximately

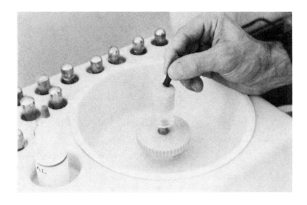

FIGURE 11-58—Removing scratches from the convex surface.

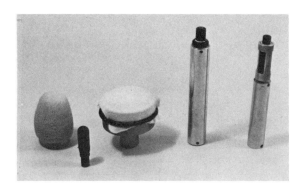

FIGURE 11-59—Tools commonly used for repowering a rigid lens.

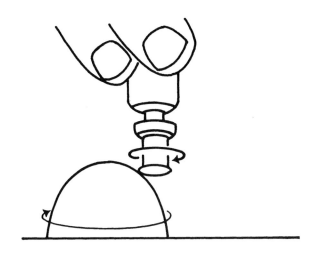

FIGURE 11-60—Use of a toepad tool and spinner for adding minus power.

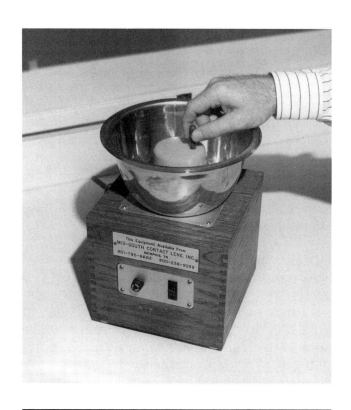

FIGURE 11-61—The use of a flat sponge tool for adding minus power.

1.0–1.5 cm from the apex of the toepad. The lens should turn freely on the spinner.[20]

Next, the lens contact with the toepad is increased by elevating the spinner so that it is perpendicular to the toepad surface. The apex of the lens should touch the toepad (Figure 11-60). The position and pressure should be held constant. The amount of power being added will depend on the amount of pressure, time, and polishing compound used. As much as 1 D may be added without changing the optics of the lens. The power should be checked every 10–15 seconds.

FLAT SPONGE TOOL

Using this method, the polishing compound is placed on the sponge tool and the lens is attached, convex side toward the tool, to a suction cup or spinner. The convex surface of the lens is held midway between the center and the periphery of the tool and rotated counterclockwise around the entire circumference of the tool (Figure 11-61). The tool should be kept moist and the power checked every 5–10 seconds. Four revolutions around the tool should produce about a –0.25 D power change.

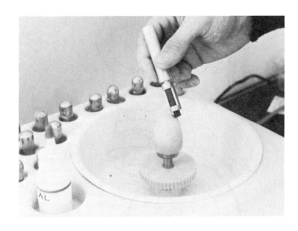

FIGURE 11-62—The position of the spinner against the toepad for adding plus power.

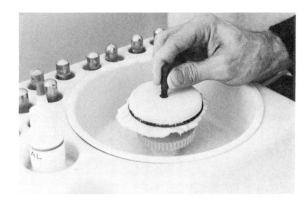

FIGURE 11-63—Adding plus power with a hollow velveteen tool.

Adding Plus Power

TOEPAD AND SPINNER

Adding plus power is accomplished in a manner similar to that for adding minus power. Once the spinner is rotating, the angle of the spinner should be lowered until approximately half of the lens is in contact with the toepad and torqued, or moved *out* of vertical alignment with the toepad (Figure 11-62). The lens rotation on the spinner should be slightly slowed. Plus power is now being added, usually at a slower rate than minus. Polishing compound should be added regularly.

HOLLOW VELVETEEN TOOL

This tool is a small, hollow cylinder with velveteen stretched over it and secured with a rubber ring. The lens is mounted concave side out on a suction cup with careful centration. The apex of the lens is then held against the center of the rotating tool, and the suction cup is rotated slightly back and forth between the fingers. Again, the lens power should be checked every 15 seconds. No more than 0.50 D of total plus power change should be expected with this procedure (Figure 11-63).

CONCLUSION

This chapter provides the paraoptometric with basic materials and design, patient instruction, verification, and modification procedures. Because the field of contact lenses is changing so rapidly, the paraoptometric is encouraged to read periodicals and other literature to keep up to date.

REFERENCES

1. Nelson PS. A short Schirmer test. Optom Monthly 1982;73:568.
2. Hamano T, Mitsunaga S, Kotani S, et al. Tear volume in relation to contact lens wear and age. CLAO J 1990;16:57.
3. Sakamoto R, Bennett E, Henry VA, et al. The phenol red thread tear test: a cross cultural study. Invest Ophthalmol Vis Sci 1993;34:3510.
4. Bennett ES, Paragina ES. Material Selection. In ES Bennett, VA Henry (eds), Clinical Manual of Contact Lenses. Philadelphia: Lippincott, 1994;32.
5. Bennett ES, Henry VA. RGP lens power change with abrasive cleaner use. Int Contact Lens Clin 1990;17:152.
6. Schwartz CA. Contact lenses: Ideas for the next generation. Rev Optom 1992;129:45.
7. Henry VA. Fitting and Evaluation. In ES Bennett, VA Henry (eds), Clinical Manual of Contact Lenses. Philadelphia: Lippincott, 1994;220.
8. Becherer PD. Soft torics: a viable modality. Contact Lens Update 1990;9:17.
9. Pence NA. The effect of monovision and driving performance. Presented at the 20th Annual North American Research Symposium on Contact Lenses, San Diego, CA, August 1993.
10. Bennett ES, Nelson JM, Henry VA. Material Selection. In ES Bennett, VA Henry (eds), Clinical Manual of Contact Lenses. Philadelphia: Lippincott, 1994;202.
11. Efron N, Veys J. Defects in disposable contact lenses can compromise ocular integrity. Int Contact Lens Clin 1992;19:8.
12. Buchler PO, Schein OD, Stamler JF, et al. The increased risk of ulcerative keratitis among disposable soft contact lens users. Arch Ophthalmol 1992;110:1555.

13. Matthews TD, Frazer DG, Minassian DC, et al. Risks of keratitis and patterns of use with disposable contact lenses. Arch Ophthalmol 1992;110:1559.
14. Bennett ES, Henry VA. Rigid Gas-Permeable Contact Lens Patient Instruction Manual. St. Louis: University of Missouri School of Optometry, 1995 (unpublished manuscript).
15. Callender M, Egan D. Verification and Inspection of Soft Contact Lens. St. Louis, 1990 (unpublished manuscript).
16. Morgan BW, Henry VA, Bennett ES. The effect of modification procedures on silicone/acrylate versus fluoro-silicone/acrylate lens materials. J Am Optom Assoc 1992;3:193.
17. Grohe RM, Caroline PJ, Norman C. The role of in-office modification for RGP surface defects. Contact Lens Spectrum 1988;3:52.
18. Gordon S. Contact Lens Adjusting Manual. Rochester, NY: UCO Optics, Inc.
19. Corns S, Carmichael B, Sorrells A. Contact Lens Modification Manual for Technicians. Bloomington, IN: Indiana University, 1981 (unpublished manuscript).
20. Lens Polisher Operating Instructions. Duffens Optical Company, Indianapolis, IN.

12/Low Vision Examination

Paul B. Freeman

A low vision examination involves a thorough optometric evaluation of a visually impaired individual. The length of the examination may vary from 45 minutes to several hours. A visual impairment, which can lead to low vision difficulties, may be caused by congenital, hereditary, traumatic, or pharmacologic factors, or it may be associated with a disease process. Successfully evaluating a low vision patient requires the integrated knowledge of optics, psychology, pharmacology, physiology, pathology, and the psychosocial impact of illness on human behavior. Although it is the optometrist who will determine the initial prescriptive recommendation for the low vision patient, it is the paraoptometric/optometrist team that will guide the patient to the successful use of the low vision prescription.[1]

To help low vision patients improve their visual quality of life, the paraoptometric assistant must first be familiar with low vision intervention.

HISTORY

As with any other examination, the low vision examination begins with a thorough medical and visual patient history. The low vision examination history tends to be more comprehensive than a routine patient history. To have a successful starting point for the examination, specific questions must be answered.[2] These questions should be based on the general areas of distance visual concerns, near visual concerns, and illumination and lighting concerns.

The responses to these questions will help frame the examination to meet the needs and goals of the patient.

Goals are the key to the patient's visual success. Generic goals such as "I want to see better" are typically unacceptable for a truly successful low vision prescription and may be indicative of a patient who has not accepted the vision loss. The unaccepting patient may insist that a conventional pair of glasses or contact lenses can return the vision loss to "normal" sight. The assistant can reinforce the optometrist's goal of providing the patient with the best vision possible by attempting to guide the patient into specific goals, such as reading, sewing, watching television, and so forth.

Goals should be task-oriented so that a demonstrated endpoint may be reached and understood by both patient and doctor. For instance, "I would like to do _____," or "I wish I could do _____ better." The low vision examination history moves from general to specific questions in order to identify the intended goal.

VISUAL ACUITY TESTING

With the history taken and a goal determined, visual acuity measurements begin. As with a conventional evaluation, a visual acuity measurement at both distance and near is the initial information obtained from the patient. The patient should be evaluated monocularly, binocularly, and with and without the current lens prescription.

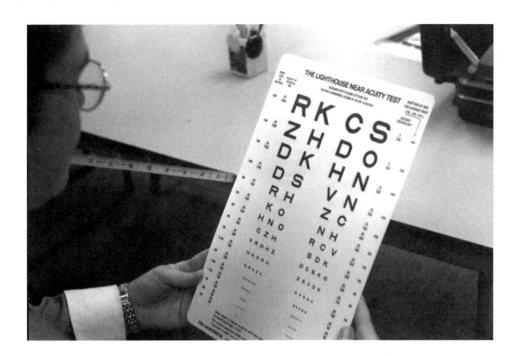

Figure 12-1—Lighthouse Near Acuity Test Chart. This is one of the many near acuity test charts. It is measured in M units but can be converted to a Snellen fraction if the tester pays attention to the distance at which the test is used.

For many low vision patients (worse than 20/400), a standard Snellen chart at a measured or equivalent 20-foot distance is inappropriate. Often, it has been previously established by other eye doctors that these patients have "failed" to see anything on the eye chart; repeating this failure only reinforces the decreased visual acuity and implications of blindness. As visual acuity testing is also an important psychological test, it is helpful to adopt a success-oriented approach.[3]

Low vision acuity testing is typically started at 10 feet but should be adapted to the individual. If acuities are far below 20/400, a closer distance of 5, 2, or 2½ feet may initially provide better results. Portable charts (e.g., the Feinbloom acuity chart, Bailey-Lovie chart,[4] etc.) should be used and set at specific distances so that achievable visual acuities may be successfully performed. Use of portable acuity charts also provides legitimate visual acuities and avoids the ambiguity of "counting fingers."

Acuities should be noted at the actual distance recorded and at the equivalent 20-foot working distance, that is, 5/200 (20/800). The 20-foot working distance is obtained by multiplying the actual numerator and denominator by the number that will provide 20 in the numerator.

$$x \times 5 = 20$$
$$x = 20/5$$
$$x = 4$$

Therefore, $5/200 \times 4/4 = 20/800$.

Near acuities should also be measured at a specific working distance. This distance, converted to diopters, in many instances will be the basis for the magnification formula that will be used to help determine the starting low vision device for near. Typically, charts with metric notation (M system) are used, as the size of these targets are standard from chart to chart. The assistant should become familiar with this system of acuity measurement (Figure 12-1).

Sometimes visual acuities will vary when using a line acuity in isolation, a letter-by-letter acuity, or a paragraph acuity. This information will be of value for later determination of starting optics and training materials. Therefore, at near, it is valuable to obtain a line or paragraph acuity which can then be compared to letter by letter acuity. You will find that these acuities do not always match.[5]

Lighting is a critical factor in both near and distance visual measurements. Lighting conditions should be recorded and may be obtained with either a light meter or by measuring the wattage of the light and the distance of the light from the task. A typoscope (line marker) may also be used to modify light/contrast involvement as well as to minimize the crowding phenomenon (i.e., words or letters appearing to run together or overlap).

INFORMATION MODIFIERS

Two tests, Contrast sensitivity function and Amsler grid, are performed with the visually impaired patient to determine how environmental vision recommendations and magnification calculations might be modified.

Contrast sensitivity function testing is used to determine the capability of distinguishing various spatial frequencies under different contrast situations or being able to distinguish figure from ground while modifying contrasting conditions.[6] This test quantifies the effect of decreased contrast in the environment on visual function. The results may help explain situations in which measured visual acuities remain the same while contrast levels change, creating difficulty in seeing. The results from this testing will also help to determine lighting and contrast necessary for visual success in the patient's everyday environment.

Amsler grid testing is used to determine the extent of central vision loss, multiple scotomas or blind areas, and distortions (metamorphopsia)[2] (see Chapter 10). The relevance of this testing is twofold: (1) If the patient has blind spots or areas of field loss, activities to train the patient to view around these spots (eccentric viewing) may be needed to help the patient maximize the remaining useful vision, both with and without low vision devices. (2) If the patient has distortion, then magnification modifications may be necessary to help minimize the distortion and maximize the remaining sight. Typically, magnification is doubled at near to accomplish this.

EYE MOVEMENT EVALUATION

Eye movement evaluation is similar to that performed in a conventional examination. Both monocular and binocular pursuits and saccadic movements should be performed to determine the integrity of the extraocular muscle system as well as the functional use of the eye movements. Convergence and divergence eye movements should be evaluated as well. These findings will be valuable in the event that binocularity can be achieved through the use of optical devices for either distance or near. Also, functionally, eye movements may have to be "trained" if proven to be erratic.

COLOR VISION AND STEREO VISION TESTING

Color vision testing and stereo testing determine the pathologic interference with color appreciation and stereo perception.

Some pathologies can cause specific color deficiencies. Red/green color deficiencies are indicative of many optic nerve disorders, and blue/yellow color deficiencies are found in many retinal disorders.[7] For example, understanding color vision would be important for the diabetic patient who is blue deficient but tries to monitor sugar levels visually using test strips that are varying shades of blue.

Binocular sensory function of an individual is evaluated through stereo perception. Stereo perception is the ability to use both eyes to see three dimensions, which can be tested with tests such as the Titmus Stereo Fly test. This is based on the disparity between images formed on the retina and is used to appreciate position in the environment. Stereo vision is the innate part of depth perception. Stereo perception should not be confused, however, with the general term *depth perception,* which is also used to describe monocular sensory function (shadow appreciation, linear perspective, clarity, etc.) and is the learned aspect of position in the environment. Both monocular and binocular information, therefore, make up depth perception.

VISUAL FIELD EVALUATION

The majority of low vision patients typically have central vision loss with good peripheral or mobility vision. However, perimetry has become a more integral part of a low vision evaluation as the incidence of head trauma, stroke, and specific diseases that cause peripheral visual field defects (e.g., glaucoma, retinitis pigmentosa, etc.) have increased.

Initial fields are usually done as a confrontation test (see Chapter 10). To monitor or diagnose a disease, however, the practitioner will typically rely on more sophisticated automated testing.

GLARE TESTING

Glare testing is important for the low vision population. A significant percentage of the visually impaired population has difficulty recovering from sudden changes in light levels. This can make the adjustment from inside to outside environment (or vice versa) frustrating.

Glare testing and recovery may be done using sophisticated equipment such as the Miller Nadler glare tester or the Brightness Acuity Tester (BAT), or by simply using a penlight. The penlight test (photostress recovery test) may be done quite simply and quickly. To perform this test, have the patient cover one eye and view a penlight, held a few inches from the eye, for 10 seconds. The patient then looks at the acuity chart and calls out the letters that can immediately be seen best. The key to the test is to see how long it takes until the acuity returns to the original measurement or close to it. Both eyes should be evaluated individually, and then the results compared to determine if one eye is affected more than the other. Longer than 50 seconds monocularly or a difference in recovery time between eyes of 20 seconds may be considered abnormal.[8] This test demonstrates light/dark difficulties to the patient and sets the stage for later discussion of a sunfilter evaluation.

OCULAR HEALTH EVALUATION

Ocular health is evaluated specifically for confirmation or identification of the disease condition(s) causing the visual impairment.

REFRACTION

The objective refraction and subjective refraction are probably the most important aspects of the evaluation of the low vision patient and should be done prior to the optical evaluation for low vision devices.

For magnification to be maximally effective, light needs to be focused on the retina properly. If not, the doctor may experience frustration at not getting the appropriate response from the patient (based on the calculated magnification information), and the patient will become frustrated because of the inability to see. An example may help to illustrate this concept.

Suppose a patient is a +10.00 D hyperope. If the doctor decides to supply a near lens that is calculated at +20.00 D and does not take into account the distance lens prescription, the patient is actually left with half the lens power (i.e., +20.00 D – +10.00 D = +10.00 D). If the prescription were accounted for, however, the total power of the lens would actually be +30.00 D (i.e., +20.00 D + +10.00 D). The opposite is true for patients with myopia. For significant astigmatism, the result is blur and distortion if the prescription is left out.

Unfortunately, some practitioners are intimidated by the presence of eye disease and as a result do not attempt to refract the visually impaired patient. Sometimes a good refraction can eliminate the need for sophisticated low vision devices. A refraction using a trial frame, trial lenses, and a retinoscope may sometimes uncover a standard lens prescription for either or both distance and near that will return the patient to a functioning visual world with conventional lenses.

Sometimes standard refractive techniques cannot be performed. In those instances, refractive techniques may be performed using variable distances. A closer distance may be called for while the patient views eccentrically (looking off to one side or the other)[9] or if there are media opacities. This technique is termed radical retinoscopy.[10]

The refractive tests should be verified in both morning and afternoon visits, especially in patients with diseases that have diurnal variations such as diabetes, glaucoma, and multiple sclerosis. Huge swings of visual acuity may be revealed by morning and afternoon refractive testing. Once the patient is aware of the variability of the eye condition, the optometric team can work to help the patient maximize this fluctuating vision while minimizing frustration.

The next area to be addressed is the evaluation of optical devices for the enhancement of visual acuities as related to the goal-oriented tasks determined in the history. To understand

```
                    FREEMAN INVERTED "V"

                    40 inches/ 100 cm

            1D      --           40 inches/ 100 cm
            2D      ----         20 inches/ 50 cm
            3D      ------       13 inches/ 33 cm
            4D      --------     10 inches/ 25 cm
            5D      ----------   8 inches/ 20 cm
            6D      ------------ 6.6 inches/ 16.6 cm
            7D      -------------- 5.7 inches/ 14.2 cm
            8D      ---------------- 5 inches/ 12.5 cm
            9D      ------------------ 4.4 inches/ 11.1 cm
           10D      -------------------- 4 inches/ 10 cm
           15D      ---------------------- 3 inches/ 6.6 cm
           20D      ------------------------ 2 inches/ 5 cm
           25D      -------------------------- 1.6 inches/ 4 cm
           35D      ---------------------------- 1.4 inches/ 2.85 cm
           40D      ------------------------------ 1 inch/ 2.5 cm
           50D      -------------------------------- .8 inch/ 2 cm
           60D      ---------------------------------- .6 inch/ 1.6 cm
           80D      ------------------------------------ .5 inch/ 1.25 cm
          100D      -------------------------------------- .4 inch/ 1 cm
```

FIGURE 12-2—The Freeman Inverted "V" is a quick reference for identifying the relationship between diopters and focal length.

---

these options, however, an appreciation of the basic principles of magnification is necessary.

MAGNIFICATION

Magnification is based on four considerations: relative size, relative distance, angular magnification, and electronic magnification.

Relative size magnification can be described as physically enlarging an object when seen at the same viewing distance. An object that is 2 inches tall when made 4 inches tall has a magnification factor of 2×. An example is large print or a big-eye needle.

Relative distance magnification is based on the apparent change in an object size based on moving the object close to the observer. If a target that is 2 inches tall at 16 inches is moved to 8 inches, it will project an image onto the retina that is twice as large as it was in its original location. A television screen that appears to become larger when the viewer moves closer to it is a good example of this.

Angular magnification is achieved by increasing the apparent size of an object at a given location through the use of sophisticated optical principles. Binoculars are an example of angular magnification. If a 2-foot target at 20 feet is enlarged through optics, such as telescope viewing, to 4 feet at the same distance, it has been magnified by a factor of 2.

Electronic magnification is a combination of relative size and relative distance magnification accomplished through the use of electronic equipment. If a target is 2 inches tall and is enlarged on a screen to 4 inches tall, when viewed at a base distance (e.g., 16 inches, 10 inches, etc.), it will result in a relative size magnification of 2×. But, when viewed at half the distance from the base distance (e.g., 8 inches, 5 inches, etc.), its apparent size as projected on the retina will be doubled, representing 4× (2× relative distance magnification × 2× relative size magnification = 4×). A closed-circuit television (CCTV) exemplifies this concept.

The magnification principles may be applied in the following systems.

Near Head-Borne Systems

A head-borne high plus lens magnification system is called a *microscope*. A microscope primarily uses the concept of relative distance magnification. The optical properties of the microscope are simply used to focus a target that is brought close to the viewer.

To be successful in the use of a microscope, the dioptric power and the focal length should be known. The Freeman Inverted "V" was developed to serve as a quick reference for either working distance or dioptric power for plus power lenses (Figure 12-2).

Figure 12-2 uses a reference point of 40 inches, or 100 cm, which is the focal length of

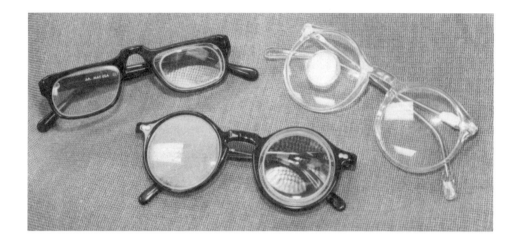

FIGURE 12-3—Head-borne microscopes can vary in design from bifocal to half eye to full diameter. The left system is a half eye, the center system is a full diameter microscope (Clear Image II). Both are from Designs for Vision (DVI). The system on the right is a UT UniVision microscopic button, which has been positioned centrally.

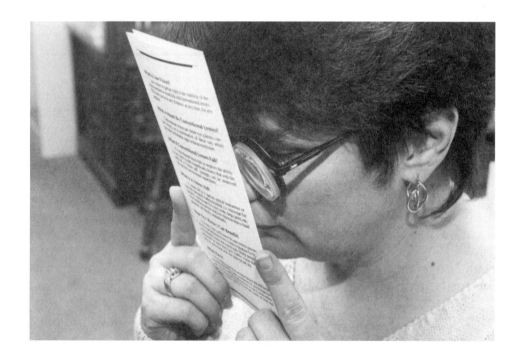

Figure 12-4—With head-borne microscopes, the primary advantage is a large field of view, whereas a disadvantage is the close working distance, Here is an example of an 8× (+32.00 D) system with a focal length of approximately 1.25 inches.

1 D. Having this information close at hand will enable you to locate the focal length of a lens quickly and easily (given the dioptric power) so you will know where to position a target. Note that to obtain these values you can either divide the focal length or the power of the lens into the apex of the inverted "V" to arrive at the complementary information. The other option is simply to look opposite to the number that you have been given, that is, 20 D = 2 inches/5 cm.

The primary advantage of a high plus lens head-mounted system is a large field of view and a somewhat familiar concept of a spectacle prescription for reading (Figure 12-3). An additional advantage is that both hands are free to hold reading materials or to perform other near activities such as threading a sewing needle, writing, and so forth. A disadvantage of this system is the close distance at which materials must be held. Because of this, it is sometimes difficult to get enough light onto the task (Figure 12-4). With specific training activities, however, the negative aspects of the working distance can be overcome so that a patient using even a +60.00 D lens can be successful.

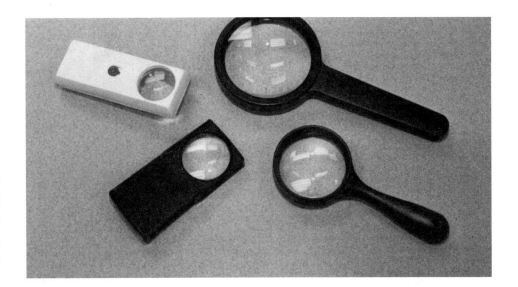

Figure 12-5—Hand-held magnifiers. Hand magnifiers vary in lens size, based mostly on the power of the optics. Some are self-illuminated, while others rely on environmental light. The magnifiers shown, from the light-colored magnifier clockwise, are the Eschenbach Self-Illuminated, Eschenbach, Coil, and Bausch & Lomb.

For example, at what distance would a patient who requires a +60.00 D microscope have to hold the material to see it clearly? What would be the total power of the lens if the patient had a distance correction of plano? An aphake with a +15.00 lens prescription? A myope with a –5.00 lens prescription? Remember the refractive information must be available to answer the question accurately. All of the patients would hold the material at a specific distance of 1.66 cm, or 0.6 inches, if the refraction were taken into account. The actual lens for each would be +60.00 D, +75.00 D, +55.00 D, respectively.

Hand-Held Magnifiers

Hand-held magnification systems are probably the most misunderstood of all magnification devices (Figure 12-5). Most people pick up a hand magnifier, hoping that it will find its own best focus. To be used properly, the magnifier should be held so that the target is at the focal length of the hand magnifier (Figure 12-6) to permit parallel rays of light to leave the hand magnifier and create the appearance of a target at optical infinity. This requires the user to have accommodation (focusing of the eye) at rest or to wear a distance lens prescription.

Bifocals do not add to the value of a properly used hand magnifier and in some instances will actually blur the image. Having to move the hand magnifier to place the image at the focal length of the bifocal will in certain situations actually subtract power from the hand magnifier.[11] If the patient keeps the target at the focal length of the hand magnifier, the magnification is constant at all viewing distances. The visual field, however, will vary, becoming larger as the hand magnifier is moved closer to the eye (see Figure 12-6).

The advantage of a hand-held magnifier is its portability and relative ease of use at any distance when using the appropriate distance lens. The key drawbacks typically are that the user may feel the need for a "third arm" when trying to hold the target and the hand magnifier, and if not held properly, the field of view and magnification may suffer. Additionally, for patients who have shaky hands (e.g., those with Parkinson's disease) or have poor hand-eye coordination, this device may be frustrating to use (see Figure 12-6).

Stand Magnifiers

Stand magnifiers are advantageous for patients who require physical stability, who may have poor dexterity, or who have hand tremors (Figure 12-7). A stand magnifier has a base that rests on the object being viewed (Figure 12-8).

Some stand magnifiers require accommodation or need to be used with a bifocal prescrip-

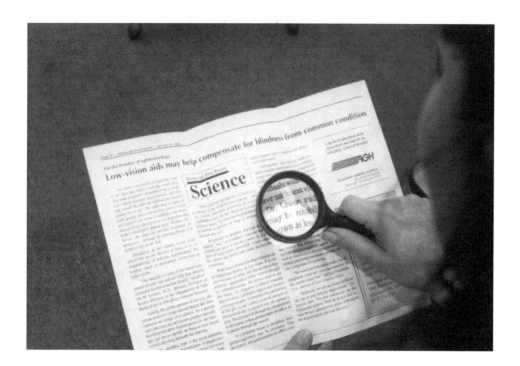

Figure 12-6—A hand magnifier is used when arm's length activities are desired. Note the field of view. This will depend on where the combination of the hand magnification/target is held in relation to the patient's face.

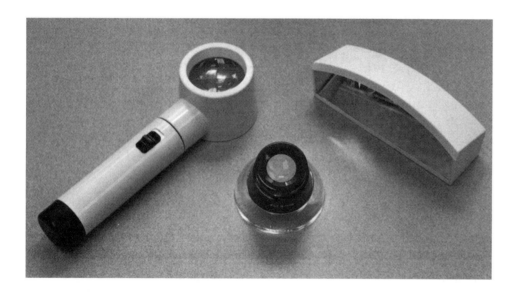

FIGURE 12-7—Stand magnifiers. Stand magnifiers vary in dimension based on lens power and design. The magnifier on the left is an illuminated Eschenbach, the middle is a Viewcraft Loupe, and the one on the right is a mirror stand magnifier.

tion. In these magnifiers, diverging rays of light leave the system and need to be converged to the retina. Some new stand magnifiers are designed to eliminate this concern by being "focusable." Two key disadvantages of stand magnifiers are illumination concerns and a limited field of view. Many stand magnifiers, however, feature internal illumination in an attempt to resolve the lighting limitations.

Electronic Video Magnifiers

CCTVs, hand camera systems, and heads-up systems such as the Bright Eye System and Magni Cam are ways to magnify information electronically. Electronic magnifiers are based on the combination of relative size and distance magnification and may be used for both reading and writing. CCTVs are designed with a television screen, moveable

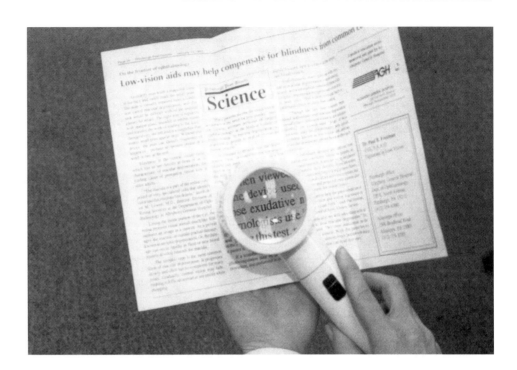

FIGURE 12-8—A stand magnifier is beneficial when stability of the device is important. This system has an internal illumination capability for enhanced lighting.

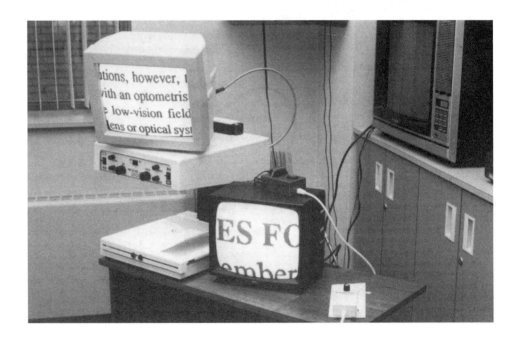

Figure 12-9—Electronic magnifiers. Most closed-circuit televisions need to be near a power source. The one on the left is an Optelec. The small hand unit in the foreground on the right, the Magni Cam, attaches to a standard television.

table, and camera with magnification capabilities (Figures 12-9 and 12-10). The camera may be integral to the system or used as a separate unit. There are also separate units that can be adapted to conventional televisions as hand camera systems. In the Bright Eye and Magni Cam systems, the viewer wears a headband with a miniature screen attached (Figures 12-11 and 12-12). A hand-held camera is used to scan the object and send the image to the screen worn by the viewer. These electronic systems enable the user to vary the magnification, some up to 60 times.

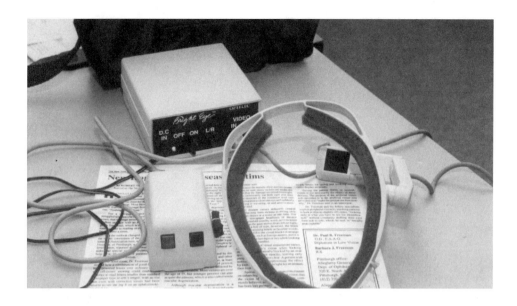

Figure 12-10—Electronic magnifiers. This heads-up unit was designed by Optelec. The camera on the left sends the image up to the small window on the right. The headband allows the viewer to use either the right or left eye.

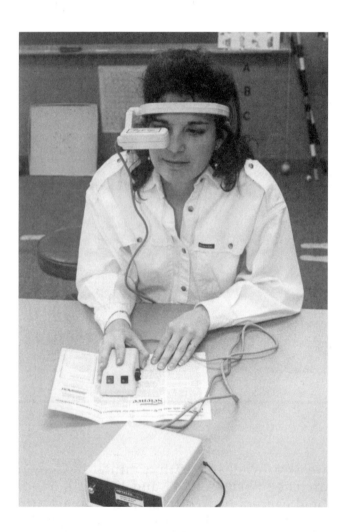

Figure 12-11—In the Bright Eye System, the viewer wears a headband with a miniature screen attached. Notice that the image produced by the hand camera must be viewed in the head-mounted "eye."

Advantages of a standard CCTV are the control of light and contrast of the targets being viewed, reverse imagery from black on white to white on black, the availability of a line guide (typoscope), and the ability to connect to computers. The primary disadvantage is decreased portability due to the weight and size of some of the devices. Also, due to divergent light leaving the screen, a near lens prescription or accommodative ability is generally needed with these systems.

A new head-mounted system has been designed to incorporate the benefits of electro-optical video magnification for distance and near application with a variable autofocus. This new system is called the Low Vision Enhancement System (LVES; affectionately called ELVIS) (Figure 12-13). It integrates all of the same properties of electro optical systems, including magnification, contrast enhancement, reverse polarity, and a large field of view. The primary disadvantage is its complexity and for some, the weight of the head unit.

Distance Magnification Devices

Distance magnification can be as simple as moving closer to what is being viewed (relative distance magnification). Optical distance magnification centers around telescopic lenses. The two types of telescopes, Galilean and Keplerian, are differentiated by the amount of light

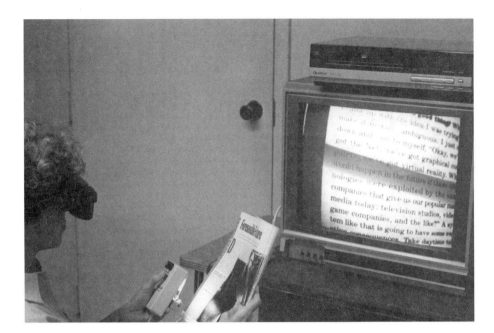

Figure 12-12—The Magni Cam is another hand-held video system that can be used either as an attachment to a standard television set or as a head-mounted system. The field of view of the head-mounted system allows for reasonable ease in its use.

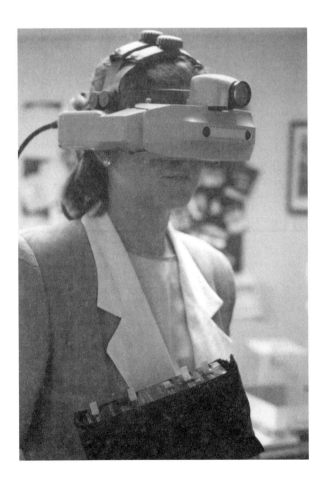

Figure 12-13—The Low Vision Enhancement System (LVES) is a video magnifier with a control panel for magnification, focusing, and lighting controls. The two small openings on the head set are for "normal" viewing, whereas the larger opening is for magnification. This can be used for viewing at a variety of distances.

allowed to pass through them, as well as where the light leaves the telescope (exit pupil). Both systems may be used as hand-held or head-mounted systems (Figures 12-14 and 12-15).

The obvious advantage of a telescope is to magnify objects in the distance. A major disadvantage can be in the cosmetics of the system. Some telescopes are very visible and may make some patients feel self-conscious about exposing their impairment. Light gathering properties may be another problem area. Because of the multiple elements in a telescope, all of the environmental light does not reach the viewer's eye. This is slightly worse in Keplerian systems than in Galilean systems, so consideration must be given to those patients who need substantial amounts of light. Finally, field of view (the stronger the system, the smaller the field of view) and general difficulty of use may create frustration. These latter disadvantages, however, can be minimized with proper training.

Field-Enhancing Devices

Field-enhancing devices may be divided into total field-enhancement systems (Figure 12-16) and field-specific enhancment systems (Figure 12-17). The former are designed for full-field enhancement through the use of reverse field telescopes or minus lenses. Reverse-field tele-

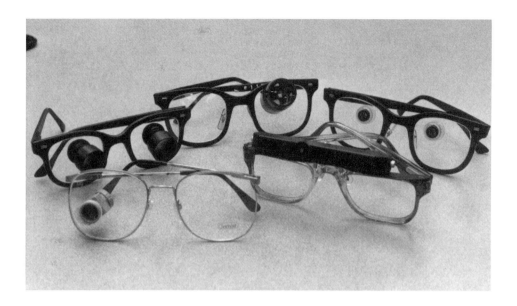

Figure 12-14—Telescopes. Telescopes may be hand-held, ring-mounted, or mounted in a frame in various positions. These shown are all mounted in a frame. Clockwise from left front are the Behind-the-Lens monocular system, Designs for Vision (DVI) Galilean binocular system, DVI monocular Keplerian system, DVI binocular microspiral Galilean system, and monocular Ocutech Vision Enhancement System.

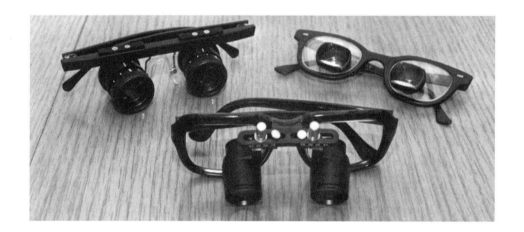

Figure 12-15—Reading telescopes. These systems allow for a longer working distance but a smaller field of view. The system in the foreground is a Shin-Nippon, the back left is an Eschenbach, and the back right is a Designs for Vision (DVI) Galilean system.

scopes are similar to a security peephole in a door. Minus lenses, as reverse-field telescopes, include more information in the field of view by minification with a minus lens. To demonstrate minification, go to a trial lens set and hold a minus lens (range –5.00 D to –10.00 D) at 10–12 inches and look through it. What you should see is a minified image with all the details of the scene it represents.

Field-specific enhancers use prisms or mirrors to direct light from a nonseeing area onto the useable part of the visual system by an eye movement into the field-specific enhancement system.[12] Information may then be identified through the use of quick, small eye movements.

Advantages of the field enhancement devices are that they help the patient to be more visually aware of the environment. The disadvantage is primarily in the change in perception of where objects are in the environment. Again, proper training in the use of these devices minimizes this disadvantage.

NONOPTICAL DEVICES

Sometimes large-print materials, modification in lighting, felt-tip marker, filters, or other nonoptical systems are used to enhance the patient's ability to see. Typically, these options are used in conjunction with optical magnifi-

Chapter 12   **291**

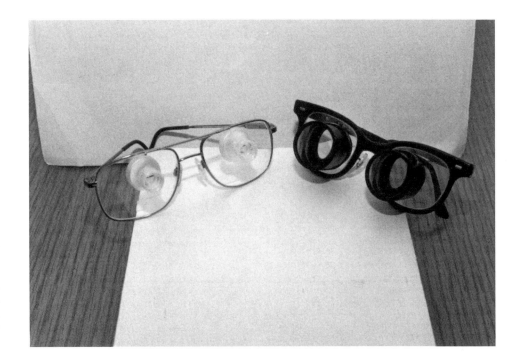

Figure 12-16—Total field enhancement systems. This system on the left is a DVI reverse field telescope mounted in a frame; the system on the right is a Designs for Vision Amorphic lens. Both are used to increase the amount of information viewed by shrinking what is seen. Another option (not shown) is a simple minus lens.

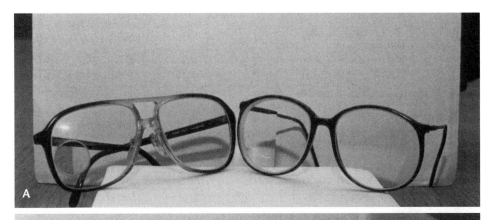

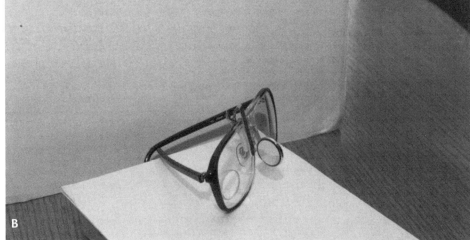

Figure 12-17—Field-specific enhancement systems. Field-specific enhancement systems are usually worn. A. The system on the left is the Gottlieb Visual Field Awareness System; the system on the right is the Onufryk Prism Image Relocator. B. A mirror system may also be used. Not shown is a Fresnel prism, which may be placed on an existing lens.

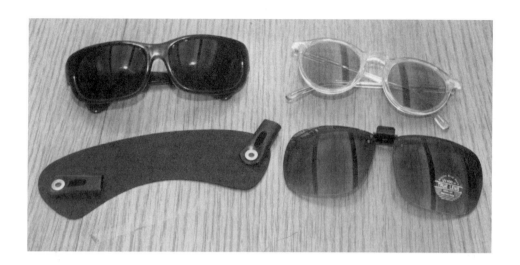

Figure 12-18—Filters. Black and white photos do not display filters well. Note, however, that they are not clear. Colors may vary both in density and wavelength absorption and transmission.

cation or by themselves when optical magnification is either not appropriate or necessary (Figure 12-18).

SUMMARY OF EXAMINATION

At the conclusion of the examination and before vision rehabilitation training with optical devices, the low vision test results should be summarized with the patient, caregiver, and/or support people. Reinforce that better sight or field awareness has been demonstrated through the course of the examination.

At this time, it is also important to confirm the patient's goals and the optical and nonoptical methods of achieving those goals. Unless the amount of work necessary to achieve the goal(s) is understood, patients may become disenchanted and frustrated. To minimize this, it helps if the patient understands that visual success is divided into two categories—optical and functional.

Optical success or improved acuity is demonstrated during the examination. *Functional success* depends on the patient's perception of success and the use of the options recommended to accomplish the goals. The assistant's input here is immeasurable. Training in the use of the device is critical to functional success. A structured, systematic, sequenced program of vision rehabilitation is key to improving the visual quality of life for vision-impaired individuals.

Low Vision Device Training

The use of a low vision device is a complex process. Success is dependent on optical experience, not necessarily on age or intelligence. Attempting to prescribe single or multiple low vision devices without providing instruction may cause confusion and discouragement for the low vision patient.

Low vision devices should be prescribed only after they have been successfully used in the office and at home. A structured program may be designed with the patient's goals in mind and should be used to acquaint the patient with the advantages and limitations of the device as well as the functional use of the system. An example of this may help further understanding.

A patient is recommended a +40.00 D lens in a head-mounted system. This will require the materials to be held approximately 1 inch, or 2.5 cm (see Figure 12-2), from the patient's face. Assume that the patient has been properly refracted and needs no additional refractive correction. In this example, the patient is plano, so the lens is actually +40.00 D. The patient should be instructed to do the following[13]:

1. Before receiving the microscope, do the following:
   a. Familiarize the patient with the 1-inch working distance by instructing the patient to train the muscles that will be used to hold the materials. To do this,

have the patient move the hands to 1 inch from the face.
  b. The patient should then move the hands in a parallel fashion in front of the eyes much the same way as the patient will be moving materials when the device is dispensed.
2. When the device is initially placed on the patient's face, the materials should be placed at 1 inch and should be larger than the patient will ultimately want to see. This should guarantee immediate optical/visual success.
3. Activities to train eye-hand movements should then be given to allow the patient the opportunity to work at the appropriate working distance, using the full field of view of the device.
4. Once this is successfully accomplished under the watchful eye of the assistant, the materials should be decreased in size until the desired size is achieved. Then, short-term reading projects and ultimately more extensive reading projects may be undertaken. This may take only one visit or may require multiple visits. If more than one visit is required, specific activities should be assigned for home training.
5. Once this is successful, other low vision devices can be explored, with the paraoptometric demonstrating various devices for different ways of viewing a task. Once the patient has an optical base from which to proceed, learning to use other devices should be easier.

This type of training to introduce the patient to devices may be done with hand-held, stand, and electronic systems as well as telescopic systems.

Psychological Impact of Visual Impairment

Any pathologic process will create a deviation from the psychological norm. It is the patient's desire to return to normal that will determine the degree of despair, frustration, discouragement, and so forth experienced by the patient. Doctors and assistants specializing in low vision may find that not all patients are willing to put in the same time or effort to achieve functional success based on the low vision recommendations. With empathy and proper structured guidance, however, most patients eventually appreciate the vision that remains and ultimately learn to take advantage of the capability to use it maximally through low vision devices. The paraoptometric is key to helping the low vision patient improve the visual quality of his or her life.

REFERENCES

1. Freeman PB. Low vision practices and the paraoptometric. J Am Optometric Assoc 1981;52:57.
2. Freeman PB, Jose RT. The Art and Practice of Low Vision. Boston: Butterworth, 1991;9.
3. Jose RT. Understanding Low Vision. New York: American Foundation for the Blind, 1983;141.
4. Bailey IL, Lovie JE. New design principles for visual acuity letter charts. Am J Optom Physiol Optics 1976;53:740.
5. Jose RT, Watson G. Increasing reading efficiency with an optical aid/training curriculum. Rev Optom 1978;115:41.
6. Wolfe JM. An Introduction to Contrast Sensitivity Testing. In M Nadler, D Miller, D Nadler (eds), Glare and Contrast Sensitivity for Clinicians. New York: Springer, 1990.
7. Borish IM. Clinical Refraction. Chicago: Professional Press, 1970;598.
8. Anstice J. Vision Care in the Home and in Institutional Settings. In A Rosenbloom, M Morgan (eds), Vision and Aging. New York: Professional Press, 1986.
9. Faye EE. Clinical Low Vision. Boston: Little, Brown, 1984;27.
10. Mehr E, Fried AN. Low Vision Care. Chicago: Professional Press, 1975;81.
11. Freeman PB. Rxing a simple reading aid for the older patient. Rev Optom 1984;121:61.
12. Gottleib D, Freeman P, Williams M. Clinical research and statistical analysis of a visual field awareness system. J Am Optometric Assoc 1992;63:581.
13. Freeman PB, Jose RT. After the Initial Examination. In PB Freeman, RT Jose (eds), The Art and Practice of Low Vision. Boston: Butterworth-Heinemann, 1991;35.

13/Binocular Vision

Karen Pollack

This chapter acquaints the paraoptometric with binocular disorders that interfere with everyday life and discusses how these disorders are treated.

During the time of the Civil War, a man named Snellen invented a chart for testing vision. The Snellen chart consists of letters of different sizes to be used to test vision at 20 feet and is a means of measuring *visual acuity*. When we measure visual acuity, we are measuring the ability of the eye to resolve detail (see Chapter 8).

Skills that give us the power or means to locate, identify, and remember what we see are known as *visual abilities*. These include keeping objects focused at different distances (including reading distance), keeping objects as single images, judging depth, locating words when reading, guiding a pencil, recognizing what is seen, and remembering what is seen. We refer to the use of these abilities as *vision*. Vision is the result of a person's ability to interpret the environment on the basis of information received through the eyes.

There are two components to vision: *visual efficiency* and *visual processing*, or visual perception. Visual efficiency includes accommodation, binocular vision, and ocular motor skills. If these skills are deficient, they may interfere with an individual's ability to gather information clearly and comfortably through the visual system. Visual processing includes directionality, visual spatial skills, visual analysis skills, and visual motor integration.

Vision, as are other abilities, is learned. The idea that vision is learned and can be taught at any age forms the basis for a form of treatment that we refer to as *vision therapy* (also known as orthoptics or vision training). Vision therapy is a process during which patients are given practice and feedback that teaches them to develop or enhance their visual abilities.

BINOCULAR VISION DISORDERS (EYE-TEAMING DISORDERS)

Binocular vision disorders, or eye-teaming disorders, refer to a variety of conditions in which the eyes drift in, out, up, or down.

There are few parts of the body that must work together with more precision than the eyes. The ability to maintain both eyes pointed at precisely the same object is *eye teaming*, or *binocularity*. Eye teaming is a crucial ability to have in order for the eyes to perform without discomfort. When both eyes are accurately aimed at the object being viewed, the information coming from the two eyes will be combined in the brain into a single image.

Fusion is the merging of the images from each eye into a single visual image. *Sensory fusion* is the process by which a single image is perceived from two separate ocular images. *Motor fusion* is the actual eye movement that occurs to keep the eyes aligned on the target of regard.

There are three degrees of motor fusion: *superimposition* (first-degree fusion) is the overlapping of two dissimilar objects; *flat fusion* (second-degree fusion) occurs when two similar images are seen as a single object; and *stereopsis* (third-degree fusion), the highest degree of fusion, is the perception of depth.

Vergence movements help align the eyes to ensure and maintain binocular vision. They are, by definition, movements of the two eyes in opposite directions. *Convergence* is the simultaneous turning in of both eyes that occurs when viewing an approaching object. There is a link between accommodation and convergence. When doing near point work, the eyes must not only focus for the plane of regard but also converge so that they both aim exactly at the same point. Even though these two systems function well independently, there must be a good relationship between them in order for near point work to proceed efficiently.

Divergence is the simultaneous turning out of both eyes when viewing an object moving away from the eyes. When a person accommodates, an amount of convergence is elicited. This is known as *accommodative convergence*. The ratio of accommodative convergence to accommodation is called the *AC/A ratio* and is expressed in units of prism diopters of convergence over diopters of accommodation (e.g., 4Δ/1 D). This ratio varies for different people and may be greater or less than the requirement for convergence of the fixation target.

A high AC/A ratio indicates a tendency for the eyes to turn in (esophoria); a low ratio indicates a tendency is for the eyes to turn out (exophoria). The convergence due to accommodation provides the initial gross change in position of the two eyes relative to the target.

Fusional vergence movements are accomplished to preserve single binocular vision. The stimulus for fusional convergence is disparate retinal images. If the eyes are aligned but slip imperceptible amounts at near, words may not pull entirely apart, but the letters may merely run together. The near point of convergence, the cover test at distance and near, measurement of the AC/A ratio, and smooth vergence ranges at distance and near are the tests routinely done in an evaluation to assess binocularity.

The purpose of the *near point of convergence test* is to assess the convergence amplitude. A remote near point of convergence with a break of more than 4 inches is considered the most consistent finding in convergence insufficiency. A penlight or transilluminator is the recommended target for testing the near point of convergence. Using a light frees the patient from accommodation.

The *cover test* is an objective method of evaluating the presence, direction, and the magnitude of the phoria (phoria is a latent deviation of the eyes which is overcome by motor fusion to result in sensory fusion) (Figure 13-1). The examiner may use multiple fixation targets to maintain attention and accommodation on the task. This may be accomplished easily using a tongue depressor with small targets on both sides of the top and bottom of the stick. The alternate cover test is performed by alternating an occluder from one eye to the other while the patient fixates the target on the tongue depressor. The examiner watches for an eye movement of the uncovered eye. At distance, the expected value is 1Δ exophoria with a standard deviation of ±1Δ. The mean expected value at near is 3Δ exophoria with a standard deviation of ±3Δ.

The purpose of measuring the AC/A ratio is to determine the change in accommodative convergence that occurs when the patient accommodates or relaxes accommodation a given amount. One way to test the AC/A ratio is to measure the phoria with the subjective distance refraction in place and then again with –1.00 D over the subjective. The difference between the two measurements is the AC/A ratio. The expected AC/A ratio is 4/1 with a standard deviation of ±2Δ.

Smooth vergence testing assesses the fusional vergence amplitude and recovery at both distance and near. The blur finding is a measure of the amount of fusional vergence free of accommodation. The break indicates the amount of fusional vergence. The recovery finding provides information about the patient's ability to regain single binocular vision after diplopia occurs. The expected findings for smooth vergence testing are found in Table 13-1.

When the eyes have no stimulus to fuse, they go to their natural resting position, the *phoric posture*. If both eyes continue to point straight ahead, even with fusion broken, their resting or phoric posture is *ortho*. If the lines of sight cross in front of the fixation point, they are *esophoric*, and if they cross behind the fixation point, they are *exophoric*. When the patient makes an attempt to fuse, the first thing that must be overcome is phoria. The type of fusional vergence used by esophores is divergence; the

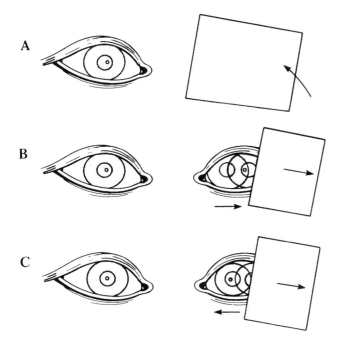

Table 13-1. Expected findings for smooth vergence testing

Smooth vergence testing	Expected finding		Standard deviation
Base out (distance)	Blur	9	±4 D
	Break	19	±8 D
	Recovery	10	±4 D
Base in (distance)	Break	7	±3 D
	Recovery	4	±2 D
Base out (near)	Blur	17	±5 D
	Break	21	±6 D
	Recovery	11	±7 D
Base in (near)	Blur	13	±4 D
	Break	21	±4 D
	Recovery	13	±5 D

Figure 13-1—A. Covering the O.S. in the first step of the cover test. B. Esophoria. Note the movement of the eye temporally to pick up fixation. C. Exophoria. Note the movement of the eye nasally to pick up fixation.

type used by exophores is convergence. The two most common binocular disorders are *convergence insufficiency* and *convergence excess*.

Convergence Insufficiency

Convergence insufficiency is a condition in which the patient has difficulty turning his or her eyes in. Some of the expected findings when performing a binocular vision exam of patients with convergence insufficiency are exophoria at near, orthophoria or low exophoria at distance, a receded near point of convergence, reduced base-out vergence, and a low AC/A ratio.

Most symptoms reported by the patient are associated with reading or other work that requires the patient to focus on something close to his or her eyes. Common complaints include eyestrain and headaches after short periods of reading, blurred vision, diplopia, sleepiness, difficulty concentrating, loss of concentration and comprehension over time, a pulling sensation behind the eyes, and movement of the words on a page. Some patients with convergence insufficiency are asymptomatic. This absence of symptoms may be due to suppression, avoidance of near visual tasks, high pain threshold, or occlusion of one eye when reading. Task avoidance is as important a reason for recommending therapy as any of the other symptoms associated with convergence insufficiency.

A vision therapy program for convergence insufficiency generally requires 12–24 office visits. The total number of therapy sessions also depends on the age of the patient, motivation, and compliance. Motivated adults can sometimes successfully complete vision therapy for convergence insufficiency in 10–12 visits. The first goal of the therapy itself is to teach the concept and feeling of converging. Once the patient can voluntarily initiate a controlled convergence movement, the other goals of the vision therapy program become much easier to accomplish. Refer to Table 13-2 and Figures 13-2 and 13-3 for treatment plan objectives for convergence insufficiency.

Convergence Excess

Convergence excess is a condition in which there is an esophoria at near, orthophoria or low to moderate esophoria at distance, reduced base in vergence, and a high AC/A ratio. The patient has difficulty with divergence.

Most symptoms are associated with reading or other work that requires the patient to focus on something close to his or her eyes. Common complaints include eyestrain and headaches

TABLE 13-2. Vision therapy objectives for convergence insufficiency
Phase 1 objectives
Develop a working relationship with the patient
Develop an awareness of the various feedback mechanisms that will be used throughout therapy
Develop voluntary convergence
Normalize positive fusional vergence amplitudes (smooth or tonic vergence demand)
Normalize accommodative amplitude and ability to stimulate and relax accommodation
Phase 2 objectives
Normalize negative fusional vergence amplitudes (smooth or tonic vergence demand)
Normalize positive fusional vergence facility (jump or phasic vergence demand)
Normalize negative fusional vergence facility (jump or phasic vergence demand)
Phase 3 objectives
Develop ability to change from a convergence to a divergence demand
Integrate vergence procedures with changes in accommodative demand
Integrate vergence procedures with versions and saccades

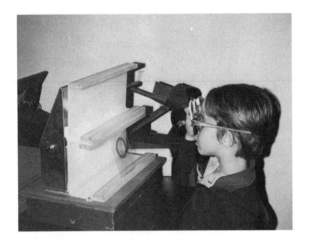

Figure 13-2—Convergence training with a topper vectogram in the polachrome trainer.

after short periods of reading, blurred vision, diplopia, sleepiness, and difficulty concentrating. Some patients with convergence excess are asymptomatic. For the same reason as for patients with convergence insufficiency, this may be due to suppression, avoidance of near visual tasks, high pain threshold, or occlusion of one eye when reading. Clinicians should always inquire about avoidance of reading or other near tasks if a patient with convergence excess reports an absence of other symptoms. Because of the high AC/A ratio, the use of plus lenses at near is an effective treatment alternative. Plus lenses relax accommodation and reduce the amount of accommodative convergence.

If negative fusional vergence is severely reduced, the magnitude of the esophoria is very large, or the patient remains uncomfortable even after wearing glasses, vision therapy should be recommended. A vision therapy program for convergence excess generally requires 12–24 office visits. If refractive correction and plus lenses are used, the number of sessions is usually less. The total number of therapy sessions also depends on the age of the patient, motivation, and compliance. See Table 13-3 for treatment plan objectives for convergence excess.

ACCOMMODATION

The ability to see objects clearly at every distance is primarily the responsibility of the accommodative system. Not only must we be able to focus quickly and effortlessly at different distances but also we must also have the ability to sustain that focusing for long periods of time. The eye is constructed so that light rays coming from a distant object will be parallel and will focus on the retina in the emmetropic eye. With objects located closer to the eye, light rays are no longer parallel and need to be acted on by the eye in order to be focused on the retina and seen clearly. This is accomplished by changes in the shape of the crystalline lens. The lens is controlled by

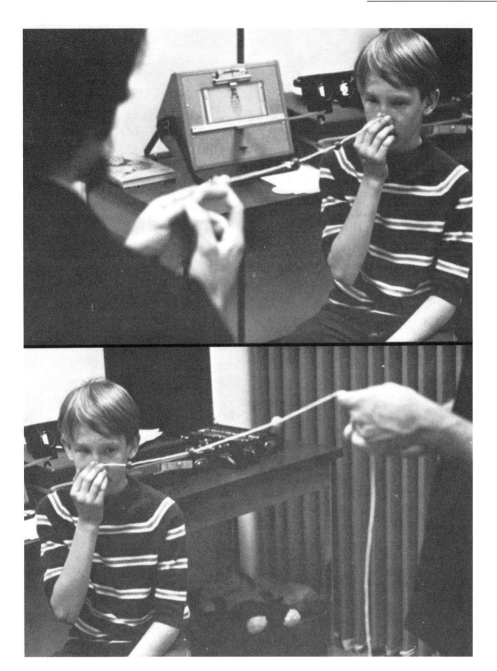

Figure 13-3—Convergence and divergence training with a brock string. (Reproduced with permission from JR Griffin, JD Grisham. Binocular Anomalies: Diagnosis and Vision Therapy [3rd ed]. Boston: Butterworth-Heinemann, 1995;363.)

contractions of the ciliary muscle of the eye. When this muscle contracts, tension is relaxed and the lens changes shape, becoming thicker and more rounded, increasing its focusing power.

It has been determined that between birth and 1 month of age, the accommodative system of a human baby is locked into the 5.00 D level. By 3 months of age, however, the system no longer appears to be locked in, and accommodation seems to vary with target distance. This also corresponds with foveal development and supports the concept of the fovea being the trigger for the accommodative system.

The evaluation of accommodative function involves measurement of the amplitude of accommodation and accommodative facility and sustainability. *Amplitude* refers to the amount of accommodation; *facility* refers to the ability to be able to change the focusing system accurately and sustain focusing for long periods of time.

The *accommodative amplitude* and *near point of accommodation tests* provide information con-

TABLE 13-3. Vision therapy objectives for convergence excess

Phase 1 objectives
    Develop a working relationship with the patient
    Develop an awareness of the various feedback mechanisms that will be used throughout therapy
    Develop voluntary convergence and divergence
    Normalize base in vergence amplitudes (smooth or tonic vergence demand)
    Normalize accommodative amplitude and ability to stimulate and relax accommodation
Phase 2 objectives
    Normalize base out vergence amplitudes (smooth or tonic vergence demand)
    Normalize base in vergence facility (jump or phasic vergence demand)
    Normalize base out vergence facility (jump or phasic vergence demand)
Phase 3 objectives
    Develop ability to change from a convergence to a divergence demand
    Integrate vergence procedures with changes in accommodative demand
    Integrate vergence procedures with versions

cerning the total limit of function of the system from relaxation of accommodation to maximal effort. The amplitude is measured under monocular conditions using either Donder's push-up test or minus lens test. A variety of norms may be used for monocular accommodative amplitude. There are tables developed by Duane and Donders that provide expected findings by age. A more commonly used system is Hofstetter's formula, which is based on Duane's figures. It is critical to measure the distance at which the patient reports a blur accurately. Even small errors in measurement may lead to large differences in results. For example, an endpoint at 2 inches suggests a 20 D amplitude, whereas a blur at 2.5 inches suggests an amplitude of 16 D. To reduce this problem, the push-up amplitude may be measured through –4.00 lenses. This modification moves the endpoint further away from the patient and allows more exact measurement of the endpoint.

The *average amplitude* at any age may be calculated using the following formula:

$$18.5 - \frac{\text{age in years}}{3}$$

The *minimum amplitude* expected for a given age may be calculated using the following formula:

$$15 - \frac{\text{age in years}}{4}$$

Accommodative facility and sustainability are both dynamic functions of the accommodative system and indicate how efficiently the system works. *Facility testing* evaluates how efficiently and quickly a person changes accommodative levels; *sustainability tests* how long a person can use the system before it fatigues. It is recommended that the doctor use a 20/30 single vertical line for this test. Testing should be done binocularly unless the patient has an accommodative or a binocular disorder. Binocular testing is an assessment of the interactions between accommodation and vergence and is not a pure measurement of accommodative facility. If a patient is binocular, the introduction of minus lenses will require the patient to stimulate accommodation to maintain clarity. As the patient accommodates, accommodative convergence will be stimulated, and the patient will lose binocularity unless he or she makes a compensatory response. To prevent the loss of binocularity, the patient must use negative fusional vergence to compensate for the accommodative convergence. As minus lenses are introduced, both the ability to stimulate accommodation and negative fusional vergence (divergence) are assessed. A normal response on binocular accommodative facility testing suggests normal function in both areas. If a patient experiences difficulty with binocular testing, monocular testing may be administered. If the patient cannot clear minus lenses binocularly, and even after occluding an eye still cannot clear

TABLE 13-4. Expected findings for accommodative facility

Age (years)	Expected finding (cycles per min)	Standard deviation (cycles per min)
Monocular accommodative facility (using a ±2.00 flipper)		
6	5.5	±2.5
7	6.5	±2
8–12	7	±2.5
13–30	11	±5
31–40	—	—
Binocular accommodative facility (using a ±2.00 flipper)		
6	3	±2.5
7	3.5	±2.5
8–12	5	±2.5
13–30	8	±5
31–40	9	±5

minus, an accommodative problem is present. If the patient fails binocularly and passes monocularly, a binocular vision problem is more likely. The expected findings for accommodative facility are found in Table 13-4.

There are three primary types of accommodative disorders: *accommodative insufficiency*, *accommodative excess*, and *accommodative infacility*.

Accommodative Insufficiency and Ill-Sustained Accommodation

Accommodative insufficiency is a condition in which the patient has difficulty stimulating accommodation. Low amplitude of accommodation is the hallmark of accommodative insufficiency.

Ill-sustained accommodation, or accommodative fatigue, has been categorized by most authors as a subclassification of accommodative insufficiency. It is a condition in which the amplitude of accommodation is normal under typical test conditions but deteriorates over time.

The most common complaints include blur, headaches, eyestrain, double vision, reading problems, fatigue, difficulty changing focus from one distance to another, and sensitivity to light. Patients may also complain of an inability to concentrate, a loss of comprehension over time, and words seeming to move on the page. All of these symptoms are associated with reading or other work that requires the patient to focus on objects near to his or her eyes. Some patients with accommodative insufficiency are asymptomatic. In such cases, the most likely explanation is avoidance of reading and other close work.

A vision therapy program for accommodative insufficiency generally requires 12–24 office visits. As with convergence insufficiency and convergence excess, the total number of therapy sessions also depends on the age of the patient, motivation, and compliance. See Table 13-5 for treatment plan objectives for accommodative insufficiency.

Accommodative Excess

Accommodative excess is a condition in which the patient has difficulty with all tasks requiring relaxation of accommodation.

Most symptoms are associated with reading or other close work. Common complaints include blurred vision, eyestrain and headaches after short periods of reading, light sensitivity, difficulty attending and concentrating on reading tasks, and diplopia. The symptom of blurred vision may be associated with both near work and distance tasks such as looking at the chalkboard, television, and driving. A characteristic of the blurred vision associated with accommodative excess is that it is often variable and worse toward the end of the day or after extensive near work.

A vision therapy program for accommodative excess generally requires 12–24 office visits. Refer to Table 13-6 for treatment plan objectives for accommodative excess.

Accommodative Infacility

Accommodative infacility is a condition in which the patient experiences difficulty changing the accommodative response level. An important characteristic of accommodative infacility is that it is a condition in which latency and speed of the accommodative response are abnormal. Thus, it is a disorder in which the amplitude is normal yet the patient's ability to make use of this amplitude quickly and for long periods of time is inadequate. This distinction between amplitude and

TABLE 13-5. Vision therapy objectives for accommodative insufficiency

Phase 1 objectives
    Develop a working relationship with the patient
    Develop an awareness of the various feedback mechanisms that will be used throughout therapy
    Normalize accommodative amplitude and ability to stimulate accommodation
    Develop voluntary convergence
    Normalize base out fusional vergence amplitudes (smooth or tonic vergence demand)
Phase 2 objectives
    Normalize ability to stimulate and relax accommodation
    Incorporate speed of response into accommodative techniques
    Normalize base in fusional vergence amplitudes (smooth or tonic vergence demand)
    Normalize base out fusional vergence facility (jump or phasic vergence demand)
    Normalize base in fusional vergence facility (jump or phasic vergence demand)
Phase 3 objectives
    Integrate accommodative facility therapy with binocular vision techniques
    Develop ability to change from a convergence to a divergence demand
    Integrate vergence procedures with versions and saccades

Table 13-6. Vision therapy objectives for accommodative excess

Phase 1 objectives
    Develop a working relationship with the patient
    Develop an awareness of the various feedback mechanisms that will be used throughout therapy
    Develop feeling of diverging
    Normalize base in vergence amplitudes at near (smooth or tonic vergence demand)
    Normalize accommodative amplitude and ability to stimulate and relax accommodation
Phase 2 objectives
    Normalize base out vergence amplitudes (smooth or tonic vergence demand)
    Normalize base in vergence facility at near (jump or phasic vergence demand)
    Normalize base out vergence facility (jump or phasic vergence demand)
Phase 3 objectives
    Normalize base in vergence amplitudes at intermediate distances
    Normalize base in vergence facility at far

facility of response is similar to that present for binocular vision anomalies.

Most symptoms are associated with reading or other close work. Common complaints are blurred vision, difficulty sustaining and attending to reading and other close work, and fatigue. The symptom most characteristic of accommodative infacility is difficulty changing focus from one distance to another.

A vision therapy program for accommodative infacility generally requires the same number of visits as the other accommodative disorders, 12–24. Since the patient already has normal amplitudes, the goal of training is to increase the speed of the accommodative response and reduce the latency. See Table 13-6 for treatment plan objectives for accommodative infacility, which are the same as for the treatment plan objectives for accommodative excess.

OCULOMOTOR DYSFUNCTION

Eye movement control develops early in a child's life. By age 2 months, a child can follow a moving target in the midplane of his or her body; by 3 months of age, a child can follow in all directions. Eye movement disorders are a diagnostic and management concern of optometrists because of the effect such problems may have on the functional capability of an individual. Accommodative and binocular vision skills reach adult levels of development very early in infancy. Clinical assessment indicates that eye movement development is considerably slower than other visual abilities. The development of eye movements continues through the early elementary school years. The long developmental process for eye movement control may leave a child with inadequate skills to meet the demands of the classroom. Difficulty with saccades and pursuits primarily interfere with performance in schoolchildren, although these problems have been reported in adults as well.

Saccades are rapid eye movements that enable us to redirect our line of sight so that the point of interest aligns with the fovea. Saccades are the fastest eye movement. Accurate saccades are important not only in the act of reading but also in almost any visual activity, including copying from the board or a book, sports, and many job-related activities.

Pursuits enable continuous clear vision of moving objects. This object-following vision reflex ideally produces eye movements that assure continuous foveal fixation of objects moving in space while keeping the object fixed on the fovea. Eye movement disorders are rarely present in isolation. They are generally found associated with accommodative, binocular, and visual perceptual dysfunctions.

Most symptoms related to saccadic dysfunction are associated with reading. These include head movement, frequent loss of place, omission of words, skipping lines, slow reading speed, poor comprehension, and short attention span.

Although pursuit difficulties have been reported in children that have reading problems, pursuit dysfunction is also likely to interfere with activities such as sports. Symptoms such as trouble catching and hitting a baseball and difficulty with other sports involving timing and following a moving object may be related to pursuit dysfunction.

Examination of eye movements involves three distinct steps: assessment of stability of fixation, saccadic function, and pursuit func-

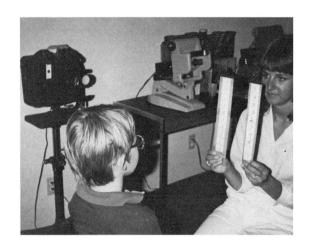

Figure 13-4—Testing saccades monocularly.

tion. Asking the patient to maintain steady fixation on a target with no observable movement of the eyes for 10 seconds is a test used to assess fixation stability.

The purpose of saccadic testing is to assess the quality and accuracy of saccadic function. Two tests used to evaluate saccades involve direct observation by the clinician or a timed/standardized test involving a visual-verbal format. Quality of movement is what is watched for when testing saccades. The patient is asked to look back and forth from one target to another in both the horizontal and vertical meridians. The examiner watches for an undershoot or overshoot, each of which looks exactly like the name given to it. The ability of the patient to pick up accurate fixation of the target is important in this test. Grading is subjective (Figure 13-4).

The Developmental Eye Movement Test is less subjective and is usually the preferred test given. The patient is asked to call off a series of numbers as quickly as possible without using a finger or pointer as a guide. The numbers are presented vertically in Tests A and B, which minimizes the need for horizontal eye movements, and in a horizontal spatial array in Test C. The response times and number of errors are then compared with tables of expecteds (Figure 13-5).

The purpose of pursuit testing is to assess the quality and accuracy of pursuit function. Direct observation of the patient's eyes following a moving target is the most commonly used clinical technique for assessing pursuits. The patient is asked to follow a target moved left to

3	4
7	5
5	2
9	1
8	7
2	5
5	3
7	7
4	4
6	8
1	7
4	4
7	6
6	5
3	2
7	9
9	2
3	3
9	6
2	4

3		7	5			9		8
2	5			7		4		6
1			4		7		6	3
7		9		3		9		2
4	5				2		1	7
5			3		7		4	8
7	4		6	5				2
9		2			3		6	4
6	3	2		9				1
7				4		6	5	2
5		3	7			4		8
4				5		2	1	7
7	9	3				9		2
1				4		7	6	3
2		5			7		4	6
3	7		5			9		8

Figure 13-5—The Developmental Eye Movement Test, tests A (left) and C (right). (Reproduced with permission from JR Griffin, JD Grisham. Binocular Anomalies: Diagnosis and Vision Therapy [3rd ed]. Boston: Butterworth-Heinemann, 1995;27.)

right, up and down, and then in a circular fashion. The movement of the target should be restricted to the circumference of the patient's head. This procedure is done monocularly.

A vision therapy program for oculomotor dysfunction generally requires 12–24 visits if vision therapy is office based. Refer to Table 13-7 for treatment plan objectives for oculomotor dysfunction.

STRABISMUS

Strabismus exists when the foveal lines of sight of the two eyes do not point to the same object in space. Strabismus is a manifest deviation of the eyes for which the system cannot compensate. This is in contrast to a phoria, which is a latent deviation held in check by fusional vergence. When fusion is broken by occluding one eye, the eyes will return to the phoric position. When the occluder is removed, the eye returns to its correct position for binocular fixation (vergence movement). If the deviation is present only when fusion is artificially broken, it is a *latent deviation*. Strabismus, on the other hand, is not held in check by fusion and becomes a *manifest deviation* (Figure 13-6).

There are several variables to consider for the determination of prognosis. The first relates to the difference between concomitant and nonconcomitant deviations. A deviation (angle of turn) is concomitant if the angle of deviation remains the same in all positions of gaze at a specified distance. In a nonconcomitant deviation, the deviation changes when the eyes move from one position of gaze to another. Nonconcomitancy may be caused by a paretic muscle, faulty muscle insertion, or cranial nerve damage.

TABLE 13-7. Vision therapy objectives for oculomotor dysfunction

Phase 1 objectives
    Develop a working relationship with the patient
    Develop an awareness of the various feedback mechanisms that will be used throughout therapy
    Develop more accurate gross saccades and fine pursuits
    Equalize gross saccadic and pursuit ability in the two eyes
    Normalize base out and base in vergence amplitudes (smooth or tonic vergence demand)
    Normalize accommodative amplitude and ability to stimulate and relax accommodation
Phase 2 objectives
    Develop more accurate fine saccades and large excursion pursuits
    Equalize fine saccadic and pursuit ability in the two eyes
    Normalize base out and base in vergence amplitudes (smooth or tonic vergence demand)
    Normalize base out and base in vergence facility (jump or phasic vergence demand)
Phase 3 objectives
    Integrate accurate saccades and pursuits with changes in vergence and accommodation
    Develop ability to change from a convergence to a divergence demand

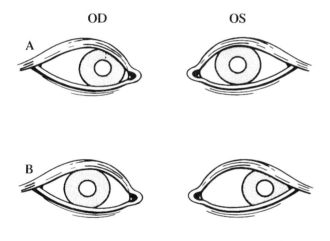

Figure 13-6—A. Right esotropia. B. Left exotropia.

The second variable is the direction of the strabismus. The direction of turn is critical. This will determine progress as well as the method of treatment. The turning in of an eye is known as *esotropia*; the turning out is known as *exotropia*. In *hypertropia*, the eye deviates up; in *hypotropia*, the eye deviates down.

The third variable, eye laterality, indicates whether the eye turn is unilateral (one eye only) or if it alternates between the two eyes.

The fourth variable in the diagnosis of strabismus is the frequency of the deviation. It is important for predicting success in alleviating the problem and in assessing binocularity. The terms used to denote frequency are *constant* and *intermittent*. When a patient presents with a strabismus, an accurate case history is vital to determine the onset of the eye turn. The onset of the eye turn will distinguish a congenital from an acquired strabismus. Any turn noted prior to 6 months of age is considered congenital, whereas those noted after 6 months are considered to be acquired.

In determining the treatment for the strabismic patient, the cause of the turn must be investigated and diagnosed. Both congenital and acquired strabismus may be the result of trauma or neurologic or disease processes. These factors must be ruled out as causes because they can be life-threatening situations that require immediate referral. Refractive errors are often a primary cause of strabismus.

There are many tests used by the optometrist to detect and diagnose strabismus. One test that is important to perform is the cover test. The cover test is one of the most useful tests in the investigation of strabismus. By occluding an eye, a latent deviation may be exposed (phoria) or the determination of a manifest deviation may be established (strabismus). The two types of cover tests are the *alternate* and the *unilateral*.

The alternate cover test is performed by alternating the occluder from one eye to the other while the patient fixates the target. The examiner watches for a versional movement of the uncovered eye, which indicates a deviation.

No movement indicates no deviation. Since only one eye is fixating at a time, fusion is never possible during the alternate cover test. Therefore, it is difficult at this time to determine whether the deviation represents a phoria or strabismus.

The unilateral cover test is used to determine whether the deviation is latent (phoria) or manifest (strabismus). The occluder is placed before one eye and then removed while the examiner watches for movement of either eye.

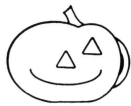

Figure 13-7—Second-degree fusion target.

Suppression and Diplopia

When a manifest deviation is present and the foveal areas of the two eyes do not point at the same object, the result will be diplopia (double vision) or confusion. Suppression is the adaptive mechanism seen most often as an attempt by the visual system to eliminate diplopia and confusion. The suppression process is an active cortical mechanism. Suppression may also occur in the nonstrabismic patient.

Simultaneous perception is considered one of the levels of sensory fusion; however, no fusion is really occurring. It occurs because of the stimulation of noncorresponding points. *Superimposition* (first-degree fusion) occurs when two dissimilar objects stimulate corresponding retinal points. *Flat fusion* (second-degree fusion) occurs when two similar objects stimulate corresponding retinal points (Figure 13-7). They have common visual directions and are perceived as superimposed. *Stereopsis* (third-degree fusion) is the highest degree of fusion and is the perception of depth due to binocular cues. No depth perception indicates a binocular problem or suppression. Commonly used tests for depth perception or stereopsis are the Titmus Stereo Fly and the Randot test.

Amblyopia

Amblyopia, or lazy eye, is the condition that exists when there is reduced visual acuity not correctable by refractive means and not attributable to obvious structural or pathologic anomalies of the eye. Vision worse than 20/30 or a two-line difference in acuity between the two eyes is considered to be amblyopia. Another indication of amblyopia is poor eye movement and possibly poor fixational abilities.

There are three types of functional amblyopia: strabismic, refractive, and form deprivation. Optometrists deal mainly with these patients.

Strabismic amblyopia arises from nonuse or prolonged suppression. *Refractive amblyopia* may be caused by an uncorrected refractive error. *Form deprivation amblyopia* usually occurs due to a physical obstruction along the line of sight such as a congenital cataract.

Careful visual acuity testing can provide information about a patient with amblyopia. When testing the normal eye, letters are consistently identified up to a certain acuity level and then consistently missed. There should be a constant cutoff of correct identification. This does not occur in the functional amblyope. This patient may identify one or two letters on each line, usually the first and last. There is no exact cutoff point for this patient. This is attributable to the *crowding phenomenon*, which is a difficulty in identifying targets close to each other. It is more pronounced in the amblyopic eye and is seen when taking visual acuities. Whole-chart acuity must be changed to single-line acuity or to single-letter acuity when testing the amblyope.

The first step in treating amblyopia is correction of the refractive error. Then occlusion therapy is recommended. Occlusion is a generally accepted procedure for the treatment of amblyopia. In occlusion therapy, the fixating eye is prevented from taking part in the act of vision so that the patient is forced to use his or her amblyopic eye. This is known as *direct patching*, which is the recommended approach. It is always important to accompany patching with activities that encourage the patient to use the amblyopic eye to help break down suppression and increase acuity. These are mainly hand-eye tasks that depend on the acuity of the patient, ranging from oculomotor exercises to accommodative exercises. The important point is that the patient actively attempts to use the eye. Binocular training begins when 20/40 acuity is attained. In-office vision therapy is also highly recommended.

Eccentric Fixation

Eccentric fixation is present under monocular conditions. The amblyopic eye fixates with a retinal area other than the fovea. If fixation is unsteady or another part of the retina is used for fixation, visual acuity is reduced. Two variables are used when assessing the fixation of a patient: central versus eccentric and the stability of the retinal area used, and steady versus unsteady. If the same point of the retina is always used, fixation is steady; if different points are used, fixation is considered unsteady. Both the amount of eccentricity and the degree of unsteadiness will determine the degree of decreased visual acuity.

Anomalous Retinal Correspondence

Each retinal point has a paired retinal point in the other eye that has the same visual direction. Images stimulating these points are interpreted as originating from the same point in space. The foveae of each eye are corresponding points and are interpreted as the straight-ahead position.

Normal correspondence results in binocular vision when corresponding retinal points are stimulated and a single percept is observed. An abnormal situation may develop where the foveae and other paired retinal points no longer have the same visual direction. The fovea, for instance, may become paired with a nasal retinal point in the esotropic patient. Stimulation of the two foveae in this patient will yield diplopia instead of a binocular image, as in the patient with normal correspondence. Single vision will occur only if the fovea of the good eye and the nasal point in the strabismic eye are stimulated. The nasal retinal point now has the straight-ahead position and acts as the new fovea. The fovea is now located temporal to the straight-ahead position and projects objects nasally

There are several variations of anomalous retinal correspondence (ARC), including harmonious ARC, unharmonious ARC, and paradoxical types I and II. Diagnosis of these will depend on the type of strabismus present and its complications, such as surgery.

Testing for ARC is always done with both eyes open. Unlike the monocular testing for eccentric fixation, ARC is a binocular phenomenon and is always tested under binocular conditions. Instruments such as the Amblyoscope, After Image Flasher, and Bagolini lenses may be used to test for ARC. Since the condition is so unpredictable, several tests are conducted and results compared to see whether the condition is embedded. A diagnosis of ARC will normally reduce the prognosis for functional success in remediating the patient.

TREATMENT PROCEDURES

The first consideration for all patients with accommodative, ocular motor, and nonstrabismic binocular anomalies is optical correction. The second is the use of additional plus or minus lenses. The use of prism to treat binocular anomalies should be the next consideration in all cases. A significant percentage of patients with binocular vision and accommodative problems cannot be successfully treated with either or both lenses and prisms alone, however. Vision therapy has been shown to be effective for accomplishing the following in accommodative, ocular motor, and nonstrabismic binocular vision disorders: increased amplitude (amount) of accommodation, increased accommodative facility (ease), eliminating accommodative spasm, increased fusional vergence amplitudes (convergence and divergence), increased fusional vergence facility, elimination of suppression, improved stereopsis, improved accuracy of saccades and pursuits, and improved stability of fixation. The type and number of procedures available for eliminating binocular problems is vast and limited only by the imagination of the doctor and therapist.

The idea that vision is learned and can be taught at any age forms the basis for vision therapy. Vision therapy is a process that relies on giving an individual feedback and practice to teach enhancement of visual abilities. Vision therapy is similar in many ways to other types of therapy that involve learning. Consequently, there are specific guidelines to facilitate learning and success. The following vision therapy guidelines and principles should be used:

- Determine a level at which the patient can perform easily. Be aware of frustration level. Use positive reinforcement.
- Maintain an effective training level.
- Emphasize to the patient that changes must occur within his or her own visual system. Make the patient aware of the goals of vision therapy.
- Use vision therapy techniques that provide feedback to the patient.
- Effort is a very important part of any therapy program. Since learning is an active process, the more the patient participates, the more he or she will derive from therapy.

Another method of treatment that may be necessary in certain cases of strabismus is extraocular muscle surgery. Surgery is considered when the angle of the strabismus is too large (30 PD or greater) to be overcome easily by fusion. Many times, surgery is recommended after therapy has been done, to improve sensory fusion. The surgery will reduce the amount of motor fusion necessary to keep the eyes straight. Surgery is normally only a cosmetic cure.

CONCLUSION

This chapter is only an introduction to binocular vision. It is important to understand the concepts presented, but competency comes only from exposure to this vast area of optometry. Vision therapy can be one of the most satisfying aspects of optometry.

SUGGESTED READING

Birnbaum M. Optometric Management of Nearpoint Vision Disorders. Boston: Butterworth-Heinemann, 1993.

Getz D. Strabismus and Amblyopia. Optometric Extension Program, Santa Ana, CA, 1990.

Griffin JR, Grisham JD. Binocular Anomalies: Diagnosis and Vision Therapy (3rd ed). Boston: Butterworth-Heinemann, 1995.

Scheiman M, Wick B. Clinical Management of Binocular Vision. Philadelphia: Lippincott, 1994.

14/Sports Vision

Shaun M. Ratchford

Float like a butterfly,
Sting like a bee
Your hands can't hit,
What your eyes can't see!!
—Muhammad Ali

Seeing is not a thing, but an act.
—Fredrick Franck, *The Zen of Seeing*

Doctors see vision as a complex learned activity of the brain.
—Jean Moyer

Most athletic teams rigorously monitor their players' diets, design demanding off-season training schedules of running and lifting, and require players to maintain their optimum physical condition. Vision, the physical sense that is crucial in athletic activities, is largely taken for granted, however. If an athlete with a well-trained body and mind is unable to use his or her eyes to full capacity in coordination with his or her physical abilities due to correctable vision problems, that athlete is not performing at 100%. In competitive situations, the visual demands placed on an athlete's eyes are far greater than those of the average person. Far too often, team coaches and management believe the ability to read the Snellen chart from 20 feet is adequate proof that their player is in top condition visually. The sports vision therapist can prove that assumption to be erroneous.

VISUAL SKILLS

There are at least 20 visual skills that make up the total visual package, and all of the 20 can be improved through testing and training with a qualified vision therapist. The goals of a sports vision training program are to remediate weaknesses, strengthen the eyes against stress or strain, and enhance the athlete's overall visual skills. The general concepts used by the vision therapist to help the athlete achieve these goals are to provide for small, incremental successes in order to avoid disappointing the athlete; to show the relevance of the visual skill to the athlete's specific sport; and to challenge the athlete's competitive nature by gradually increasing the time and difficulties of the exercises.

The basic premise underlying the practice of sports vision therapy is that the eyes "feed" the brain and that the brain interprets the data, which in turn sets the body in motion. Ninety percent of the information accumulated in the brain is collected through the eyes. If the data acquired by the brain are incorrect, incomplete, or not received in a timely manner, performance suffers. All visual skills, whether strong or weak, may be enhanced through training and performance thereby improved.

The sports vision therapist must know and understand the visual demands of the athlete's individual sport before beginning the training. Mastery of the visual requirements of the sport is most important in designing an effective remediation program, and especially in winning the trust of the athlete.

The *American Optometric Association Guidebook* lists 17 visual skills and explains how and if any of the skills apply to a specific sport. The book also offers a general overview of the sport, a list of relevant testing and training equipment, a list of the most common eye injuries encountered by athletes, and a list of protective eye wear. For therapists who are not members of the American Optometric Association (AOA)—Sports Vision Section and for those who do not have the guidebook, an option is to take the list of 20 visual skills from this chapter and use it as a checklist while observing the athlete in action.

If possible, the therapist should arrange to watch the athlete as he or she practices or competes in his or her sport. This observation can provide the therapist with the perfect opportunity to develop a rapport with the athlete and begin gaining trust. Meeting the athlete in her or his arena also invites her or him to begin a dialogue about her or his visual strengths and weaknesses.

The specific visual skills to test and train (which are followed by examples of the skill used in a sport) include the following:

Acuity, dynamic: The ability to see an object clearly when it is moving, you are moving, or both are moving (e.g., a batter picking up the spin rotation of a pitch as it approaches the plate)

Anticipation time: the ability to use visual clues to predict where and when something will happen or move (e.g., the center fielder seemingly moving on the fly ball before it is hit)

Acuity, static: The ability to read clearly the 20/20 row of letters on an eye chart 20 feet away (e.g., a rifle shooter's ability to see the bull's eye target clearly through the scope)

Central/peripheral vision: The speed at which you can change your awareness from a straight-ahead position to the outer extremes of your visual field (e.g., the point guard in basketball leading a three-on-one fast break and passing the ball off with a no-look pass as the defender steps up to make a defensive play)

Color vision: The ability to see the hues and vibrance of color (e.g., the home team wearing away colors to try to confuse a color-blind quarterback)

Depth perception: The ability to judge quickly and accurately either or both the distance and speed of an object in space or as it moves through space (e.g., the ability of the golfer or caddie to judge the distance of a drive, approach shot, or putt)

Eye dominance: The eye that processes the information a split second before the other eye (e.g., a shooter mounting the gun on the side of the dominant eye so that cross firing does not occur)

Eye-hand/foot/body coordination: The ability to get your hands, feet, or body to react to what the eyes see (e.g., the hockey goalie reacting to a shot on goal)

Eye motility (pursuit): The ability of the eyes to track or follow an object smoothly (e.g., the tennis player keeping his or her eye on a serve)

Eye teaming: The ability of the eyes to point and aim together to give the brain a clear single picture (e.g., the soccer goalie following a shot on goal)

Glare recovery: The ability of the eyes to adjust to bright lights or flashes (e.g., the shortstop's ability to pick up the infield fly after it comes out of the sun)

Night vision: The ability to see in dim illumination (e.g., the race car driver driving the night portion of the 24 hours of a LeMans race)

Saccade: The ability of the eyes to make jump movements (e.g., a quarterback looking from the primary receiver to the secondary receiver to the tertiary receiver)

Spatial localization: The ability to sense where you are relative to other objects in space (e.g., the swimmer hitting the underwater turn perfectly to win the race)

Speed of focusing: The ability of the eyes to focus clearly on objects moving at and away from them (e.g., the badminton player receiving and returning a volley)

Speed of recognition: The time it takes the brain to get the body to respond after the brain perceives something (e.g., the trap shooter moving the gun toward the clay target)

Visual concentration: The ability to endure visual noise and distracters without affecting performance (e.g., the free throw shooter seeing only the rim and not the sea of hands waving behind the blackboard trying to distract him or her)

Visual memory: The ability to take information that the eyes feed the brain and use it for future decisions (e.g., the quarterback recognizing the blitz after seeing the defensive alignment at the line of scrimmage)

Visual reaction time: The time it takes the eyes to get the brain to get the body to move (e.g., the drag racer letting off the clutch as soon as the light turns green)

Visualization: The ability to create a mental picture that preprograms the body to achieve its maximum potential (e.g., the diver who has dived the perfect dive moments after visualizing each motion of the dive)

All visual skills, whether weak or strong, can be enhanced through training. The information gathered from a sports vision workup may be used to predict athletic performance and provides very useful information for the athlete as well as the coach, general manager, or trainer. The key to optimum improvement lies in accurately matching the needs of the athlete with a training program that is sports specific. Improvement is the result of a sports vision training program.

SPORTS VISION THERAPY

Sports vision therapy is a two-part program designed to identify the strengths and weaknesses of an individual's visual makeup and to devise a regimen of individualized training exercises that enhance visual potential. The first component of the program is a 2-hour sports vision workup. This evaluation is necessary to assess those visual skills that are critical to athletic success. A sports vision workup includes a standard eye exam—refractive condition, ocular skills, and visual health—with the additional testing of such specifically athletic visual skills as eye-hand coordination, peripheral awareness, response and reaction time, visual concentration, and balance. An in-depth report follows the workup explaining the results of each test, ranking the results according to national norms, and listing specific recommendations for the patient.

The second component of the sports vision program is the actual sports vision training. The training program generally consists of three phases. In the first phase, visual training builds a strong foundation by strengthening the visual skills of the patient. These include accommodation, ocular motilities, and binocularity skills. This phase of the training usually lasts 3–4 weeks. Phase two involves working on the sports specific skills such as balance, quickness, peripheral awareness, eye-hand/foot coordination, and speed of recognition skills. This phase lasts approximately 5–8 weeks. Phase three teaches the mind to visualize the positive results desired, both on and off the playing field. This final phase usually takes 2–4 weeks.

The initial step in the program involves an office visit of 2.0–2.5 hours, during which a complete sports vision workup is done. Results of the testing and recommendations for a training program are provided to the patient. If the patient then chooses to begin training, he or she can expect the program to last a minimum of eight 1-hour weekly visits. If the patient's time is short, it is possible to customize the training by giving priority to the two or three skills most crucial for the patient's success in his or her sport. Shortening the time given to training usually means that the patient is highly motivated and can be counted on to practice the skills and apply the learning to his or her performance without supervision.

For most patients, the most important aspect of the program is the home training. During the weekly office visits, the sports vision therapist prepares the patient for the practice routine. Typically, one to three exercises are prescribed for the patient each week. The sports vision therapist reviews the home training techniques during the office visit to assure the patient's understanding of the procedures and comfort with them. Some of the exercises require equipment which is loaned to the patient. Commonly, a Brock string, peg rotator, vectogram, tachistoscope, stereoscope, flipper, peripheral awareness trainer, and saccadic fixator are used in the home training program. A $50–100 deposit in addition to the normal fees to cover the cost of any damage done to the equipment at home is often required by the therapist. Because many patients find that particular pieces of equipment are important in maintaining the level of skill gained, some will even purchase equipment at the conclusion of their training program. Expensive equipment is *not* necessary in sports vision therapy, however.

The equipment used in training can vary from homemade and inexpensive, such as a rotating disk and loose lenses, to the very sophisticated and expensive. Please contact the companies listed in Table 14-1 for information on their equipment and listings of their prices.

A practice thinking of getting involved in sports vision should eventually have a piece of equipment that can address all of the visual skills previously listed.

Home therapy exercises are practiced daily on a set schedule and should take a patient a minimum of 20 minutes per session. Patients can be asked to keep records of scores or notes on any difficulty that they have with the exercises. In addition, it is important to advise the patient of the probability of reaching a plateau at some point in her or his training. Although they occur regularly, plateaus may be broken by using yoked prisms, balance boards, and a strobe light. These visual and physical distracters increase the difficulty of the skill so that returning to the original version eases the challenge for the patient and the bottleneck is broken.

As with most motor skills learning, the commitment and motivation of the learner is paramount to a successful training program. If the patient is unwilling to practice the homework daily, the benefits of the program are greatly diminished. The therapist can help in keeping the athlete motivated by stressing the relevance of the homework to a specific skill in the patient's game and by predicting gains that result from steady practice.

As with many recreational and even some professional athletes, the person in need of sports vision training often feels the pressure of failing to live up to their athletic potential despite hours of practice and physical training. Often overlooked by them is the real cause of their inadequate performance. They misread such symptoms as bad hands, poor reactions (too early or too late) and balance, squinting, and inconsistency, failing to recognize that these are the signs of an athlete with visual problems.

TABLE 14-1. Companies that supply sports vision equipment

Academic Therapy Publications
20 Commercial Blvd.
Novata, CA 94947

Bernell Corporation
750 Lincolnway E
South Bend, IN 46634-4637
(800) 348-2225

Lafayette Instruments
P.O. Box 5729
Lafayette, IN 47903
(800) 428-7545

Vistech, Inc.
1372 N. Fairfield Road
Dayton, OH 45432

Franel Optical Supply
P.O. Box 96
Maitland, FL 32751
(800) 327-2070

Efficient Seeing Publications
7510 Soquel Drive
Aptos, CA 95003

Computer Orthoptics
Distributed by RC Instruments, Inc.
99 W. Jackson St.
Cicero, IN 46034
(800) 346-4925

Tempo Instruments
87 Modular Ave.
Commack, NY 11725

Biofeedtrac, Inc.
26 Schermerhorn St.
Brooklyn Heights, NY 11201

Visiontronics
1519 Spring Garden Way
Forest Grove, OR 97116

GTVT
18807 10th Place West
Lynwood, WA 98036
(800) 848-8897

Wayne Engineering
1825 Willow Road
Northfield, IL 60093
(708) 441-6940

PATIENT AND PRACTICE BENEFITS

The benefits of sports vision therapy are many. Sports vision therapy offers a new and unique service to patients. No longer will patients' visual needs be left untreated or referred to other therapists. Sports vision can provide the practice with new areas of income, especially if the training is done by a therapist and not the doctor. Sports vision creates great opportunities for public relations and exposure.

Sports vision can help anyone interested in improving his or her visual skills. This includes young and old, male and female, as well as the "weekend warrior" and professional athlete. Athletes from the following sports seem to show the strongest interest in participating in and benefiting from sports vision testing and training: shooting, shotgun and rifle (trap, skeet, sporting clay, small bore, and large bore), golf, tennis, baseball, softball, basketball, football, volleyball, soccer, skiing, lacrosse, swimming, badminton, and auto racing.

The bulk of training patients will come directly from current patient load. Pictures on the wall, pamphlets in the waiting room, and a protective eye guard display in your dispensary can create a patient's awareness and interest in the training.

Sports screenings are the second area that generates patients for the practice. Screenings may be done in house, with the athletes coming to the office, or may be done out of the office at the athlete's school or site. Screenings done at the office are the most efficient and productive because the equipment is already set up, the layout is familiar, and experienced staff is at your disposal.

Screenings done outside the office at the gymnasium or the team's practice site involve a lot more time and organization but are a great source of new patients. It is very important to make contact with the person at the site—usually the trainer or athletic director—who will be in charge of setting up equipment and getting the athletes there in a timely and orderly fashion and who will act as the liaison between the therapist and the school, league, or team. It is imperative that the therapist and the staff get to the site early to check and set up equipment so that the screening will flow smoothly. Screenings done on the road are just that, screenings, and usually are not as involved as testing done in the office. This means that some of the athletes may be asked to come to the office or may be referred out for further testing.

FURTHER INFORMATION

The following organizations can provide information and the *American Optometric Association Guidebook*, as well as videos and news of conferences:

American Optometric Association (AOA)
Sports Vision Section
243 North Lindbergh Blvd.
St. Louis, MO 63141
(800) 365-2219

International Academy of Sports Vision (NASV)
7699 Palmilla Drive, Suite 3120
San Diego, CA 92122
(213) 936-1684

College of Vision Development (COVD)
11365 Sunset Hills Road
Reston, VA 22090-5221
(703) 471-4600

Optometric Extension Program Foundation (OEPF)
1921 East Carnegie Ave., Suite 3L
Santa Ana, CA 92705
(714) 250-8070

SUGGESTED READING

Gregg J. Vision and Sports: An Introduction. Boston: Butterworth, 1987.
Loren DF, MacEwen CJ. Sports Vision. Boston: Butterworth-Heinemann, 1995.

15/Ocular Emergencies and Triage

Frank L. Galizia

The first contact a patient makes with an eye care office is usually by telephone. The first person this patient comes into contact with is usually the technical support staff. Obviously, the paraoptometric does not want to overlook a true emergency. It may be very detrimental to a busy practice's schedule to "squeeze" someone in for a "mild irritation," however.

This chapter reviews many of the more common eye emergencies and considers ways to ensure that a serious case is not mistaken for something trivial.

WHAT IS AN EYE EMERGENCY?

An emergency is defined as a sudden, generally unexpected occurrence or set of circumstances demanding immediate action. A broken temple on a patient's glasses is probably not an emergency. A corneal ulcer is an emergency. The difficulty lies in deciding where to draw the line for eye problems that are not so obvious and clear cut.

The presence of either one of two principal conditions or of both helps determine the level of an emergency: *vision loss* and *pain*. If a patient complains of either of these symptoms, he or she must be seen as soon as possible.

COMFORT ZONE

Everyone involved with eye care has what is referred to as a "comfort zone." This is a zone in which a person feels comfortable handling, diagnosing, and treating patients. If you are dealing with a patient whose problem makes you edgy, uncertain, or uncomfortable, you are outside of your comfort zone.

Only with time and experience do you enlarge this zone. Eye care is a vast science. Everyone has limits, so never feel embarrassed to admit you are unsure. Take the opportunity to broaden your knowledge base whenever possible, but never work in doubt. Do not hesitate to ask the other members of your office team if you are ever unsure or uncomfortable with handling an emergency case.

If a patient calls with a problem that falls outside your comfort zone, check with your doctor or other members of the office staff to determine whether the patient should be seen that day. If this is not possible, make sure the patient is seen that day. Always err on the side of safety for your patients.

TIME

Eye emergencies have no respect for time. They can occur at any time of the day, and your office must be ready for them around the clock. Anyone who has practiced eye care for any length of time is aware that most emergencies and difficult cases seem to present right before lunch or right about closing time. It has been said with a humorous slant that 75% of all retinal detachments present at 4:30 P.M. on Fridays.

THE GOLDEN RULE

As always, each emergency patient should be treated the way you would want to be treated or the way you would want your relative to be treated. Because emergency patients are often worked into a schedule, they tend to make you feel rushed to stay on that schedule. No matter what the symptoms are, remember there was enough reason for the patient to call your office. Although many emergencies turn out to be routine, the patient usually does not see it that way. Above all else, treat the patients the way you would wish to be treated.

THE GREAT DETECTIVE

Once it is decided to see a patient due to an apparent emergency, the most important part of the examination begins: the case history. It can be said that "if you do not know where you are going after the history is taken, you are truly lost."

Taking an accurate history may be the paraoptometric's job. Being thorough and complete, asking the right questions, and properly recording the patient responses will be critical in assisting the doctor in diagnosing and creating a treatment plan.

First, record the patient's version of what exactly happened or how the patient came to notice something was wrong. Make sure this includes *onset, frequency,* and *duration* of all the patient's reported symptoms.

Onset should tell you when, where, and possibly how the symptoms began, especially if they are the result of an injury. Frequency qualifies how often the symptoms are present. Duration is the length of time the symptoms last. This helps to determine whether or not any pattern exists with the patient's symptoms.

Be sure to allow enough time for the patient to describe the symptoms that sent them to your office. Another important question that needs to be asked is whether or not vision has been affected. If so, this individual symptom will also need to be assessed for onset, frequency, and duration.

Now let's take a look at some of the more common emergencies, how the patient may present them to the office, and how they are managed. These include corneal abrasions, anterior uveitis, foreign bodies, conjunctivitis, episcleritis, glaucoma attack, flashes and floaters, and neurologic conditions.

Corneal Abrasions

When the cornea is injured, it presents with three major calling cards: *pain, photophobia*, and *lacrimation*. Since pain is involved, the patient should automatically be fit into the schedule.

Most abrasions are superficial and involve only the epithelial layer of the cornea. It is the concentration of nerves in this region that yields such painful symptoms. If the cornea is scratched or abraded, there will be pain. Therefore, these patients may come into the office wearing crude patches over the eye, holding their hand over the eye, or squinting. There is also a tendency for the eye to be watering (lacrimation). The patient may also be sensitive to light, or photophobic.

The patient will most likely have an obvious history of injury and can supply ample detail as to what happened. Abrasions are often the result of improper contact lens insertion or removal (Figure 15-1). It is exceptionally rare to have an abrasion go all the way through the cornea. When this type of corneal injury occurs, suturing or corneal glue may be necessary. These procedures are best performed at an ambulatory surgery center.

Under the slit lamp, an abrasion appears as a break in the epithelial layer, or outer layer of the cornea. An abrasion will stain using fluorescein dye and viewed through a slit lamp with a cobalt blue filter. Treatment for superficial abrasions usually includes a cycloplegic agent, such as 5% homatropine, to prevent a secondary condition known as uveitis and an antibiotic, such as fluoroquinolones, gentamicin, or tobramycin. The eye is then *pressure patched* (Figure 15-2) and the patient is scheduled for a follow-up visit in 24 hours.

Recent studies have questioned whether pressure patching is favorable in such cases. More severe cases seem to benefit from patching; however, mild cases seem to do well with cold compresses to relieve the pain. Moderate corneal abrasions also benefit by use of a soft contact lens referred to as a *bandage lens*. Unlike

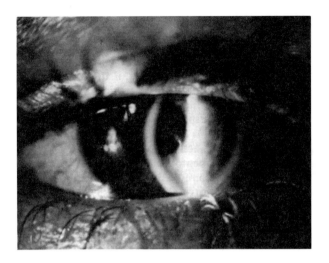

Figure 15-1—Corneal abrasion caused by a mascara brush. (Reprinted with permission from JD Bartlett, SD Jaanus. Clinical Ocular Pharmacology [2nd ed]. Boston: Butterworth-Heinemann, 1989:601.)

pressure patches, bandage contact lenses allow the patient to use the eye while it is healing.

It is wise to advise the patient to wear sunglasses because of photophobia. You may want to have disposable sunglasses available for these patients. Even if a patch is worn, bright light in the nonabraded eye will cause pain to the abraded eye from the sympathetic response. The use of a cycloplegic in the abraded eye reduces this effect.

Resolution time of the abrasion depends on the extent of the injury. When the patient reports the eye is starting to feel better, they are usually on the road to recovery. Most epithelial abrasions heal within 24–48 hours. There is usually no scarring. Scarring can occur when the injury goes as deep as the stromal layer (the middle layer) of the cornea.

Anterior Uveitis

A patient with uveitis will usually present with the same symptoms as someone with a corneal abrasion. Since the symptoms are identical, the differential diagnosis is made by the slit-lamp examination. Corneal abrasions are obvious under the magnification of the biomicroscope, or slit lamp, especially with fluorescein staining (Table 15-1). A case of uveitis will present an intact cornea. The anterior chamber, which is the area directly behind the cornea but in front of the iris, will have white blood cells (leukocytes) and proteins floating in the aqueous. This is referred to as *cells and flare*.

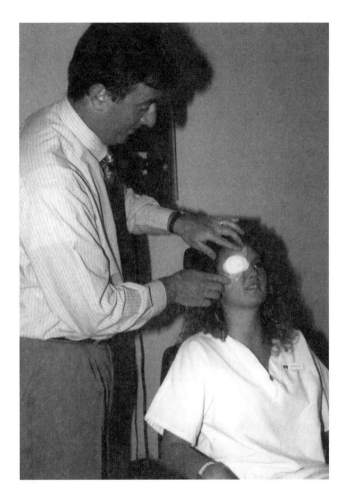

Figure 15-2—A typical pressure patch.

TABLE 15-1. Various injection presentations of red eyes

1. Uveitis or corneal problem
2. Conjunctivitis
3. Episcleritis

The case history of a patient with uveitis is a little less exacting than that for abrasions. The patient will probably note an eye irritation or pain which started a few days earlier and just kept getting worse over time. An eye with uveitis also looks more red near the limbus (the junction between the sclera and cornea). This is different from conjunctivitis, where the redness

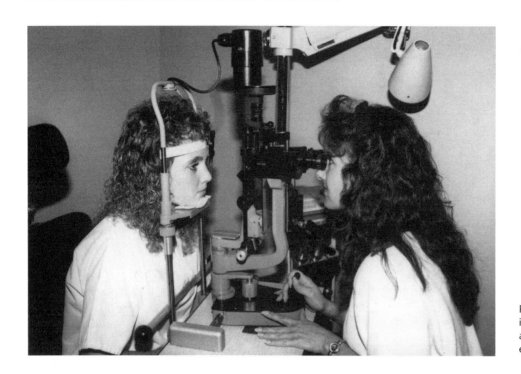

Figure 15-3—Slit-lamp examination is a valuable step in making an accurate diagnosis of any ocular emergency.

is predominantly in the fornices (the junction between the lids and the sclera) (Figure 15-3).

Treatment usually involves a *cycloplegic agent* (5% homatropine) for comfort and a *steroidal agent* (1% prednisolone or 0.1% dexamethasone) to relieve the inflammation. Follow-up visits are usually scheduled at 48–72 hours.

The underlying cause of uveitis is usually not found. In chronic cases, an underlying systemic problem may be found from extensive lab testing. Systemic causes include sarcoidosis, ankylosing spondylitis, rheumatoid arthritis, and other inflammatory diseases.

Foreign Body

Corneal foreign bodies usually present with moderate to extreme pain. Since the eye usually accommodates foreign bodies, such as contact lenses, the actual foreign body is not what brings the patient into the office (Figure 15-4). Instead, it is the rust that forms in the cornea approximately 24–48 hours afterwards or the ensuing inflammatory response that forces the patient to have his or her eye checked (Figure 15-5).

The scenario most often seen is a mechanic working with a drill or grinder or someone working in construction without safety eye wear protection. Since a foreign body is a form

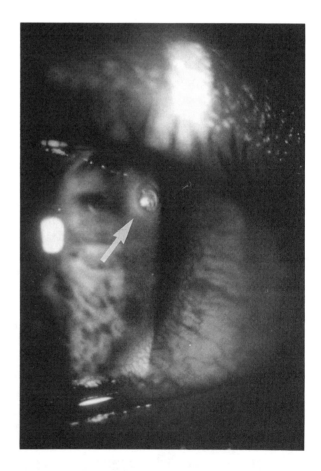

Figure 15-4—A metallic foreign body embedded on the cornea. (Reprinted with permission from JD Bartlett, SD Jaanus. Clinical Ocular Pharmacology [3rd ed]. Boston: Butterworth-Heinemann, 1995;687.)

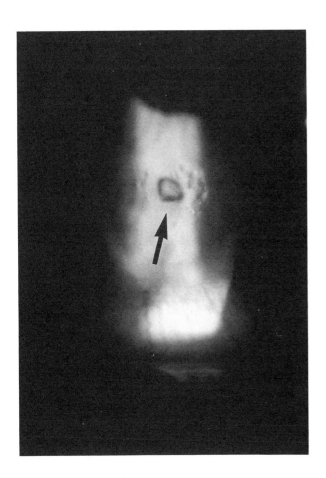

Figure 15-5—Rust ring (arrow) that develops from a metallic foreign body. (Courtesy of Olee J. Olsen, O.D.) (Reprinted with permission from JD Bartlett, SD Jaanus. Clinical Ocular Pharmacology [3rd ed]. Boston: Butterworth-Heinemann, 1995;689.)

of a corneal injury, you may expect symptoms of pain, photophobia, and lacrimation.

It is critical to record in the case history what the patient was doing when the foreign body was lodged in the eye. If any high-speed machinery was being used, an x-ray of the globe may be necessary to rule out any intraocular foreign body.

Most foreign bodies are trapped by the "sticky" nature of the corneal or conjunctival epithelium. To remove them, topical anesthetic drops are applied first. Then one of several different instruments may be used to "peel" the foreign body away. These instruments include a spud (which looks like a cooking spatula when placed under a microscope), a bent 20-gauge hypodermic needle, or even a fish-line loop attached to a handle (Bailey's loop) (Figure 15-6).

If the foreign body was nonmetallic, the patient is ready for patching after the foreign body is removed. Once a foreign body is removed, the cornea has a resultant abrasion. The treatment is identical to that of a corneal abrasion, as outlined earlier.

If the foreign body is metallic, there is a possibility that rust has begun to form within the layers of the cornea. Rust will usually cause an immune reaction, which includes swelling (edema) and pain. Therefore, the rust is usually removed after the foreign body has been peeled away.

The rust may either be removed with a bent hypodermic needle or more appropriately "brushed" away with an Algerbrush (Figure 15-7). Once all of the rust has been removed, the cornea is once again treated as though it were a corneal abrasion. Follow-up visits for most foreign body removals are usually at 24 hours.

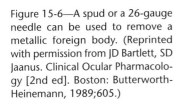

Figure 15-6—A spud or a 26-gauge needle can be used to remove a metallic foreign body. (Reprinted with permission from JD Bartlett, SD Jaanus. Clinical Ocular Pharmacology [2nd ed]. Boston: Butterworth-Heinemann, 1989;605.)

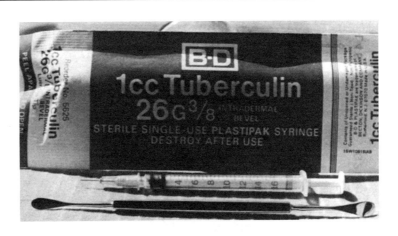

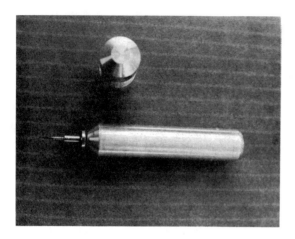

Figure 15-7—An Algerbrush is effective and safe in removing corneal rust rings. (Reprinted with permission from JD Bartlett, SD Jaanus. Clinical Ocular Pharmacology [2nd ed]. Boston: Butterworth-Heinemann, 1989;606.)

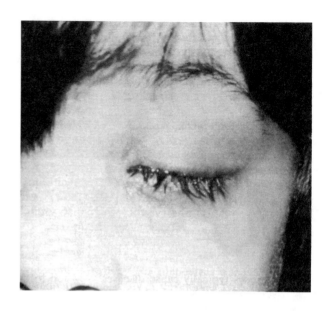

Figure 15-8—Watery discharge in primary herpes simplex blepharoconjunctivitis. (Reprinted with permission from JD Bartlett, SD Jaanus. Clinical Ocular Pharmacology [2nd ed]. Boston: Butterworth-Heinemann, 1989;539.)

Conjunctivitis

Just about everyone would agree that conjunctivitis is not an emergency. It is definitely a case you will often see in an emergency setting, however (Figure 15-8).

Conjunctivitis will cause irritation at best and should not have a significant impact on vision. Hence, a person with symptoms of conjunctivitis need not be seen immediately. But remember, there was enough concern for the patient to call, so when possible, these patients are quite grateful to be worked in.

A patient with conjunctivitis usually states that his or her eye (or eyes) is red and irritated. The patient may also report that he or she has "pink eye." The onset is usually 1–3 days prior to the call, and there is concern because it does not seem to be getting any better.

With conjunctivitis, the redness seems to be in the fornices, unlike a corneal abrasion or uveitis, in which the redness appears at the limbus. There may be increased drainage from the eye. A mucopurulent discharge usually accompanies bacterial conditions, whereas a watery discharge usually accompanies viral or allergic conditions.

Treatment is based on the diagnosis of bacterial, viral, or allergic conjunctivitis. Although a broad-spectrum antibiotic is used most specifically for bacterial conditions, there is some value in prescribing this for viral conditions, too. Antiviral medications are very specific for viral conditions, especially when treating the herpes simplex virus. Allergic conditions are usually treated with cold compresses, vasoconstrictors, and possibly mild anti-inflammatory agents (Table 15-2).

If conjunctivitis of any sort should involve the cornea, it is referred to as a *keratoconjunctivitis*. Corneal involvement is usually simple to diagnose on the basis of pain. Remember, conjunctivitis does not cause pain; corneal problems do.

Keratoconjunctivitis is usually treated the same as conjunctivitis, however, a cycloplegic (5% homatropine) may be added to prevent secondary uveitis. Follow-up on all types of conjunctivitis and keratoconjunctivitis is based on the severity of each case but usually falls between 48–72 hours.

Episcleritis

A case of episcleritis is simple to diagnose. The patient will call and usually state that his or her eye has been red for about 1–2 weeks and now is starting to hurt. The vision is usually not affected, but the onset of the ache or pain will bring them into the office (Figure 15-9).

This case is simple because it usually presents with a "sector" of the sclera involved. To the naked eye, this condition may be confused for a

TABLE 15-2. Treatment for conjunctivitis	
Type of conjunctivitis	Treatment
Bacterial	Gentamicin (Garamycin)
	Trimethoprim/polymyxin B (Polytrim)
Viral	1% Trifluridine (Viroptic)
Allergic	Naphazoline/pheniramine (Naphcon-A, Albalon-A) (available over the counter)

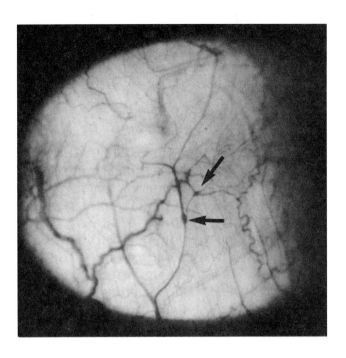

Figure 15-9—Diffuse episcleritis demonstrating vessel injection, tortuosity, and saccular dilatations (arrows). (Reprinted with permission from JD Bartlett, SD Jaanus. Clinical Ocular Pharmacology [3rd ed]. Boston: Butterworth-Heinemann, 1995;764.)

subconjunctival hemorrhage. Subconjunctival hemorrhages do not hurt, however, and the slit lamp examination of episcleritis reveals several engorged, deep vessels on the sclera, not blood from a hemorrhage.

Episcleritis is usually an eye problem with an underlying systemic problem, usually a form of arthritis. A patient presenting with episcleritis should be asked about the presence of any arthritic condition, and the results should be recorded in the chart.

Treatment involves a medium- to high-strength steroid (1% prednisolone or 0.1% dexamethasone). Since resolution usually takes 1–3 weeks, a follow-up visit should be scheduled at approximately 1 week.

Glaucoma Attack (Narrow Angle, Angle Closure)

Someone having a glaucoma attack will report a great deal of pain from within the eye that seems to radiate outward. The patient will also report a reduction in vision and possibly note an upset stomach or nausea. The redness in the eye will be concentrated near the limbus, just as it is for a corneal injury or uveitis.

The pain is so great that the patient will report soon after the original symptoms were first noted. The deciding factor in the diagnosis will obviously be an extremely high intraocular pressure. On a Goldmann tonometer, the pressure is usually higher than 40 mm Hg and may even be higher than 60 mm Hg.

These high pressures allow the aqueous humor to seep into the cornea, which causes the cornea to swell (edema). This will cause decreased vision and pain. This edema goes away once the pressure is brought under control.

To "break" the attack, either or both a miotic agent (2% pilocarpine) and a beta-blocker agent (betaxolol) may be used, along with oral carbonic anhydrase inhibitors such as acetazolamide or methazolamide. If these agents fail, oral hyperosmotic agents (glycerol) are usually attempted. Oral hyperosmotics usually make the patient vomit shortly afterward, so be prepared by having an emesis pan available.

Occasionally, the above in-office medications fail, and the patient may need to be admitted to a hospital, where intravenous hyperosmotics can be administered. Fortunately, this step is extremely successful at bringing the intraocular pressure to normal or even subnormal levels.

Once a glaucoma attack is brought under control, no matter by what means, the job is still not finished. The patient is then placed on a glaucoma treatment regimen until laser surgery can be performed to correct the problem more permanently.

It should be noted the glaucoma attack described above is not to be confused with the more common "open-angle" glaucoma. *In "open-angle" glaucoma, there is rarely a symptom to alert the patient that a problem exists.* So the type of glaucoma seen on an emergency basis is most often of a narrow-angle variety.

Flashes and Floaters

The patient with either or both flashes and floaters in their vision usually calls in relatively soon after the onset of symptoms to report them. This call is usually sparked by a fear that a retinal detachment has occurred. Although retinal detachments give symptoms of either or both flashes and floaters, chances of a retinal detachment, tear, or hole remain small. Since early detection of these retinal conditions is imperative if repair is going to be successful, however, all flashes and floater symptoms must be treated as a retinal detachment until proven otherwise.

Although there is no pain associated with flashes and floaters, and the vision change might be a mere obscuration, patients with these symptoms should be seen without delay. Careful detail should be made as to the onset, frequency, and duration of these symptoms.

Flashes and floaters are always a symptom of a problem or change "within" the eye. Therefore, the examination must include a dilated fundus examination. Retinal holes, tears, or detachments can be found relatively easily with a binocular indirect ophthalmoscope or with a gonioscopic lens.

With retinal holes, tears, or detachments, the flashes are caused by the physical stimulation of the retina or loose portions of a retinal flap within the vitreous. The floaters are caused by either or both nonfunctioning retina and blood elements floating within the vitreous. Referral to a retinal specialist should be made immediately to avoid further deterioration to the retina.

Once a retinal problem has been ruled out, which is usually the case, symptoms of flashes and floaters are then associated with either a posterior vitreous detachment or an ophthalmic migraine. Most commonly a separation has occurred between the vitreous and the retina. This is called a *posterior vitreous detachment* (PVD) and should not be confused with a retinal detachment, even though they sound similar.

With a PVD, the flashes are caused by the vitreous physically pushing against the retina. The floaters are the result of proteins coagulated in the center of the vitreous. PVDs usually occur spontaneously, however, they can be brought on by physical exertion or injury.

Severe PVDs may also develop into a retinal hold, tear, or detachment. This is why a patient diagnosed with PVD is asked to return in 6 weeks to rule out a retinal problem. The chances of a retinal problem are small, but the patient should be reminded to return to the office if his or her symptoms increase.

Neurologic Conditions

In general, neurologic conditions are those that occur either along the optic nerve or within the brain itself. Therefore, these cases involve problems that occur in places that cannot be seen without the help of sophisticated equipment such as a computerized axial tomography scan or magnetic resonance imaging scan.

Because of this, eye care professionals usually do not treat these types of patients, but instead play a critical role in diagnosing where the problem may be. Once a diagnosis is made, the patient may then be referred to a neurologist or neurosurgeon for treatment.

Ophthalmic migraines are a neurologic condition much like a conventional migraine headache. Symptoms of an ophthalmic migraine are usually very time specific. Flashes of light appear in an arc-like fashion, starting centrally and working their way peripherally until they finally disappear after approximately 20–30 minutes.

Ophthalmic migraines may or may not be followed by a migraine headache. They pose no threat to the health or vision of the eye, and the patient should be made aware of this. This condition is repetitive and recognized as an irritating phenomenon. It generally will improve over time. Patient education is the only treatment and must be handled appropriately to alleviate patient concern and apprehension.

Since the neural pathways within the brain are in such tight quarters, a cranial lesion of any sort would probably have at least some impact on the visual system. This is why it is so critical to monitor pupil functions, extraocular muscle coordination, and visual field findings.

Emergency neurologic cases usually report with sudden or gradual loss of vision in one or both eyes. The presence or absence of pain is very critical to determine because it plays an integral part in determining the diagnosis.

Since a clinician cannot usually view the actual problem, neurologic cases demand more than ever that a complete and accurate history be taken and recorded. These cases are usually diagnosed before the history is completed. The diagnosis is then "proven" by clinical testing.

Since either or both vision loss and pain is involved, these patients should have no trouble getting in to see the doctor. Since these problems may have serious, life-threatening origins, however, everyone involved in patient care must be careful not to make any foregone conclusions or volunteer an irresponsible prognosis.

Every office should have a good working relationship with both a neurologist and a neurosurgeon to facilitate a speedy referral for neurologic cases.

CONCLUSION

No matter what emergency case you are involved with, you must remember to treat the patient as if he or she were a relative and forget about the clock on the wall. A patient reporting pain or vision loss is an emergency, and every attempt must be made to get the patient into the office for evaluation.

The importance of a complete and accurate history cannot be stressed enough. With any symptom, make sure to determine the circumstances of onset, frequency, and duration.

Make sure each patient has a full understanding of their condition and their treatment regimen before leaving the office. Facilitate appropriate follow-up appointments or referrals to a specialist's office.

Above all, never work in doubt. Always work within your "comfort zone." The challenges created by emergency eye care will provide you with the satisfaction of participating in a very noble profession.

SUGGESTED READING

Collum DR, Chang B. The Wills Eye Manual Office and Emergency Room Diagnosis of Eye Disease (2nd ed). Philadelphia: Lippincott, 1994.

APPENDIXES

APPENDIX A

Infection Control Guidelines for the Optometric Practice*

Optometrists are now providing an expanded scope of service in the treatment and management of eye diseases and eye injuries. This may include the use of techniques and procedures that pose an increased risk for transmission of infectious diseases within optometric practices. Additional attention needs to be focused on the use of appropriate office hygiene procedures and universal precautions to prevent either or both exposure to and transmission of disease (Table A-1). The Primary Care and Ocular Disease Committee of the American Optometric Association has developed this report to provide recommendations to optometrists for the prevention of in-office disease transmission.

Most optometric procedures are considered low risk for the transmission of disease. Under some circumstances, however, for example, when instruments come in direct contact with an infected patient, when exposure to blood occurs, or when eye cultures are taken, there exists the potential for the transmission of disease.

Although considerable attention has been directed toward the transmission of the human immunodeficiency virus (HIV) and the hepatitis B virus (HBV), these are certainly not the only pathogens for which precautions need to be taken in the optometric practice. Adenovirus, herpes, tuberculosis, *Pseudomonas*, *Staphylococcus*, and others also need to be considered. Transmission of these pathogens generally can be prevented through the use of universal precautions and standard disinfection procedures in the optometric practice.

The report is divided into two sections. Section one applies to all optometric practices. It provides basic recommendations for infection control to protect patients and optometric staff. Section two applies to optometric practices where there is a risk of exposure to bloodborne pathogens. It provides a review of the requirements of the Occupational Safety and Health Administration (OSHA) Bloodborne Pathogens Standard and a sample exposure control plan for use in optometric practices. A copy of the complete OSHA Bloodborne Pathogens Standard (29 CFR 1910.1930) can be obtained from the U.S. Government Printing Office, Washington, DC 20402. Request Occupational Exposure to Bloodborne Pathogens, Order No. 069-001-00040-8. The cost is $2.

Based on procedures in your practice, you will need to determine whether only section one (universal precautions) applies or if both section one and section two (OSHA standards) are applicable. If both sections apply, all aspects of this report including the OSHA standards must be met.

SECTION ONE

With the increased prevalence of acquired immune deficiency syndrome (AIDS), hepatitis, and other bacterial and viral diseases in the United States, it is likely that some patients carrying these diseases will be encountered in optometric practice. It is impractical to try to identify all patients who may be carrying infectious agents. As a result, the following procedures should be routinely used by optometrists and their staffs for all patients seen in their practices. These guidelines have been developed based on the recommendations of the Centers for Disease Control (CDC) as "universal precautions" to prevent the transmission of disease within health care practices.[1,2,3]

Hand Washing

Proper hand washing represents one of the most effective means of preventing the transmission of disease. Many eye diseases are manually transmissible, and it is the responsibility of optometrists and their staffs to practice effective hand washing before and after examinations and procedures.

---

*This appendix was reprinted with permission from American Optometric Association Primary Care and Ocular Disease Committee. Infection control guidelines for the optometric practice. J Am Optom Assoc 1993;64:853.

TABLE A-1. Definitions of key terms	
Bloodborne pathogens	A pathogenic microorganism that is present in human blood and can cause disease in humans
Exposure incident	A specific eye, mouth, other mucous membrane, nonintact skin, or parenteral contact with blood or other potentially infectious materials
Occupational exposure	Reasonably anticipated skin, eye, mucous membrane, or parenteral contact with blood or other potentially infectious materials that may result from the performance of an employee's duties
Personal protective equipment	Specialized clothing or equipment, such as gloves, gowns, masks, and eye protection, worn by an employee for protection
Potentially infectious materials	Include blood, semen, vaginal secretion, cerebrospinal fluid, pericardial fluid, peritoneal fluid, amniotic fluid, saliva in dental procedures, and any body fluid visibly contaminated with blood (Tears are not considered to be potentially infectious materials under the Occupational Safety and Health Administration standard unless they contain visible blood.)
Universal precautions	An approach to infection control that treats all blood and body fluids as if they are infectious; precautions include hand washing, the wearing of gloves (as appropriate), and the sterilizing of instruments

Hands should be thoroughly washed with soap and water and thoroughly dried with a fresh cloth towel or with disposable paper towels.

Fingernails should be of reasonable length and clean. Hands should be frequently inspected for cuts, abrasions, or breaks in the skin.

Disposable Latex Gloves

All health care workers should routinely use appropriate barrier precautions to prevent skin and mucous membrane exposure when in contact with blood or other potentially infectious materials (this does not include tears, unless they contain visible blood). If an open wound or weeping lesion is present on the patient or the hands of optometrists or their staffs, disposable gloves should be worn.

Disposable gloves should be readily available for use by optometrists and their staffs when needed. All staff members should be instructed as to their proper use, particularly noting the following:

1. Gloves are not a substitute for hand washing.
2. Gloves are for single use only and must be discarded after each patient use.
3. Hands should be washed after gloves are removed.

Gowns and Masks

Gowns and masks are normally unnecessary for routine optometric procedures. In cases in which optometrists or their staffs may be in close contact with a patient with a known or suspected pathogen that may be transmitted by airborne means, masks should be used. If optometrists or their staffs are infected with a pulmonary disease or other disease that is transmitted by airborne means, masking is necessary to protect the patient.

Gowns and masks should be used as a barrier precaution whenever the possibility of splattering or splashes of blood or other body fluids contaminated with blood or other infectious materials may occur.

Protective Eye Wear

Protective eye wear is normally unnecessary except in situations in which blood or contaminated fluids may be splashed into the eyes of optometrists or their staffs. Either goggles or eye glasses with solid side shields may be used for protection.

Handling of Tissue

In the course of a patient evaluation, it may be necessary to handle the eyelids or surrounding facial tissue, thus coming in contact with potentially infected surfaces. Effort should be made to minimize contact with these tissues, particularly in the presence of a known infection, by using gloves, finger cots, or "no-touch" techniques involving the use of cotton tipped applicators.

Handling of Sharp Instruments

Precautions must be taken to prevent injuries caused by needles, syringes, or other sharp instruments. To prevent needle-stick injuries, used needles should not be bent, broken, or recapped by hand. After they are used, disposable syringes, needles, and other sharp items must be placed in appropriate infectious waste containers for disposal. Nondisposable sharps should be placed in puncture-resistant containers for sterilization. These containers must be readily accessible.

Instrument Disinfection

All instruments that come in contact with the patient should be wiped clean and either or both thoroughly disinfected and sterilized as appropriate after each use. Most ophthalmic instruments can be disinfected by immersion for 10 minutes in one of the following solutions:

1. 3% Hydrogen peroxide
2. A 1/10 dilution (0.5% solution) of common household bleach (sodium hypochlorite)
3. 70% Ethanol or isopropyl alcohol

The device should be thoroughly rinsed in tap water and air dried before reuse.

Special care may need to be taken to protect tonometer tips from damage. Two reports have noted that isopropyl alcohol, although effective in removal of viruses, may damage Goldmann applanation tonometer tips over time.[4,5] One study comparing all three disinfection solution procedures has recommended the use of 3% hydrogen peroxide as the method of choice for Goldmann tonometers.[6]

The tip of a digital pneumotonometer may be cleaned with an alcohol swab and allowed to air dry. Alternately, a disposable latex cover may be placed over the tonometer tip.

For effective disinfection the Schiötz tonometer must be disassembled between uses in order to clean the barrel. Since the noncontact tonometer does not make contact with the cornea or tears, it does not require routine disinfection. The front surface may be wiped with an alcohol swab if it should accidentally touch the eye, however.

Contact Lens Disinfection

Optometrists and their staffs involved in the fitting and dispensing of contact lenses should be familiar with proper disinfection techniques for in-office use. Lenses should be applied or removed only after proper hand washing. All trial lenses must be disinfected after each patient use using one of the following CDC-recommended procedures[7]:

1. Hard lenses (polymethylmethacrylate [PMMA]) can be disinfected with a commercially available hydrogen peroxide system currently approved for use with soft contact lenses. Also, most hard lenses can be disinfected using the standard heat treatment regimen used for soft lenses (78–80°C) for 10 minutes.
2. Rigid gas permeable (RGP) lenses can be disinfected using a commercially available hydrogen peroxide system approved for use with soft contact lenses. RGP lenses should not be heat disinfected as the lenses may warp.
3. Soft contact lenses can be disinfected with an approved hydrogen peroxide system. Some soft lenses have also been approved for heat disinfection.

Infectious Waste Disposal

The Environmental Protection Agency (EPA) and the CDC, as well as many state, county, and city governments, have developed guidelines that govern the disposal of either or both hazardous and infectious waste. Optometrists should be familiar with the requirements they may need to meet.

Infectious waste has been defined by the EPA as "wastes that in all probability contain pathogenic agents that, because of their type, concentration, and quantity, may cause disease in persons exposed to the waste."

TABLE A-2. *Infection control guidelines checklist*

The following universal precautions should be followed for the care of all patients in an optometric practice.

Hand washing
  Hands and other skin surfaces should be washed before every patient contact and immediately after contact with blood or other potentially infectious materials.
  Hands should also be washed immediately after gloves are removed.

Protective equipment
  Use appropriate barrier precautions to prevent exposure to blood or other potentially infectious materials.
  Disposable latex gloves should be used for touching blood, mucous membranes, or nonintact or infected skin of patients.
  Wear gloves if you have any open wound or cuts on your hands.
  Gloves must be disposed of after contact with each patient.
  Protective eyewear should be worn during procedures that are likely to generate splattering of blood or other potentially infectious materials.
  Masks should be worn during procedures when the transmission of airborne diseases exists.
  Gowns should be worn during procedures that are likely to generate splashes of blood or other potentially infectious materials.

Handling of sharp instruments
  To prevent injuries, all disposable needles, syringes, and other sharps must be handled and disposed of properly. Never try to bend, break, or recap a used needle by hand.
  All nondisposable sharps must be placed in puncture proof containers and disinfected or sterilized after each use.
  Proper puncture-resistant containers must be available for use in disposal of sharps.

Instrument disinfection
  All instruments that come in contact with the patient should be wiped clean and disinfected or sterilized after each use.

Contact lens disinfection
  All trial contact lenses must be disinfected after each use using either a chemical (hydrogen peroxide) or heat disinfection system.

Infectious waste disposal
  All infectious waste must be placed in appropriate containers and disposed of according to federal, state, and local regulations.

Although a number of categories of infectious waste exist, optometric practices would most likely need to be concerned with the following items:

1. All used disposable gloves need to be discarded as hazardous waste.
2. All sharps used in patient care should be considered potentially infectious waste and placed in appropriate infection control containers for disinfection or disposal.
3. All disposable items (e.g., tissues, gauze, etc.) contaminated with blood or other infectious materials should be disposed of in clearly marked infectious waste receptacles.
4. All infectious waste must be placed in appropriate containers and disposed of according to federal, state, and local regulations.

Infection Control Guidelines Checklist

To assist in the review of the universal precautions discussed above, Table A-2 contains an infection control guidelines checklist. This can be a helpful guide for staff training and for delineating appropriate office procedures.

SECTION TWO: OCCUPATIONAL SAFETY AND HEALTH ADMINISTRATION BLOODBORNE PATHOGENS STANDARD

The infection control guidelines in section one relate to general precautions that should be taken in the care of all patients within optometric practices. OSHA has also developed specific regulations that relate to the prevention of the transmission of bloodborne diseases to health care workers as well. The Bloodborne Pathogens Standard, which became effective March 6, 1992, requires employers to ensure that any of their employees who may be at risk for exposure to blood and other potentially infectious materials are appropriately protected.[8]

The likelihood of exposure to bloodborne diseases in most optometric practices is limited. OSHA does not consider individuals coming in contact with tears, unless they contain visible blood, to have occupational exposure. However, before you dismiss these requirements as not relating to your practice, be sure to do a careful review of all staff duties and procedures. If it can be reasonably anticipated that any of your employees may come in contact with blood or other potentially infectious materials (as defined in this regulation) as part of his or her routine duties, you must comply with all aspects of this standard.

Exposure Control Plan

The standard requires that all employers whose employees may experience occupational exposure must develop and implement a written exposure control plan. A copy of the plan should be accessible to employees, reviewed at least annually, and updated when needed. The following sections list the elements that must be included in the plan.

Exposure Determination

A list of all job classifications, tasks, and procedures having potential exposure must be developed.

Methods of Compliance

1. The use of universal precautions (as described in section one) shall be observed to prevent contact with blood or other potentially infectious materials. Precautions include hand washing, the wearing of gloves (as appropriate), and the sterilizing of instruments.
2. Engineering and workplace controls shall be used to eliminate or minimize employee exposure. This may include the following:
    a. Providing hand-washing facilities that are readily accessible to employees, or if unavailable, antiseptic hand cleanser and clean towels.
    b. Ensuring that employees wash their hands immediately after removal of gloves or other personal protective equipment or after contact with blood or other potentially infectious materials.
    c. Ensuring that needles or other contaminated sharps shall not be bent or recapped except as allowed by the standard.
    d. Prohibiting eating, drinking, smoking, applying cosmetics or lip balm, and handling contact lenses in work areas where there is a reasonable likelihood of occupational exposure.
3. Personal protective equipment shall be used where occupational exposure remains after institution of engineering and workplace controls. Masks in combination with eye protection devices such as goggles or glasses with solid side shields or chin length face shields shall be worn whenever splashes, spray, spatter, or droplets of blood or other potentially infectious materials may be generated and eye, nose, or mouth contamination can be reasonably expected. Gowns should be worn during procedures that are likely to generate splashes of blood or other potentially infectious materials.
4. Employers shall ensure that the worksite is maintained in a clean and sanitary condition. All equipment and working surfaces shall be cleaned and decontaminated after contact with blood or other potentially infectious materials. Waste materials containing liquid or semiliquid blood or other potentially infectious materials shall be placed in containers that are closeable, constructed to prevent leakage, labeled, and color-coded for identification.

Contaminated laundry shall be placed in and transported in bags or containers labeled or color coded for identification.

Hepatitis B Vaccination

Employers shall make available HBV vaccinations to all employees who have occupational exposure. These must be provided at no cost to the employee. The vaccination must be started within 10 working days of the employee's initial assignment. Should an employee refuse the vaccine, he or she must sign a declination form using specific language requested by OSHA.

Postexposure Follow-Up

Postexposure follow-up and evaluation must be made available to all employees who have had an exposure incident.

The evaluation and follow-up should include the following:

1. Documentation of the route of exposure and circumstances under which the exposure occurred
2. Testing of the individual's blood, after consent, to determine HBV and HIV infectivity

Information and Training

Employers shall ensure that all employees with occupational exposure participate in a training program that must be provided at the time of initial assignment to tasks where occupational exposure may take place and at least annually thereafter. The training shall include the following:

1. A copy of the OSHA standard and an explanation of its contents
2. A general explanation of bloodborne diseases and their mode of transmission
3. An explanation of your practice's exposure control plan
4. An explanation of the appropriate methods of recognizing tasks that may involve exposure and the use and limitations of methods to prevent exposure
5. Information on the selection and use of personal protective equipment
6. Information on the HBV vaccine
7. An explanation of procedures to follow if an exposure incident occurs and for postexposure evaluation

Records of training sessions need to be maintained for 3 years and shall include dates provided, summary of training, and names of person(s) conducting the training.

Medical Records

Employers shall establish and maintain confidential medical records for each employee with occupational exposure to include name and Social Security number, employer hepatitis vaccination status, and results of any medical examinations or testing.

The methods by which your office will comply with these requirements must be included in a written exposure control plan that should be available for all employees to review. A sample exposure control plan is presented in Figure A-1. Before finalizing your exposure control plan, you should review and understand the complete OSHA Bloodborne Pathogen Standard (29 CFR 1910.1930).

Additional information and guidance for employee training can be found in the OSHA publication, "Occupational Exposure to Bloodborne Pathogens," Order No. 3127. A copy can be obtained without cost from your regional OSHA office or from the OSHA Publications Office, 200 Constitution Ave., N.W., Room N3101, Washington, DC 20210. Enclose a self-addressed label.

RESPONSIBILITY TO PATIENTS

Optometrists have a moral and ethical responsibility to care for all patients.[9] With proper precautions, optometrists and their staffs are at low risk of contracting infections in the course of routine clinical practice. The risk of contracting HIV infection in the ophthalmic health care disciplines is considered to be remote. To date there is no evidence that the virus can be contracted from tears, contact lenses, or routine patient contact.

It must be remembered, however, that optometrists and their staffs will come in contact with many types of patients with a variety of potentially infectious conditions. It is the legal and ethical responsibility of all optometrists to be knowledgeable about and to practice effective techniques to prevent disease transmission between patients, staff, and themselves. An infection control plan tailored to the specific needs of your practice should be developed and implemented.

As optometry continues to assume a greater role in providing primary eye care services, it

Exposure control plan

Practice name: _____
Date: _____

In compliance with the Occupational Safety and Health Administration (OSHA) Bloodborne Pathogens Standard, 29 CFR 1910.1030, the following exposure control plan has been developed. This plan shall be reviewed and updated annually or whenever necessary to accommodate new tasks or procedures or to reflect new OSHA standards.

A. Purpose
   The purpose of this Exposure Control Plan is to
   1. Minimize or eliminate occupational exposure to blood or other potentially infectious body fluids; and
   2. Comply with 29 CFR 1910.1030 OSHA Bloodborne Pathogen Standard.

B. Exposure determination
   OSHA requires each employer to develop a listing of all job classifications in which employees may incur occupational exposure to blood or other potentially infectious materials. This listing is to identify all at-risk employees so proper training in safe work practices and procedures can be completed.

   In this office, the following job classifications may incur occupational exposure to blood or other potentially infectious materials:

   _____ _____ _____
   _____ _____ _____

   Tasks and procedures that might cause employees to have occupational exposure include the following:

   Job classification   Tasks/procedures
   _____   _____
   _____   _____
   _____   _____

C. Methods of compliance
   The following procedures will be followed in this office to minimize or eliminate occupational exposure to blood or other potentially infectious materials:

   1. Universal precautions
      Since not all individuals with infectious diseases can be identified, all human blood and certain human body fluids shall be treated as if infectious for HBV, HIV, and other bloodborne pathogens; therefore, the same infection control procedures and practices will be used with all individuals.
   2. Engineering and workplace controls
      Engineering and work practice controls will be used to eliminate or reduce exposure to infectious materials. If occupational exposure remains after institution of these controls, personal protective equipment shall be provided and used.

      The following engineering and workplace controls will be used:
      _____

      (continued)

FIGURE A-1—Sample exposure control plan. The plan presented in this figure is an example only. Consult the complete Occupational Safety and Health Administration Bloodborne Pathogens Standard to ensure compliance.

The above-mentioned controls will be examined and maintained on a regular schedule.

In work areas where there is reasonable likelihood of exposure to blood or other potentially infectious materials, employees will not eat, drink, apply cosmetics or lip balm, smoke, or handle contact lenses. Food and beverages will not be kept where blood or other infectious materials are present.

3. Personal protective equipment

    All personal protective equipment (PPE) used will be provided without cost to employees. PPE will be chosen based on reasonably anticipated exposure to blood or other potentially infectious materials.

    The following procedures will require the use of PPE:
    _____

    All PPE will be cleaned, laundered, and disposed of without cost to the employee. Repairs and replacements will also be made at no cost to the employee. Any garments penetrated by blood or other infectious material shall be removed immediately or as soon as feasible. All PPE will be removed prior to leaving the work area. After removal, PPE shall be placed in a designated and appropriate area or container for storage, washing, decontamination, or disposal.

    Gloves will be worn when it is reasonably anticipated that the employee will have contact with blood or other potentially infectious materials or when handling or touching contaminated items or surfaces. Disposable gloves are not to be washed or decontaminated for reuse and are to be replaced as soon as practical when their function as a barrier to exposure is compromised.

    Masks, eye protection, or combination face shields are required whenever splashes, splatters, or droplets of blood or other potentially infectious materials may be anticipated and contamination may occur.

4. Housekeeping

    All contaminated surfaces and equipment will be decontaminated immediately or as soon as feasible after any spill of blood or contact with other potentially infectious material.

    Decontamination will be accomplished using the following materials:
    _____   _____   _____
    _____   _____   _____

    Contaminated disposable equipment and supplies shall be discarded in appropriate containers that are labeled and color coded (fluorescent orange or orange-red). These containers shall be easily accessible and located as close as possible to the work area.

    When moving regulated waste containers, the containers shall be closed before removal or replacement to prevent spillage during handling, storage, transport, or shipping. If leakage is possible, the container shall be placed in a properly color coded second container with a label attached to identify its contents. Reusable containers shall not be opened, emptied, or cleaned in any manner that would expose the employee to the risk of injury or contamination.

    Note: Disposal of regulated waste shall be in accordance with applicable federal, state, and local regulations. Laundry contaminated with blood or other potentially infectious materials shall be handled as little as possible. Such laundry will be placed in appropriately marked (biohazard labeled or color coded) bags at the location where it was used.

(continued)

D. Hepatitis B vaccine

Hepatitis B vaccinations shall be made available to all employees who may have occupational exposure, and postexposure follow-up will be provided to employees who have had an exposure incident.

All medical evaluations and procedures including the hepatitis B vaccinations and postexposure follow-up will be:

1. Available at no cost to the employee;
2. Available at a reasonable time and place;
3. Performed by or under the supervision of a licensed physician or by or under the supervision of another licensed healthcare professional; and
4. Provided according to U.S. Public Health Service recommendations.

Hepatitis B vaccination shall be made available after the employee has received training in occupational exposure and within 10 working days of initial assignment for all employees who have occupational exposure unless the employee has previously received the complete hepatitis B vaccination series, antibody testing has revealed immunity, or a medical contraindication is indicated.

If an employee initially declines hepatitis B vaccination but at a later date decides to accept the vaccination, the vaccination shall then be made available. All employees declining the hepatitis B vaccination shall sign the OSHA-required waiver indicating refusal.

If a routine hepatitis B vaccine booster is recommended by the U.S. Public Health Service at a future date, such booster injections shall be made available.

E. Postexposure evaluation and follow-up

All exposure incidents shall be reported, investigated, and documented. When an employee incurs an exposure incident, it shall be reported to _____.

After a report of an exposure incident, the exposed employee shall immediately receive a confidential medical evaluation and follow-up, including at least the following elements:

1. Route of exposure documentation;
2. Circumstances under which exposure incident occurred;
3. Identification and documentation of source individual, unless identification is infeasible or impossible.
4. If source individual is known, then a blood test shall be done as soon as feasible to determine HIV/HBV infectivity.

Results of the source individual's testing shall be made available to the exposed employee, and the employee shall be informed of applicable laws and regulations concerning disclosure of the identity and infectious status of the source individual.

Collection and testing of blood for HBV and HIV serologic status will comply with the following:

1. Exposed employee's blood shall be collected and tested as soon as feasible after consent is obtained;
2. Employee will be offered the option of having his or her blood tested for HIV/HBV serologic status.

All employees who incur an exposure incident will be offered postexposure evaluation and follow-up in accordance with the OSHA standard.

(continued)

> F. Information and training
>
> Training will be provided at the time of initial assignment to tasks where occupational exposure may occur and shall be repeated within twelve months. It should include the following:
>
> 1. A copy and explanation of the OSHA standard;
> 2. Discussion of the epidemiology and symptoms of bloodborne diseases;
> 3. Explanation of the modes of transmission of bloodborne pathogens;
> 4. Explanation of the Bloodborne Pathogen Exposure Control Plan and method for obtaining a copy;
> 5. Identification of tasks that may involve exposure;
> 6. Explanation of use and limitations of methods to reduce exposure, for example, work practices, engineering controls, and PPEs;
> 7. Information on types, use, location, removal, handling, decontamination, and disposal of PPE;
> 8. Information on the hepatitis B vaccination, including efficiency, safety, administration, and benefits;
> 9. Information and explanation for appropriate action if exposure incident occurs; and
> 10. Explanation and identification of appropriate signs, labels, and color-coding systems.
>
> Additional training shall be provided when there is a change of tasks or procedures.
>
> G. Evaluation and review
>
> _____ shall be responsible for annually reviewing this program and its effectiveness and updating it as needed.

also must assume greater responsibility in safeguarding public health. The OSHA Bloodborne Pathogens regulation is another example of additional requirements that some optometric practices will need to meet. It provides guidance that all optometrists should consider in order to enhance infection control procedures in their offices as well.

REFERENCES

1. Centers for Disease Control. Recommendations for preventing possible transmission of human T-lymphotropic virus type III/lymphadenopathy associated virus from tears. MMWR 1985;34:533.
2. Centers for Disease Control. Recommendations for prevention of HIV transmission in health-care settings. MMWR 1987;36:3.
3. Centers for Disease Control. Update: Universal precautions for prevention of transmission of human immunodeficiency virus, hepatitis B virus, and other bloodborne pathogens in health-care settings. MMWR 1988;37:377.
4. Chronister C, Russo P. Effects of disinfecting solutions on tonometer tips. Optom Vis Sci 1990;67:818.
5. Clinical Alert 2/4. Updated recommendations for ophthalmic practice in relation to the human immunodeficiency virus. Ophthalmology 1989;96:1.
6. Lingel N, Coffey B. Effects of disinfecting solutions recommended by the Centers for Disease Control on Goldmann tonometer biprisms. J Am Optom Assoc 1992;63:43.
7. Centers for Disease Control. Recommendations for prevention of HIV transmission in health-care settings. MMWR 1987;36:IV.
8. Department of Labor, Occupational Safety and Health Administration. 29 CFR Part. 1910.1030, Occupational exposure to bloodborne pathogens; Final rule. Federal Register, 1991;58;64175–64182.
9. American Optometric Association, House of Delegates. Resolution 9 of 1991. Human Immunodeficiency Virus (HIV) Infection, June 25, 1991.

APPENDIX B

Common Pharmaceuticals Used in Eye Care

Commonly used cycloplegics, mydriatics,* and topical anesthetics

Generic name	Example of trade name	Concentration	Onset/duration of action
Cycloplegics and mydriatics			
Phenylephrine	AK-Dilate	2.5% and 10% solutions	30–60 min/3–5 hrs
	Mydfrin	2.5% solution	
	Paremyd	1% solution	15–60 min/4 hrs
Hydroxyamphetamine			
Tropicamide	Mydriacyl	0.5% and 1% solutions	20–40 min/4–6 hrs
Cyclopentolate	AK-Pentolate	1% solution	30–60 min/2 days
	Cyclogyl	0.5%, 1%, and 2% solutions	
Homatropine	Isopto-Homatropine	2% and 5% solutions	30–60 min/3 days
Scopalomine	Isopto-Hyoscine	0.25% solution	30–60 min/4–7 days
Atropine	Isopto-Atropine	0.5%, 1%, 2%, and 3% solutions	45–120 min/7–14 days
Topical anesthetics			
Proparacaine	Ophthetic, Alcaine	0.5%	10–30 sec/15–20 min
Tetracaine	Tetracaine	0.5%	

*Cycloplegics and mydriatics are used for pupil dilation and ciliary muscle suppression.

Commonly used ophthalmic antibacterial agents

Generic name	Example of trade name	Formulation
Individual antibiotics		
Bacitracin	AK-Tracin	Solution and ointment
Chloraphenicol	Chloroptic	Solution and ointment
Ciprofloxacin	Ciloxan	Solution
Gentamicin	Garamycin	Solution and ointment
Norfloxacin	Chibroxin	Solution
Ofloxacin	Ocuflox	Solution
Sulfacetamide	Bleph-10	Solution and ointment
Tetracycline	Achromycin	Solution
Tobramycin	Tobrex	Solution and ointment
Combinations and mixtures		
Polymyxin B/bacitracin	Polysporin	Ointment
Polymyxin B/neomycin/gentamicin	Neosporin	Solution and ointment
Polymyxin B/trimethoprim	Polytrim	Solution
Antiviral agents		
Trifluridine	Viroptic	Solution
Vidarabine	Vira-A	Ointment

Commonly used ocular anti-inflammatory agents

Generic name	Trade name	Concentration (%)
Steroids		
Dexamethasone	Decadron (solution)	0.1
	Decadron (ointment)	0.05
Fluorometholone	FML	0.1
	Flarex	0.1
Medrysone	HMS	1
Prednisolone	Pred Mild	0.12
	Pred Forte	1.0
Nonsteroidal anti-inflammatory drugs		
Diclofenac	Voltaren	0.1
Flurbiprofen	Ocufen	0.03
Ketorolac	Acular	0.5

Commonly used antiglaucoma medications

Generic name	Trade name	Concentration (%)
Pilocarpine	Pilocar, Pilostat, Isoptocarpine, Pilopine Gel Ointment 4%	0.5, 1, 2, 3, 4, 6
Dipivefrin	Propine	0.1
Betaxolol	Betoptic-S	0.25
Carteolol	Ocupress	1
Levobunolol	Betagan	0.25, 0.5
Metipranolol	Optipranolol	0.3
Timolol	Timoptic	0.25, 0.5
Apraclonidine	Iopidine	0.5, 1
Dorzolamide	Trusopt	2

GLOSSARY

A-scan Instrument that uses sound waves to measure the length of the eyeball
Absolute scotoma An area in which vision is entirely absent
Accommodation The ability of the eye to focus
Accounts receivable Money owed by the office
Acquired immune deficiency syndrome (AIDS) A syndrome of the human immune system caused by infection with human immunodeficiency virus
Algerbrush A device to remove a rust ring from a corneal foreign body
Amblyopia Reduced visual acuity with no apparent cause and not correctable by refractive means
Ammetropia The refractive condition that exists when accommodation is relaxed; parallel light rays entering the eye do not focus on the retina
Amsler grid A test to evaluate the integrity of central vision
Angle of incidence The angle that is formed by the light ray and the surface of the medium
Angular magnification Magnification expressed as a ratio of the angle subtended by the image to that subtended by the object with respect to a viewing point of reference
Aniseikonia A difference in the size of the two retinal images
Anisometropia An unequal refractive state of the two eyes
Ankylosing spondylitis An arthritic disease linked to uveitis
Aphakia Absence of the crystalline lens
Applanation tonometry A tonometer that measures the intraocular pressure by flattening a small portion of the cornea; example: Goldmann tonometer
Aqueous humor Clear fluid that is produced in the ciliary processes and fills the space from the posterior cornea to the anterior vitreous; maintains the intraocular pressure, nourishes the cornea, iris, and lens
Artificial tears Topical eye drops for use in the eye formulated to relieve the symptoms of dry eyes
Astigmatism Optical defect in which the light entering the eye does not form a single point focus but forms two focal points; corrected by use of cylindrical eyeglasses or contact lenses (spherical or toric)
Axial length The length of the eyeball from the cornea to the posterior pole
B-scan Instrument that uses sound waves to provide a cross section of the eye tissue; used to evaluate structures that cannot be viewed directly
Back vertex power (BVP) The vergence power expressed with reference to the posterior surface of a lens
Base curve Measurement of the back curvature of a lens
Benzalkonium chloride (BAK) A preservative used in topical eye drop preparations
Beta-blocker A drug whose topical effects lower intraocular pressure and whose systemic effects include slowing of heart rate
Bifocal A lens that provides both distance and near correction
Binocular Simultaneous use of both eyes
Bitoric lenses A lens having toroidal surfaces on both sides; used to correct astigmatism and aniseikonia
Blending A technique used to render the edges of a bifocal almost invisible
Blink rate The amount a person blinks in a given unit of time
Campimetry Investigation of the integrity of the field of vision
Cataract An opacity of the crystalline lens capsule
Chief complaint Patient's reason for the office visit
Chlorhexidine A preservative used in rigid contact lens solutions
Computerized axial tomography (CAT) scan An x-ray technique used to visualize internal structures
Concave lens A lens that is thinner in the center and thicker at the edges; parallel light passing through this type of lens is diverged, or refracted, away from the midline; also known as a minus lens
Confrontation fields A technique used to screen for visual field defects using the fingers of the examiner
Conjunctiva Mucous membrane covering the sclera of the eye
Contrast sensitivity test A test that measures the patient's perception of the difference between the compared stimuli
Convergence Simultaneous turning in of both eyes that occurs when viewing an approaching object
Convex lens A lens that is thicker in the center and thinner at the edges; parallel light rays passing through this type of lens are refracted by each surface to converge toward the midline behind the lens; also known as a plus lens
Corneal sensitivity Testing the sensitivity of the cornea to external stimuli
Crowding phenomenon The increased difficulty in identifying targets that are closely adjacent to other targets
Cycloplegic A parasympatholytic pharmacologic agent that paralyzes the ciliant body, causing loss of accommodation and, by sphincter paralysis, dilation
Decongestants Pharmaceuticals that cause vasoconstriction and subsequent nasal relief
Diopter Unit of refractive power; abbreviated "D"
Diplopia Double vision
Disinfection To destroy harmful bacteria and viruses
Divergence Ability of both eyes to move laterally simultaneously
Double vision Appreciation of two disparate retinal images
Eccentric fixation Fixation with a retinal area other than the fovea
Edema Swelling of tissues due to fluid influx
Emmetropia The power of the cornea and the lens at rest correspond with the axial length of the eye, so parallel light rays are appropriately refracted to focus on the retina
Episcleritis Inflammation of the episclera
Epithelium Top layer of the cornea
Eso In
Ethylenediaminetetraacetic acid (EDTA) Eye drop preservative
Exo Out
First-degree fusion Superimposition
Fluorescein A dye used topically to evaluate corneal integrity and intravenously to evaluate blood vessel integrity
Focal length The distance from the lens to the point where the light rays meet on the midline
Fovea Central (1.5 mm) area of the macula; responsible for the sharpest vision, fine discriminations, and high visual acuity; area of highest concentration of cone cells and no blood vessels; also called fovea centralis
Front surface toric lenses A lens with toricity on the front surface
Fundus Interior portion of the eyeball that can be seen on ophthalmoscopy or photography. Includes the retina and optic disc.
Fusion The merging of the images from each eye into a single visual image
Galilean telescope A refracting telescope that produces an erect, virtual image
Glare test A test for glare induced by cataract
Glaucoma Intraocular pressure disease
Hepatitis B Inflammation of the liver caused by the hepatitis B virus
Hofstetter's formula $A = 18.5 - 0.15Y$, where A is the average amplitude of accommodation and Y is age
Hydrogen peroxide Chemical disinfectant used for contact lens disinfection
Hydrophilic Related to having a strong attraction to water
Hyper Up
Hyperopia A refractive condition in which, when accommodation is relaxed, parallel light rays entering the eye focus behind the retina; also known as farsightedness

Hyperosmotic A solution with a greater osmotic gradient than surrounding tissues
Hypo Down
ICD-9-CM Diagnosis Codes for Optometry Codes used for billing
Indentation tonometry A tonometry that measures the intraocular pressure by indenting a small portion of the cornea; example: Schiotz tonometer
Index of refraction A number that indicates the speed of light through a medium compared with the speed of light in a vacuum
Indirect ophthalmoscope An instrument used to take stereoscopic views of the fundus
Intraocular pressure Fluid pressure maintained in the eye by the aqueous humor; measured with a tonometer
Isopter A contour line in visual fields representing connecting points of retinal sensitivity
Keplerian telescope An astronomic telescope
Keratoconjunctivitis Inflammation of the cornea and conjunctiva
Keratometry Measurement of the corneal curvature; measured with a keratometer
Lacrimation Tearing of the eye
Lenticular A design used on lenses to reduce thickness and weight
Limbus The area of the eye dividing the cornea from the sclera
Low tension glaucoma Intraocular pressure within the normal range but either or both the optic nerve and visual field are damaged
Macula Central portion of the retina surrounding the fovea; responsible for acute central vision
Macular degeneration A disease of the eye involving loss of structure and function of the macula
Magnetic resonance imaging scan A noninvasive diagnostic technique that produces computerized images of the internal structures of the body
Magnification An increase in apparent size of an image or object
Malingering Feigning or deliberately giving false test responses indicating illness or disability for personal gain
Metamorphopsia Distortion of vision
Microscope A magnifying optical instrument
Minus lens A lens that diverges light
Monocular Use of only one eye
Monovision Technique that sets one eye for distant vision and one eye for near vision
Myopia A refractive condition in which, when accommodation is relaxed, parallel light rays entering the eye focus in front of the retina; also known as nearsightedness
Neurologist A physician who specializes in the study of the nerves
Optical infinity The distance where light rays become parallel (20 feet, or 6 m)
Ortho Referring to the eyes being in perfect or straight alignment
Orthokeratology A treatment for myopia that uses a series of progressively flatter contact lenses to flatten the cornea
Over-refraction Refraction of a patient wearing a contact lens
Oxygen permeability (Dk) The ability for oxygen to penetrate a contact lens

Palpebral aperture The space between the eyelid margins
Pantoscopic tilt The angle that the frame front makes with the temples when viewed from the side
Papilla A small, nipple-shaped elevation
Perimetry The study of the visual fields
Peripheral vision The visual fields representing side vision
Phoria Tendency of an eye or eyes to deviate from the ortho
Photophobia Symptom causing pain on viewing a light; light sensitive
Photopic Pertaining to daylight vision
Physiologic blind spot The area of scotoma associated with the optic nerve head
Plus lens A lens that converges light
Polymethylmethacrylate (PMMA) A clear plastic material used for rigid contact lenses; first material used after glass
Posterior vitreous detachment The detachment of the vitreous from its attachment on the retina and producing symptoms of a floater
Presbyopia The condition in which lost elasticity of the lens leads to the inability to accommodate
Pressure patch Placement of a patch over the eye in some cases of corneal abrasion
Prism A lens that bends light
Pseudoaphakia Term used for the aphakic correction after a lens implant
Pursuits Eye movements as they follow a moving target; smooth eye movements
Radiuscope An instrument that measures the curvature of a contact lens
Refraction Altering of the pathway of light as it passes from one medium to another
Retina The light-sensitive tissue lining the back of the eye
Retinoscope An instrument used to perform refraction
Saccades Eye movements when looking from one target to another; jumping, two-eyed movements
Scotoma Area of absent vision or an area of depressed sensitivity in the visual field
Second-degree fusion Flat fusion
Seconds of arc Measurement units for recording stereopsis results
Slit-lamp examination Examination of the eye performed using a biomicroscope
Stereopsis Ability to see or appreciate depth using both eyes; highest degree of depth perception
Stereo vision Use of two eyes in looking at an object to gain stereopsis
Sterilization To free objects from living microorganisms by subjecting the objects to intense heat or chemical action
Steroid A drug used to reduce inflammation
Tear break-up time The amount of time it takes for the tear film on the cornea to break up
Thimerosal A mercury-based preservative used in contact lens solution
Third-degree fusion Stereopsis
Trifocal A lens that provides correction for distance, intermediate, and near
Tropia Constant or actual deviation of an eye
Uveitis Inflammation of the uveal tract
Vergence Movements of the two eyes in opposite directions

INDEX

A-Scan ultrasonography, 69, 196–197
AA, 68, 176
AC/A ratio, 296
Academic Therapy Publications, 312
Accommodation, 68, 298–302
    amplitude of (AA), 68, 176
    definition, 175
    disorders, 301–302
    near point of (NPA), 175–176, 299
    testing, 299–300
Accommodative amplitude, 299, 300
Accommodative convergence, 296
Accommodative excess, 301
Accommodative fatigue, 301
Accommodative infacility, 301–302
Accommodative insufficiency, 68, 301
Accommodative reserve, 68
Accounting, 15–25
    accounts payable, 17
    accounts receivable, 24–25
    bank statements, 18
    billing and collections, 24–25
    billing statements, 22, 25
    cash receipts, 15
    check-writing system, 15–17
    computer systems and, 34–35
    credit card payments, 23
    daily control sheet, 20
    fee slip, 24
    ledger card, 20
    past-due accounts, 25
    patient fees, 20, 23–24
    payment policies, 20, 23–24
    payment receipts, 20, 22, 23
    payroll, 17–18
    pegboard system, 19, 21
    petty cash, 18
    recording charges or payments, 18–20
Accounts payable, 17
Accounts receivable, 24–25
Achromatism, 171
Acquired aniseikonia, 81
Acquired immune deficiency syndrome (AIDS), 327
Acuity
    dynamic, 310
    static, 310
Adenovirus, 327
After Image Flasher, 307
AIDS, 327
Air sinuses, 39–40
Alternating cover test, 177
Amacrine cells, 55
Amblyopia, 82, 306–307
    form deprivation, 306
    functional, 82
    refractive, 82, 306
    strabismic, 82, 306
    treatment, 82
Amblyopia ex anopsia, 82
Amblyoscope, 307

American National Standards Institute (ANSI), 122, 140–143, 147–150
    add power standards, 142, 148
    attenuation tolerance standards, 150
    base curve standards, 148
    center thickness standards, 149
    cylinder axis standards, 141, 148
    distance refractive power standards, 147
    eyewire closure standards, 149
    geometric tolerance standards, 149
    impact resistance standards, 149
    impact resistance test method, 150
    localized error standards, 148–149
    localized error test method, 150
    mechanical tolerance standards, 149
    optical tolerance standards, 147–149
    physical quality standards, 150
    prism standards, 142–143, 148
    segment horizontal location standards, 149
    segment positioning standards, 142
    segment size standards, 149
    segment tilt standards, 149
    segment vertical location standards, 149
    sphere and cylinder power standards, 141
    transmission tolerance standards, 150
    ultraviolet protection standards, 150
    warpage standards, 148
American Optometric Association (AOA), 1, 313
    address and phone number, 37
    code of ethics, 2
    Diagnosis Codes for Optometry, 27
    infection control guidelines, 327–336
    membership information, 37
    Optometric Procedures, Diagnosis and Treatment, 27
Ametropia, 77
    axial, 70
    refractive, 70
    vs. emmetropia, 69–70
Amplitude of accommodation (AA), 68, 176
Amsler grid, 203, 205–206, 281
Aneurysm, 58
Angle of incidence, 63–64
Aniseikonia, 81–82
Anisometropia, 81
Annulus of Zinn, 59
Anomaloscope, 170
Anomalous retinal correspondence (ARC), 307
Anomalous trichromat, 171
ANSI. *See* American National Standards Institute (ANSI)
Anterior uveitis, 51, 317–318
Anticipation time, 310
Antimetropia, 81
AOA. *See* American Optometric Association
Aphakia, 78–81
    binocular, 81
    definition/description, 78
    monocular, 80
    treatment, 79–80

Aphakic lenses, 79–80, 99, 136
    power measurement for, 115–116
Applanation tonometry, 190
Aqueous humor, 51
ARC, 307
Arc perimeter, 206–207
Arteries
    central retinal, 52
    ophthalmic, 52
Arthritis, 52
Aspheric lenses, 135–136
Association fibers, 58
Astigmatism, 73–76, 229
    against-the-rule, 74
    compound, 74
    compound myopic, 74
    compound hyperopic, 74
    corneal, 74
    definition/description, 73–74
    irregular, 74
    measuring, 74
    mixed, 74
    oblique, 74
    ocular, 74
    residual, 74, 75
    simple, 74
    surgical treatment of, 76
    symptoms, 75
    treatment, 75
    types, 74
    with-the-rule, 74
Audiovisual presentations, 31, 33
Auto-Plot Tangent Screen, 205
Auxiliary prism, 116
Axial ametropia, 70
Axial anisometropia, 81
Axial length, 69

B-scan ultrasonography, 197–198
Bagolini lenses, 307
Balance lenses, 99
Bandage lenses, 316
Bank statements, 18
Basic secretors, 45
Bernall Corporation, 312
Bernell Stereo Reindeer test, 172
Bevels, 134–135
    hide-a-bevel, 134
    nylon suspension grooved, 134
    peripheral, 223
    pin, 134
    rimless, 134
    safety, 134
    V, 134
Bifocal lenses, 78, 114, 136–140
    annular, 231
    aspheric progressive addition, 232
    blended, 137
    contact, 231–232
    double segment, 98
    executive, 97
    Franklin, 97
    full-width, 97
    invisible, 136–140
    kryptok, 97
    order verification, 136–140
    parameter verification, 265
    power measurement for, 114
    progressive addition, 138–140
    round, 96–97
    soft contacts, 241
    straight-top, 96
    translating segmented, 231–232
Binasal hemianopsia, 58
Binocular vision, 295–308
    accommodation. *See* Accommodation
    disorders, 295–298
    oculomotor dysfunction, 302–304
    treatment procedures, 307–308
Biofeedtrac Inc., 312
Bipolar cells, 55
Bitemporal hemianopsia, 58
Bitoric lenses, 231
Blepharitis, 45
Blepharoconjunctivitis, 45
Blepharospasm, 41
Blind spot, 53
    physiologic, 199
Blindness, causes of, 210
Blink rate, contact lenses and, 215
Blood pressure, 181–182
Bloodborne pathogens, 330–336
Blur point, 175
Blurred vision, 51, 70, 75
Bones, 42
    ethmoid, 39, 40
    frontal, 39, 40
    lacrimal, 39, 40
    maxilla, 39, 40, 41
    maxillary, 40
    palatine, 39, 41
    sphenoid, 39, 40
    zygomatic, 39, 40
Bowman's membrane, 48
Boxing system, 121–122, 143
Break point, 176
Breaking fusion, 175
Bridge size, 122
Bridge types, 145
Brightness Acuity Tester, 194, 282
Broad H test, 177–178
Brodman's area 8, 17, 58
Bruch's membrane, 52, 53
Bulbar conjunctiva, 44
Bullous keratopathy, 242
Burton screener, 203–204
Business management, 1–38. *See also* Office procedures; Personnel
    code of ethics, 2
    community involvement, 37
    computer systems, 34–35
    office communications, 36–37

policy/procedure manuals, 36–37

Campimetry, 200
Canal of Schlemm, 51
Canaliculi, 46
Capsule, 56
Cataracts, 56, 210
    congenital, 78, 82
    cortical, 79
    definition/description, 78
    infantile, 78
    nuclear, 79
    power measurement for lenses, 115–116
    senile, 79
    subcapsular, 79
    traumatic, 78
Centers for Disease Control (CDC), 327
Central corneal clouding (CCC), 224
Central retinal artery, 52
Central vision, 310
Chalazion, 44
Chemosis, 44
Chiasm, optic, 57
Choriocapillaris, 52
Choroid, 52–53
Ciliary body, 51–52
Ciliary muscle, 51, 56, 76
Circles of eccentricity, 199, 202
Code of ethics, 2
Collagen, 48
College of Vision Development (COVD), 313
Colmascope, 129
Color vision, 168–171, 310
    classifications, 171
    evaluating, 169
    testing, 169–171, 281
Common tendinous ring, 59
Compound anisometropia, 81
Compound astigmatism, 74
Compound hyperopic astigmatism, 74
Compound myopic astigmatism, 74
Computer Orthoptics, 312
Computer systems, 34–35
    data storage and backup, 34
    hardware, 34
    office applications, 34–35
    software, 34
    video display terminal, 34
Concave lenses, 65, 71, 84
Cone cells, 54, 69, 171
Confrontation testing, 201–202
Congenital cataract, 78, 82
Conjunctiva, 44–45
Conjunctivitis, 44, 50, 320
    giant papillary, 218
    keratoconjunctivitis, 320
Consultation letters, 27–28
Contact lenses, 15, 75, 78, 213–277
    bifocal, 78, 231–232, 241
        annular, 231
        translating segmented, 231–232
    aspheric progressive addition, 232
    bitoric, 75, 231
    care and handling, 245–261
    cases for, 248, 256
    disinfecting, 329
    disposable, 244–245
    extended-wear. See Extended-wear lenses
    flexible. See Flexible lenses
    front surface toric lenses, 231
    hard, 75. See also RGP lenses
    history, 213
    industry, 213
    inserting, 248–249, 256–258
    modifying, 267–276
    order form, 224, 225, 237
    parameter verification, 261–265, 265–267
    patient instructions, 251–254, 259–261
    prefitting evaluation, 213–220
        blink rate and type, 215
        corneal evaluation, 217
        corneal sensitivity, 215
        eyelids, 217–218
        keratometry, 218
        lid considerations, 214–215
        patient case history, 213–214
        patient hygiene, 218
        pupil considerations, 214–215
        tear film, 215–216
    pregnancy and, 214
    purpose/scope, 213
    recentering, 251
    removing, 249–251, 259
    rigid. See RGP lenses
    soft. See Flexible lenses
    tolerance standards, 266
    toric, 75, 236–239
    toric base curve lenses, 231
    toric peripheral curve lenses, 231
    trifocal, 232
Contrast sensitivity, 193
Contrast Sensitivity Function, 281
Convergence, 61, 296
    accommodative, 296
    definition, 175
    near point of (NPC), 175–176, 296
Convergence excess, 297–298
Convergence insufficiency, 297
Convex lenses, 65, 84
Cornea, 46–50
    contact lens sensitivity and, 215
    damage to, 48–49
    evaluating, 217
    flat, 69
    function/purpose, 46
    layers, 46–48
    monkey's, 48
    nervous supply, 46
    optics of, 66–67
    steep, 69
Corneal abrasions, 316–317
Corneal astigmatism, 74

Corneal curvature, 67
Corneal foreign bodies, 318–319
Corneal neovascularization, 46
Corneal reflection system, 208
Corneal transplant, 49
Correspondence
    consultation letters, 27–28
    contact lens patient referral form, 30
    greeting cards, 29, 31
    patient referral letter, 29
    patient referral thank-you letter, 31
    school vision report forms, 29
    thank you notes, 28–29
Cortex, 56
Cortical cataract, 79
Cover tests, 176–177, 296, 305–306
CR-39 plastic lenses, 91–93
Cross-eye, 61
Crowding phenomenon, 306
Crown glass, 91
Crystalline lenses, 67–69, 78
Cycloplegics, 51
Cylindrical lenses, 75, 85, 86

DBL, 122
Decentration, 90
Dendrite, 54
Depth perception, 310
Descemet's membrane, 48
Deuteranomalous anomalous trichromat, 171
Deuteranope dichromat, 171
Developmental Eye Movement Test, 303
Deviation
    latent, 304
    manifest, 304
Diabetes, 71, 210
Dial-thickness gauge, 128–129
Dichromat, 171
Dichromatism, 171
Dilator muscle, 50
Diopters, 65
    prism, 85
Diplopia, 79, 176, 306
Direct patching, 306
Disposable contact lenses, 244–245
    benefits, 244–245
    implementing, 245
    problems with, 245
Distance between lenses (DBL), 122
Divergence, 61, 296
Dress code, 2–3
Dynamic acuity, 310
Dystrophy, 242

Eccentric fixation, 307
Eccentricity, circles of, 199, 202
Ectropion, 42
Educational materials, 31, 33
Efficient Seeing Publications, 312
Eikonometer, 81
Emergencies. *See* Medical emergencies

Emmetropia, vs. ametropia, 69–70
Endothelium, 48
Entropion, 42
Environmental Protection Agency (EPA), 329
Epiphora, 46
Episclera, 49–50
Episcleritis, 50, 320–321
Epithelium, 47, 48
    nonpigmented, 50
    pigmented, 51
Equator, 59
Esophoric, 177, 296
Esotropia, 305
Ethmoid air sinuses, 39, 40
Ethmoid bone, 39, 40
Ethmoiditis, 40
Examination, 161–182. *See also* Patients; Tests and testing
    amplitude of accommodation (AA), 176
    blood pressure, 181–182
    color vision, 168–171
    contact lens prefitting evaluation, 213–220
    cover tests, 176–177
    eye dominance, 180–181
    interpupillary distance (PD), 178–180
    low vision, 279–293
    near point of accommodation (NPA), 175–176
    near point of convergence (NPC), 175–176
    patient history, 161–164, 213–214
        checklist format, 163
        family medical history, 163–164
        greeting the patient, 162
        open-ended approach, 162
        outline method, 162–163
        techniques in obtaining, 162–164
    pursuit eye movements, 177–178
    recording methods, 161
    role of paraoptometric in, 161
    saccadic eye movements, 177–178
    stereoacuity, 171–175
    stereopsis, 171–175
    testing location, 161
    testing method, 161
    testing sequence, 161
    visual acuity data, 164–168
    visual skills, 182
Exophoric, 177, 296
Exotropia, 305
Extended-wear lenses, 241–244
    contraindications, 242–243
    for aphakics, 242
    for children, 242
    for medical patients, 242
    for myopic patients, 242
    high–water content, 243
    history, 241–242
    low–water content, 243–244
    medium–water content, 243
    rigid gas-permeable (RGP), 244
    silicone elastomer, 244
    types of, 243–244
External limiting membrane, 54

Extraocular muscles, 58–61
　agonist pairs in two eyes, 61
　antagonist pairs in one eye, 61
　facts regarding, 60
　oblique muscles, 58–61
　rectus muscles, 58–59
Eye. *See also* Ocular anatomy; Vision
　optical components of, 66–69
　refractive status of, 63–82
Eyeball, 47–50
　anterior chambers, 46
　cross section of, 47
　fibrous tunic, 46–50
　length of, 69
　nervous tunic, 46, 53–55
　posterior chambers, 46
　vascular tunic, 46, 50–53
Eye dominance, 180–181, 310
Eye emergencies. *See* Medical emergencies
Eye-hand-foot-body coordination, 310
Eyelid, 40–43
　conjunctiva, 44
　contact lenses and, 214–215, 217–218
　external structure, 43
　glands in, 44–45
　layers of tissue, 43
　levator palpebrae superioris, 43
　meibomian, 44
　Mueller's muscle, 44
　orbicularis oculi, 43
　problems associated with, 42
　structure, 43–44
　subcutaneous areolar layer, 43
　submuscular areolar layer, 43
　tarsal glands, 44
　tarsal plate, 43–44
Eye motility, 310
Eye movements
　disorders, 303–304
　evaluating in low vision patients, 281
　pursuit, 177–178, 303
　saccadic, 177–178, 303, 310
　testing, 61
Eyestrain, 75
Eye teaming, 310
　disorders, 295–298
Eyewire groove tips, 121

Farnsworth D-15 Dichotomous Test, 169
Farnsworth Lantern Test, 170
Farnsworth-Munsell 100 Hue Test, 169
Farsightedness. *See* Hyperopia
Fibrous tunic, 46–50
　cornea, 46–50, 66–67
　sclera, 49–50
Filing, 12–13
Fixation, eccentric, 307
Fixation methods, 208–209
　corneal reflection system, 208
　direct visualization of the pupil, 208
　Heijl-Krakau method, 208

Flashes and floaters, 322
Flat fusion, 295, 306
Flexible lenses, 75, 80, 232–241
　advantages, 235
　bifocal, 241
　care and handling, 254–261
　cases, 256
　chemistry, 234–235
　cleaning, 255–256
　daily wear, 234
　disadvantages, 235
　disinfecting, 254–255
　extended wear. *See* Extended-wear lenses
　fitting, 235–236
　follow-up care, 235–236
　history, 232–233
　inserting, 256–258
　manufacturing techniques, 233–234
　order form, 237
　parameter verification, 265–267
　　base curve radius, 266
　　center thickness, 266–267
　　diameter, 267
　　edge inspection, 267
　　power, 265–266
　　surface inspection, 267
　patient instructions, 259–261
　presbyopic correction, 239–241
　removing, 259
　tints, 235
　toric, 236–239
Fluoro-silicone/acrylate (F-S/A), 225–226
Focal length, calculating, 84
Focimeter, 107
Focusing, speed of, 310
Food and Drug Administration (FDA), 106, 225
Foramen, 39, 42
Form deprivation amblyopia, 306
Forms
　appointment reminder, 11
　appointment sheets, 9, 10
　billing statement, 22
　checkwriting system, 16, 17
　contact lens order form, 225, 237
　contact lens patient referral, 30
　contact lens progress check, 231
　exposure control plan, 333–336
　fee slip, 24
　fee statement, 25
　optical order form, 106, 107
　payroll check system, 19, 20
　pegboard system, 21
　preliminary evaluation for contact lenses, 219
　quick claim form receipt, 27
　receipt, 22
　receipt/charge slip, 23
　school vision report, 33
Fornix, 44
Fovea, 54, 56–57, 199
Fovea centralis, 69
Foveola, 54

Frame eyesize, 121, 143
Frames, 14–15, 151–160
   adjusting, 155–158
   aligning, 155, 152
   boxing system, 121–122
   bridge size, 122
   care and handling of, 158
   dispensing to children, 159–160
   dispensing to elderly patients, 158–159
   fitting, 151
   follow-up adjustments, 158
   order verification, 143–145
      bridge type, 145
      color, 144–145
      quality, 145
      shape, 145
      size, 143
      temple type, 145
   parameter information, 144
   temple length, 144
Franck, Fredrick, 309
Franel Optical Supply, 312
Franklin, Benjamin, 78
Fresnel Press-On membrane lenses, 99
Frontal air sinuses, 40
Frontal bone, 39, 40
Functional amblyopia, 82
Fundus photography, 195–196
Fusion, 295
   categories, 306
   degrees of, 295
   flat, 295, 306
   motor, 295
   sensory, 295, 306
Fusional vergence movements, 296

Galilean telescope, 288
Ganglion cell layer, 55
Ganglion cells, 55, 57
Giant papillary conjunctivitis (GPC), 218
Glands
   goblet cells, 44
   Krause, 44, 45
   lacrimal, 45
   Moll, 45–46
   sebaceous, 44
   Wolfring, 44, 45
   Zeis, 44–45
Glare recovery, 310
Glare testing, 193–194
   in low vision patients, 282
Glass lenses, 126
   absorptive, 100–101
   chemical tempering, 94
   coatings, 130–132
   colored, 102
   crown, 91
   different types of, 92
   heat tempering, 94
   photochromic, 103
   tempering, 94, 129

   tints, 129–130
Glasses. *See* Frames; Lenses
Glaucoma, 190, 210, 321–322
Globe. *See* Eyeball
Goblet cells, 44
Goldmann bowl perimeter, 207–208
GPC, 218
Greeting cards, 29, 31

Haller's layer, 52
Hardware, 34
Harrington Flocks Visual Field Screener, 203–204
HBV, 327, 331–332
Headaches, 75
   migraine, 322
Heijl-Krakau method, 208
Hemianopia, 57
Hemianopsia, 57
   binasal, 58
   bitemporal, 58
Hemorrhage, subconjunctival, 50
Hepatitis B virus (HBV), 327, 331–332
Herpes, 327
Heterophoria, 61
Hide-a-bevel, 134
High-index plastic lenses, 93, 126
High–water content lenses, 243
HIV, 327
Hofstetter's formula, 300
Holmgren Wool Test, 171
Homonymous, 57
Horizontal cells, 55
Human immunodeficiency virus (HIV), 327
Hydrogen peroxide, 255
Hydrophilic contact lens. *See* Flexible lenses
Hypermetropia, 72
Hyperopia, 68, 72–73
   behavioral signs of, 72
   physical signs of, 72
   surgical treatment of, 76
   treatment, 73
Hypertension, 182
   ocular, 51
Hypertropia, 305
Hypotension, ocular, 51
Hypotropia, 305

Ill-sustained accommodation, 301
Incidence, angle of, 63–64
Indentation tonometry, 190
Index of refraction, 64, 83
Induced prism, 89–90
Industrial safety lenses, 94
Infantile cataract, 78
Infection control guidelines, 327–336
   bloodborne pathogens, 330–336
   checklist, 330
   contact lens disinfection, 329
   definitions of key terms relating to, 328
   disposable latex gloves, 328
   exposure control plan, 331–336

gowns, 328
hand washing, 327–328
infectious waste disposal, 329–330
instrument disinfection, 329
masks, 328
protective eye wear, 328
responsibility to patients, 332
sharp instrument handling, 329
tissue handling, 328–329
Infectious waste disposal, 329–330
Inferior oblique muscle, 58, 61
Inferior rectus muscle, 58, 59
Inherent aniseikonia, 81
Inner nuclear layer, 55
Inner plexiform layer (IPL), 55
Insurance, 25–26
Internal limiting membrane, 55
International Academy of Sports Vision (NASV), 313
Interpupillary distance (PD), 106, 133–134, 171
   distance PD measurement, 178–179
    monocular PD measurement, 180
   near PD measurement, 179
   testing, 178–180
Interpupillary distance rule, 154
Interval of Sturm, 74
Intraocular pressure (IOP), 189, 190
IOL, 80
IOP, 189, 190
IPL, 55
Iris, 50–51
Irregular astigmatism, 74
Iseikonic lenses, 82

K readings, 185
Keplerian telescope, 288
Keratoconjunctivitis, 320
Keratoconus, 48, 71
Keratometer, 67, 185, 218, 262
Keratometry, 185–189, 218, 229
   definition/description, 185
   locating the cylinder axis, 186, 188
    measuring the power of major meridians, 188
   patient testing, 185–186
   recording findings from, 188–189
   test equipment, 185
Keratopathy, bullous, 242
Keratoplasty, 49
Keratotomy, radial, 76
Krause glands, 44, 45

Lacrimal bone, 39, 40
Lacrimal fossa, 40, 45
Lacrimal sac, 46
Lacrimal system, 45–46
Lafayette Instruments, 312
LARS principle, 238
Laser surgery, 76
Latent deviation, 304
Lateral geniculate body, 58
Lateral geniculate nucleus (LGN), 58
Lateral rectus muscle, 58, 59

Lazy eye. *See* Amblyopia
Left optic tract, 57
Lens Analyzer, 118
Lens clock, 127–128
Lens order verification, 122–143
   base curve, 127–128
   bevel, 134–135
   calibration, 128
   center thickness, 128–129
   centration, 122–124
   coatings, 129–132
   design, 126–127
   high-power, 136
   invisible bifocals, 136–140
   materials, 125–126
   moderate-power aspheric, 135–136
   multifocal, 132–134
   near interpupillary distance, 133–134
   optical quality, 135
   power, 122, 124–125
   prism, 122–124
   progressive addition, 138–140
   segment alignment, 133
   segment height, 132–133
   segment type, 132
   segment width, 133
   spectacle measurement, 125
   tempering, 129–130
   tints, 129–132
   warpage, 128
Lenses, 56
   ANSI standards. *See* American National Standards Institute (ANSI)
   aphakic, 79–80, 99, 115–116, 136
   aspheric, 135–136
   balance, 99
   bifocal. *See* Bifocal lenses
   coatings for, 100–101
   concave, 65, 71, 84
   concepts of light and, 83–85
   contact. *See* Contact lenses
   convex, 65, 84
   cylindrical, 75, 85, 86
   designs, 94–99
   dispensing thinnest possible, 93
   E/D style occupational, 98
   forms of, 85–86
   Fresnel Press-On membrane, 99
   glass, 91, 126, 129
   high-power, 136
   impact resistance, 93–94
   industrial safety, 94
   iseikonic, 82
   laboratory considerations, 99–100
   materials for, 91–93, 125–126, 159
   measuring power of, 65
   minus. *See* Concave lenses; Lenses, concave
   multifocal, 90, 94–98, 110–114, 132–134
   myodisc, 99
   ophthalmic, 91–104
   optical cross, 87–88

Lenses *(continued)*
    order verification. *See* Lens order verification
    ordering from optical laboratory, 105–107
    photochromic, 130
    planocylindrical, 94
    plastic, 91–93, 126, 129, 159
    plus. *See* Convex lens; Lenses, convex
    polarized sun, 104
    progressive addition, 138–140
    progressive addition multifocal, 95–96
    quadrifocal, 98
    single-vision, 110–114
    spherical, 75, 85, 94, 111
    spherocylindrical, 75, 86, 87–88, 94, 112
    Technica progressive addition, 98–99
    tints for, 101–104
    trifocal, 78, 90, 97, 114–115
    using a lensometer. *See* Lensometer
Lensometer, 107–121, 265
    automatic, 124
    auxiliary prism, 116
    calibration check, 108
    corona-and-crossline target, 117
    diagram, 109
    eyepiece focus position scale, 110
    eyepiece reticle, 110
    focusing, 108
    in-focus target, 110
    manufacturers of, 107–108
    out-of-focus target, 110
    parts of, 108
    power measurement for
        aphakic lens, 115–116
        bifocal lens, 114
        multifocal lens, 110–114
        single-vision lens, 110–114
        sphere lens, 111
        spherocylinder lens, 112
        trifocal lens, 114–115
    power measurement with
        automatic, 117–118
        with various, 116–117
    prism measurement, 118–121, 124
    spectacles position on, 110
    target lines, 112
Lensometry, principles of, 107–121
Lenticular opacification, 78
Lesions, 57–58
Letters. *See* Correspondence
Levator palpebrae superioris, 43
LGN, 58
Light
    optics of, 63–66
    speed of, 83
Light rays, 63–65, 83
Light waves, 83
Low-tension glaucoma, 190
Low vision, 279–293
Low Vision Enhancement System (LVES), 288
Low–water content lenses, 243–244
LVES, 288

Macula lutea, 54, 69
Macular degeneration, senile, 210
Macular sparing, 58
Magni Cam, 289
Magnification, 283
Magnifiers
    device training, 292–293
    distance magnification devices, 288, 289
    electronic video, 286–288
    field-enhancing devices, 289–290
    hand-held, 262, 285
    head-borne systems, 283–285
    nonoptical devices, 290, 292
    projection, 264
    stand, 285–286
Mail, 26–31. *See also* Correspondence
Major reference point (MRP), 120
Management, business, 1–38
Manifest deviation, 304
Maxilla bone, 39, 40
Maxillary air sinuses, 40
Maxillary bone, 40
Medial rectus muscle, 58, 59
Medicaid, 26
Medical emergencies, 315–323
    anterior uveitis, 317–318
    conjunctivitis, 320
    corneal abrasions, 316–317
    definition, 315
    episcleritis, 320–321
    flashes and floaters, 322
    foreign body in eye, 318–319
    glaucoma attack, 321–322
    neurologic conditions, 322–323
    obtaining case history, 316
    patient treatment, 316
    time factor, 315
    treatment comfort zone, 315
Medicare, 26
Medications, 50–51, 337–338
Medium–water content lenses, 243
Meibomian, 44
Melanocytes, 52
Memory, visual, 311
Mesothelium, 48
Microscope, 283–285
Migraine, ophthalmic, 322
Miller Nadler glare tester, 282
Mixed anisometropia, 81
Mixed astigmatism, 74
Moll glands, 45–46
Monochromatism, 171
Monovision technique, 78
Motor eye fields, 58
Motor fusion, 295
MRP, 120
Mucin layer, 45
Mueller cells, 55
Mueller's muscle, 44
Multifocal lenses, 90, 94–98
    bifocal. *See* Bifocal lenses

E/D style occupational, 98
occupational types, 97–98
order verification, 132–134
power measurment for, 110–114
progressive addition, 95–96
quadrifocal, 98
Technica progressive addition, 98–99
trifocal, 78, 90, 97, 114–115, 232
Muscles
ciliary, 51, 56, 76
dilator, 50
extraocular, 58–61
inferior oblique, 58, 61
inferior rectus, 58, 59
lateral rectus, 58, 59
medial rectus, 58, 59
Mueller's, 44
oblique, 58–61
paralytic, 61
paretic, 61
rectus, 58–59
superior oblique, 58, 59, 61
superior rectus, 58, 59
Mydriatics, 50–51
Myodisk lenses, 99
Myopia, 70–71
extended-wear lenses for patients with, 242
pathologic, 71
physiologic, 70
surgical treatment of, 76
treatment for, 71

Nasal canthus, 45
NASV, 313
National Paraoptometric Registry, 37
NCT, 191
Near point of accommodation (NPA), 175–176, 299–300
Near point of convergence (NPC), 175–176, 296
Nearsightedness. *See* Myopia
Needle-nose pliers, 156
Nerve, optic, 55, 57
Nerve fiber layer, 55
Nervous tunic, 46, 53–55. *See also* Retina
Neural retina, 54
Neurologic conditions, 322–323
Neurotransmitter, 54
Night vision, 310
Noncontact tonometer (NCT), 191
Nonpigmented epithelium, 50
Nonuniform cobblestone appearance (NUCA), 218
NPA, 175–176, 299–300
NPC, 175–176, 296
NUCA, 218
Nuclear cataract, 79
Nylon-jawed pliers, 156
Nylon suspension grooved bevel, 134

Oblique muscles, 58–61
Occluder, 168
Occupational Safety and Health Administration (OSHA), 330–336

Ocular anatomy
anatomic directions, 39, 40
definition/description, 39
external structures, 40–45
extraocular muscles, 58–61
eyeball, 46–50
eyelid, 40–43
globe, 46–50
lacrimal system, 45–46
lens, 56
orbits, 39–40
visual pathway, 56–58
Ocular astigmatism, 74
Ocular health, 282
Ocular hypertension, 51
Ocular hypotension, 51
Oculomotor dysfunction, 302–304
OEP, 313
Office manager, 36
Office procedures, 3–31
appointments, 7–12
confirming by telephone, 8
emergency situations, 7–8. *See also* Medical emergencies
follow-up/recall, 10–12
gathering data from patients, 8–9
offering various choices, 7
scheduling, 7–8
writing down, 7
reminder card, 11
correspondence, 26–31
consultation, 27–28
contact lens patient referral form, 30
greeting cards, 29, 31
patient referral letter, 29
patient referral thank-you letter, 31
school vision report forms, 29
thank-you notes, 28–29
filing, 12–13
financial records. *See* Accounting
forms. *See* Forms
greeting patients, 9–10
insurance coverage, 25–26
mail, 26–31
reception area, 3–4
supplies. *See* Office supplies
telephone technique, 4–6
answering, 4–5
elements of courtesy, 4
handling complaints, 6
patient requesting information, 5
requests for cost information, 6–7
screening calls, 4–6
taking messages, 5–6
Office supplies, 13–15
business, 13
contact lenses, 15
educational materials, 31, 33
examination room, 13–14
frames, 14–15
optical, 14

Office supplies *(continued)*
  solutions and drugs, 14
Oily layer, 45
Oblique astigmatism, 74
Ophthalmic artery, 52
Ophthalmic dispensing, 151–160. *See also* Frames
Ophthalmic migraines, 322
Ophthalmic ultrasonography, 196–198
Ophthalmometer, 67, 185
OPL, 55
Optic chiasm, 57
Optic nerve, 55, 57
Optic radiations, 58
Optic tract, 58
Optical center, 65
Optical cross, 87–88
Optical infinity, 63
Optical laboratory
  lens order verification, 122–143
  ordering contact lenses from, 224, 225, 236
  ordering lenses from, 105–107
Optometric Extension Program Foundation (OEP), 313
Optometry, promoting the field of, 37
Ora serrata, 53
Orbicularis oculi, 43
Orbits, 39–40
  bones in, 39, 42
  composition, 39
  definition/description, 39
  floor of, 40
  foramen in, 39, 42
  lacrimal fossa, 40
  walls of, 40–40
Ortho, 177, 296
Orthokeratology, 71
Orthophoric, 177
OSHA, 330–336
Outer nuclear layer, 54
Outer plexiform layer (OPL), 55

Pad-angling pliers, 156
PAL, 106, 138–140
Palatine bone, 39, 41
Palpebrae, 40–41
Palpebral aperture, 41, 214
Palpebral conjunctiva, 44
Panuveitis, 52
Papillae, 217–218
Paralytic muscle, 61
Paranasal sinuses, 40
Paraoptometric, definition, 1
Paretic muscle, 61
Pars optica, 53
Pathologic myopia, 71
Patients
  communicating with, 1–2
    children, 35
    disabled, 35
    elderly, 35
  confidentiality and, 2
  corresponding with. *See* Correspondence
  dispensing frames to
    children, 159–160
    elderly, 158–159
  educational materials for, 31, 33
  examination. *See* Examination
  fees charged to, 20, 23–24
  greeting, 9–10
  handling complaints by, 6
  insurance coverage, 25–26
  medical emergencies. *See* Medical emergencies
  obtaining information from, 8–9
  optometrist communications with, 35–36
  records, 2
  requesting information by telephone, 5
PD. *See* Interpupillary distance (PD)
PD rule, 143
Perimetry, 200
Peripheral bevel, 223
Peripheral vision, 310
Personnel
  code of ethics, 2
  dress code, 2–3
  office manager, 36
  payroll, 17–18
  personal phone calls, 2
  policy manuals, 36–37
  staff meetings with, 36
Petty cash, 18
Phenol Red Cotton Thread test, 216
Phoria, 61, 177
Phoric posture, 296
Photochromic glass, 103
Photochromic lenses, 130
Photochromic plastic, 103–104
Photophobia, 51, 193, 317
Photopigments, 53
Photoreceptors, 53, 54, 69
Physiologic blind spot, 199
Physiologic myopia, 70
Pigmented epithelium, 51
Pin bevel, 134
PIP, 169
Pituitary adenomas, 58
Planocylindrical lenses, 94
Plastic lenses, 126
  coatings, 129–130
  CR-39, 91–93
  different types of, 92
  high-index, 93, 126
  photochromic, 103–104
  tempering, 129
  tinted, 102, 129–130
Pliers, 155–157
PMMA, 224
Polariscope, 129
Polarized lenses, 104
Polishing compounds, 267–268
Polycarbonate lenses, 93
Polymethylmethacrylate (PMMA), 224
Posterior synechia, 51
Posterior uveitis, 52

Posterior vitreous detachment (PVD), 322
Potential acuity meter, 194–195
Prentice's rule, 89
Presbyopia, 51, 68, 76–78, 239
    definition/description, 76
    patient case history, 77
    patient factors, 76–77
        age, 76
        ametropia, 77
        environmental conditions, 77
        general health, 76
        self-image, 77
        stature, 77
        visual demand, 76–77
    progression, 78
    symptoms, 77
    treatment, 77
Prescriptions. *See also* Lenses
    decentration, 90
    multifocal, 90
    prism, 89–90
    sphere equivalent, 89
    transposing plus cylinder into minus cylinder, 88–89
Pressure patch, 316
Prism, 89–90, 264
    ANSI standards, 142–143, 148
    auxiliary, 116
    horizontal, 123, 125
    induced, 89–90
    level reference point, 123
    measuring, 118–121, 124
    order verification, 122–124
    Risley auxiliary, 116
    vertical, 124
Prism diopters, 85
Prism power, 84–85, 89
Prism reference point (PRP), 120–121
Progressive addition lenses (PALs), 106, 138–140
Progressive addition multifocal lenses, 95–96
Protanope dichromat, 171
Protoanomalous anomalous trichromat, 171
PRP, 120–121
Pseudoisochromatic plate (PIP), 169
Pseudomonas, 327
Ptosis, 42
Puncta, 45, 46
Pupil, 50
    constriction, 175
    direct visualization of, 208
    contact lenses and, 214–215
Pupillary frill, 51
Pupillary testing, 50
Pursuit eye movements, 177–178, 303
PVD, 322

Quadrantanopia, 57
Quadrantanopsia, 57
Quadrants, 56
Quadrifocal lenses, 98

Radial keratotomy, 76

Radial meridians, 199, 201
Radiuscope, 261–262, 266
Randot test, 306
Recognition, speed of, 310
Recovery point, 175, 176
Rectus muscles, 58–59
Recurrent erosion, 242
Refraction, 282–283
    index of, 64, 83
Refractive amblyopia, 82, 306
Refractive ametropia, 70
Refractive anisometropia, 81
Refractive status, 63–82
Residual astigmatism, 74, 75
Reticle, 262
Retina, 50, 53–55
    cone cells, 54, 69, 171
    layers, 53–56
    location, 53
    optics of, 69
    rod cells, 54, 69, 171
Retinal detachments, 210
Retinitis pigmentosa, 53
Retinoscopy, 72
RGP lenses, 220–224
    back vertex power (BVP), 221
    base curve radius (BCR), 221
    basic principles, 220–224
    bifocal, 231–232
    bitoric, 231
    cases for, 248
    disinfecting, 329
    edge and center thickness, 223–224
    extended wear, 244
    inserting, 248–249
    keratometer diopter conversion to millimeters, 222
    materials for, 224–227
        fluoro-silicone/acrylate (F-S/A), 225–226
        polymethylmethacrylate (PMMA), 224
        silicone elastomer, 227
        silicone/acrylate (S/A), 225
        SoftPerm, 226–227
    modifying, 267–276
        adding minus power, 274–275
        adding plus power, 276
        applying intermediate/peripheral curves, 270–272
        edge shaping, 272
        polishing, 272–273
        polishing compounds, 267–268
        reducing lens diameter, 268–270
        removing scratches, 273–274
        spindle unit, 267
    optical zone diameter (OZD), 221
    overall diameter (OAD), 220–221
    parameter verification, 261–265
        base curve radius, 261–262
        bifocal designs, 265
        center thickness, 263
        diameter, 262–263
        edge evaluation, 263–264
        peripheral curve widths, 263

RGP lenses *(continued)*
    power, 261
    prism, 264
    surface evaluation, 263–264
    tolerances, 265
    toric base curves, 264
  patient instructions, 251–254
  patient progress evaluation, 227–229
    case history, 227
    form for, 229, 231
    keratometry, 229
    over-refraction, 227
    postrefraction, 229
    slit lamp exam with lenses off, 227, 229
    slit lamp exam with lenses on, 227
    visual acuity with lenses on, 227
  patient wear symptoms, 228–229
  peripheral curves, 221–223
  recentering, 251
  removing, 249–251
  solutions, 246–248
    artificial tears, 247
    cleaning, 246–247
    lubricants, 247
    multipurpose, 247
    preservatives, 247–248
    wetting and soaking, 246
  tints, 224
  toric base curve, 231
  toric peripheral curve, 231
  trifocal, 232
  vertex distance chart at 12 mm, 222
Right optic tract, 57
Rigid gas-permeable (RGP) lenses. *See* RGP lenses
Rimless bevel, 134
Risley auxiliary prism, 116
Rod cells, 54, 69, 171
Roll-and-polish process, 134–135
Round-flat jawed pliers, 156
RPE detachments, 52

Saccadic eye movements, 177–178, 303, 310
Safety bevel, 134
Sarcoidosis, 52
Sattler's layer, 52
Schirmer test, 216
Schlemm, canal of, 51
School vision report forms, 29
Sclera, 41, 49–50
  composition, 49
  inflammations of, 50
Scleral spur, 49
Scleritis, 50
Scotoma, 57, 199, 200, 209
Sebaceous glands, 44
Secretors, basic, 45
Senile cataract, 79
Senile macular degeneration, 210
Sensory fusion, 295, 306
Service contracts, 26
Silicone elastomer lenses, 227, 244

Silicone/acrylate (S/A), 225
Silsoft lenses, 227
Simple anisometropia, 81
Simple astigmatism, 74
Simultaneous perception, 306
Sinuses, 39–40
  air, 39–40
  paranasal, 40
Slot gauges, 263
Smooth vergence testing, 296
Snellen chart, 280
SoftPerm, 226–227
Software, 34
Spatial disorientation, 75
Spatial localization, 310
Speed of focusing, 310
Speed of recognition, 310
Sphenoid air sinuses, 40
Sphenoid bone, 39, 40
Sphere equivalent, 89
Spherical lenses, 75, 85, 94, 111
  biconcave, 86
  biconvex, 85
  meniscus, 86
  plano concave, 86
  plano convex, 85
  power measurement for, 111
Spherocylindrical lenses, 75, 86, 94
  optical cross of, 87–88
  power measurement for, 112
Sphincter, 50
Sphygmomanometer, 181
Spindle unit, 267
Sports vision, 309–313
  equipment suppliers, 312
  organizations related to, 313
  skills, 309–311
  therapy, 311–312
  therapy benefits, 313
Squinting, 61, 70, 75
Staphylococcus, 327
Static acuity, 310
Static threshold, 199
Stereoacuity. *See* Stereopsis
Stereopsis, 171–175, 295, 306
  definition/description, 171–172
  distance, 175
  fine, 173
  gross, 173
  intermediate, 173
  tests for, 172
Stereo vision, testing, 281
Stethoscope, 181
Stimulus depravation, 82
Strabismic amblyopia, 82, 306
Strabismus, 61, 214, 304–307
Stroma, 48, 50
Sty, 44
Subcapsular cataract, 79
Subconjunctival hemorrhage, 50
Subcutaneous areolar layer, 43

Submuscular areolar layer, 43
Superimposition, 295, 306
Superior oblique muscle, 58, 59, 61
Superior rectus muscle, 58, 59
Supplies, office, 13–15
Suppression, 306
Suprathreshold, 199
Suprathreshold screening, 204
Sutures, 39
Synapse, 54, 55
Synechia, posterior, 51

Tangent screen, 204–205
Tarsal conjunctiva, 44
Tarsal glands, 44
Tarsal plate, 43
Tear film
    contact lenses and, 215–216
    layers, 45
Technica progressive addition lenses, 98–99
Telephone, 4–6
    answering, 4–5
    confirming patient appointments, 8
    elements of courtesy, 4
    personal phone calls, 2
    recalling patients for follow-up visits, 11
    requests for cost information, 6
    requests for patient information, 5
    screening calls, 4–6
    taking messages, 5–6
Telescopes, 288–289
Tempering, 129–130
Temple types, 145
Templing angle pliers, 155
Tempo Instruments, 312
Test equipment
    A-Scan ultrasonography, 69
    After Image Flasher, 307
    amblyoscope, 307
    Amsler grid, 203, 205–206, 281
    anomaloscope, 170
    arc perimeter, 206–207
    Auto-Plot Tangent Screen, 205
    automated perimeters, 208
    automated screeners, 204
    Bagolini lenses, 307
    Brightness Acuity Tester, 194
    Burton screener, 203–204
    colmascope, 129
    dial-thickness gauge, 128–129
    eikonometer, 81
    focimeter, 107
    fundus photography, 195–196
    Goldmann bowl perimeter, 207–208
    hand-held magnifier, 262
    Harrington Flocks Visual Field Screener, 203–204
    interpupillary distance (PD) rule, 154
    keratometer, 67, 185, 218, 262
    Lens Analyzer, 118
    lens clock, 127–128
    lensometer, 107–121, 265
    occluder, 168
    ophthalmic ultrasonography, 196–198
    ophthalmometer, 67, 185
    PD rule, 143
    polariscope, 129
    potential acuity meter, 193–194
    projection magnifier, 264
    pseudoisochromatic plate (PIP), 169
    radiuscope, 261–262, 266
    reticle, 262
    retinoscope, 72
    Snellen chart, 280
    sphygmomanometer, 181
    spindle unit, 267
    stethoscope, 181
    tangent screen, 204–205
    thickness caliper, 128–129
    Tono-Pen, 192–193
    tonometer, 189
    transmittance meters, 131–132
    typoscope, 281
    Vertexometer, 116–117
Tests and testing
    accommodation, 175–176
    accommodative facility, 299
    accommodative sustainability, 300
    Bernell Stereo Reindeer test, 172
    blood pressure, 181–182
    Brightness Acuity Tester, 282
    Broad H test, 177–178
    color vision, 168–171, 281
    confrontation, 201–202
    contrast sensitivity, 194
    Contrast Sensitivity Function, 281
    convergence, 175–176
    cover tests, 176–177, 305–306
    Developmental Eye Movement Test, 303
    eye dominancy, 180–181
    eye movements, 61
    Farnsworth D-15 Dichotomous Test, 169
    Farnsworth-Munsell 100 Hue Test, 169
    Farnsworth lantern test, 170
    glare, 193–194, 282
    Holmgren Wool Test, 171
    interpupillary distance (PD), 178–180
    keratometry, 185–189
    Miller Nadler glare tester, 282
    Phenol Red Cotton Thread test, 216
    Randot test, 306
    Schirmer test, 216
    smooth vergence, 296
    specialty tests, 185–198
    stereo vision, 281
    Titmus Stereo Fly test, 172, 173, 306
    Titmus Stereotest, 172
    tonometry, 189–193
    visual acuity, 164–168, 279–281
    visual fields, 208–210, 281–282
    visual skills, 182
Therapy, vision. *See* Vision therapy
Thickness caliper, 128–129

Titmus Stereo Fly test, 172, 173, 306
Tono-Pen, 192–193
Tonometer, 189–190
Tonometry, 189–193
    applanation, 190
    definition/description, 189
    indentation, 190
    test equipment, 189–191
Toric base curve lenses, 231
Toric lenses, 236–239
    candidates for, 238
    determining angle of rotation, 237–238
    parameter verification, 264
    stabilization, 236–237
Toric peripheral curve lenses, 231
Transmittance meters, 131–132
Traumatic cataract, 78
Trichromatism, 171
Trifocal lenses, 78, 90, 97
    contact, 232
    power measurement for, 114–115
Tritanomalous anomalous trichromat, 171
Tritanope dichromat, 171
Trochlea, 59
Tropia, 177
Tuberculosis, 52, 327
Typoscope, 281

Ultrasonography, 196–198
    A-scan, 69, 196–197
    B-scan, 197–198
Ultraviolet protection, 100–101, 103–104, 130–132
    ANSI standards, 150
Unilateral cover test, 177
Uveitis, 210
    anterior, 51, 317–318
    posterior, 52

V bevel, 134
Vacuole, 56
Vascular disease, 210
Vascular tunic, 46, 50–53
    choroid, 52–53
    ciliary body, 51–52
    iris, 50–51
Vergence movements, 296
    fusional, 296
Vergences, testing, 61
Vertexometer, 116–117
Vertical divergence, 61
Video display terminal, 34
Vision
    binocular, 295–308
    blurred, 51, 70, 75
    central, 310
    color, 168–171, 281, 310
    low, 279–293
    night, 310
    peripheral, 310
    sports, 309–313
Vision Service Plan, 26
Vision therapy, 295
    for accommodative excess, 302
    for accommodative insufficiency, 302
    for amblyopia, 306–307
    for binocular disorders, 307–308
    for convergence excess, 298, 300
    for convergence insufficiency, 297
    for oculomotor dysfunction, 304
    sports, 311–312
Visiontronics, 312
Vistech Inc., 312
Visual acuity, 164–168
    charts for, 164–165
    definition/description, 164
    testing low vision, 279–281
    testing sequence, 165–166
    testing technique, 165–168
    with rigid lenses on, 227
Visual concentration, 310
Visual cortex, 56, 57
Visual efficiency, 295
Visual fields, 56, 57, 199–211
    circles of eccentricity, 199, 202
    confrontation testing, 201–202
    defects, 57–58
    definition/description, 199
    radial meridians, 199, 201
    testing in low vision patients, 281–282
    testing instruments, 203–208
    testing procedures, 208–210
Visual impairment, psychological impact of, 293
Visualization, 311
Visual memory, 311
Visual pathway, 56–58
Visual processing, 295
Visual reaction time, 311
Visual skills, 295, 309–311
    testing, 182
Vitamin A, 53

Walleye, 61
Watery layer, 45
Wayne Engineering, 312
Wide-jawed hinge angling pliers, 156
Wolfring glands, 44, 45

Zeis glands, 44–45
Zonula adherens, 54
Zonular fibers, 56
Zygomatic bone, 39, 40